WITHDRAWN
WRIGHT STATE UNIVERSITY LIBRARIES

Thyroid Ultrasound and Ultrasound-Guided FNA Biopsy

Thyroid Ultrasound and Ultrasound-Guided FNA Biopsy

edited by

H. Jack Baskin, M.D.

Florida Thyroid and Endocrine Clinic
Orlando, Florida, USA

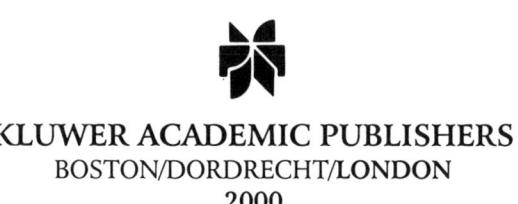

KLUWER ACADEMIC PUBLISHERS
BOSTON/DORDRECHT/LONDON
2000

Distributors for North, Central and South America:
Kluwer Academic Publishers
101 Philip Drive
Assinippi Park
Norwell, Massachusetts 02061 USA
Telephone (781) 871-6600
Fax (781) 871-6528
E-Mail <kluwer@wkap.com>

Distributors for all other countries:
Kluwer Academic Publishers Group
Distribution Centre
Post Office Box 322
3300 AH Dordrecht, THE NETHERLANDS
Telephone 31 78 6392 392
Fax 31 78 6546 474
E-Mail <services@wkap.nl>

Electronic Services <http://www.wkap.nl>

Library of Congress Cataloging-in-Publication Data

Thyroid ultrasound and ultrasound-guided FNA biopsy / edited by H. Jack Baskin.
    p. ; cm.
    Includes bibliographical references and index.
    ISBN 0-7923-8662-0 (alk.paper)
    1. Thyroid gland--Diseases--Diagnosis. 2. Thyroid gland--Ultrasonic imaging.
3. Thyroid gland--Needle biopsy. I. Baskin, H. Jack.
    [DNLM: 1. Thyroid Diseases--diagnosis. 2. Biopsy, Needle--methods. 3. Thyroid
Gland--ultrasonography--methods. WK 200 T5485 2000]
    RC655.5 .T56 2000
    616.4'407543--dc21
                                        99-047121

Copyright © 2000 by Kluwer Academic Publishers

All rights reserved. No part of this publication may be reproduced, stored in a retrieval system or transmitted in any form or by any means, mechanical, photo-copying, recording, or otherwise, without the prior written permission of the publisher, Kluwer Academic Publishers, 101 Philip Drive, Assinippi Park, Norwell, Massachusetts 02061

Printed on acid-free paper.

Printed in the United States of America

Contents

List of contributors...vii

Preface..ix

Acknowledgments..xi

1. **History of Thyroid Ultrasound**
   H. Jack Baskin..1

2. **Principles of Ultrasound Technique**
   Dara Treadwell..9

3. **Method of Performing Ultrasonography of the Neck**
   Manfred Blum and Joseph Yee..35

4. **Comparison of Ultrasound with Other Types of Thyroid Imaging**
   H. Jack Baskin..59

5. **Ultrasound of Thyroid Nodules**
   H. Jack Baskin..71

6. **Neck Ultrasound and the Endocrine Surgeon**
   Edward Paloyan, Regina P. Walker, and Ann M. Lawrence 87

7. **Thyroid Fine Needle Aspiration Biopsy**
   Hossein Gharib..103

8. **Ultrasound-Guided Fine Needle Aspiration Biopsy of Thyroid Nodules**
   Richard S. Haber...125

9. **Techniques of Ultrasound-Guided FNA Biopsy**
   Tomotsu Yokuzawa, Kanji Kuma, and Masahiro Sugawara....137

10.	The Role of Ultrasound in Managing Thyroid Cancer H. Jack Baskin..155
11.	**Percutaneous Ethanol Injection of Benign Thyroid Nodules and Cysts Using Ultrasound** Enrico Papini and Claudio M. Pacella...............................169
12.	**Color Flow Doppler Sonography of the Thyroid** Fausta Bogazzi, Luigi Bartalena, and Professor Enio Martino..215

Index..239

Contributors

H. Jack Baskin, M.D.
2921 North Orange Avenue
Orlando, FL 32804, USA

Luigi Bartalena, M.D.
Instituto di Endocrinologia
University of Pisa
Via Paradisa, 2
56124, Pisa, Italy

Fausta Bogazzi, M.D.
Instituto di Endocrinologia
University of Pisa
Via Paradisa, 2
56124, Pisa, Italy

Manfred Blum, M.D.
Professor of Clinical Medicine and Radiology
New York University
School of Medicine
New York, NY 10016, USA

Hossein Gharib, M.D.
Mayo Clinic
200 First Street SW
Rochester, MN 55905, USA

Richard Haber, M.D.
Mount Sinai Hospital
Box 1055
5th Avenue & 100th Street
New York, New York 10029, USA

Kanji Kuma, M.D.
Kuma Hospital
Kobe, 650-0011, Japan

Ann M. Lawrence, M.D., Ph.D.
Loyola University Medical Center
Maywood, IL 60153 USA

Professor Enio Martino
Instituto di Endocrinologia
University of Pisa
Via Paradisa, 2
56124, Pisa, Italy

C.M. Pacella, M.D.
Department of Endocrine, Metabolic and Digestive Diseases
Ospedale Regina Apostolorum
00041, Albano, Rome, Italy

Edward Paloyan, M.D.
827 Taft Road
Hindale, IL 60521-4836, USA

Enrico Papini, M.D.
Department of Endocrine, Metabolic and Digestive Diseases
Ospedale Regina Apostolorum
00041, Albano, Rome, Italy

Masahiro Sugawara, M.D.
VA Medical Center & UCLA School of Medicine
West Los Angeles, CA 90073, USA

Dara R. Treadwell, B.S.
100 North Park Avenue
Apopka, FL 32703-4146, USA

Regina P. Walker, M.D.
Loyola University Medical Center
Maywood, IL 60153 USA

Joseph Yee, M.D.
Professor of Clinical Medicine and Radiology
New York University
School of Medicine
New York, NY 10016, USA

Tomotsu Yokozawa, M.D.
Kuma Hospital
Kobe, 650, Japan

Preface

Over the past two decades ultrasound has undergone numerous advances in technology such as gray-scale imaging, real-time sonography, high resolution 7.5-10 Mtz transducers, and color-flow Doppler that make ultrasound unsurpassed in its ability to provide very accurate images of the thyroid gland quickly, inexpensively, and safely. However, in spite of these advances, ultrasound remains drastically underutilized by endocrinologists. In part, this is due to a lack of understanding of the ways in which ultrasound can aid in the diagnosis of various thyroid conditions and to a lack of experience in the ultrasound technique by the clinician.

The purpose of this book is to demonstrate how ultrasound is integrated with the history, physical examination, and other thyroid tests (especially FNA biopsy) to provide valuable information that can be used to improve patient care. Numerous ultrasound examples are used to show the interactions between ultrasound and tissue characteristics and explain their clinical significance. Also presented is the work of several groups of investigators worldwide who have explored new applications of ultrasound that has led to novel techniques that are proving clinically useful.

In order to reach its full potential, it is critical that thyroid ultrasound be performed by the examining physician. This book instructs the physician how to perform the ultrasound at the bedside so that it becomes part of the physical examination. Among the new developments discussed are the new digital phased-array transducers, which allow ultrasound and FNA biopsy to be combined in the technique of ultrasound-guided FNA biopsy. Over the next decade, this technique will become a part of our routine clinical practice and a powerful new tool in the diagnosis of thyroid nodules and in the follow-up of thyroid cancer patients.

Acknowledgement

Special thanks and appreciation are accorded to
Mrs. Kathryn Holsinger who provided expert secretarial
assistance during the preparation and editing of this textbook.

Thyroid Ultrasound and Ultrasound-Guided FNA Biopsy

1

HISTORY OF THYROID ULTRASOUND

H. Jack Baskin, M.D., F.A.C.E.
Florida Thyroid and Endocrine Clinic
Orlando, FL 32804 USA

INTRODUCTION

Ultrasound technology evolved following World War II as an outgrowth of the research used in developing radar. Subsequently it was introduced into medicine in the early 1960's. I recall first using an ultrasound machine in 1965 as an intern in the emergency room of Grady Memorial Hospital in Atlanta. Its purpose was to examine patients who had undergone head trauma to detect a possible "pineal shift", diagnostic of a subdural hemorrhage. With this early "A-Mode" (amplitude mode) ultrasound, the sound waves from the transducer placed behind the patient's ear were reflected as echoes or vertical spikes along a horizontal axis on a Cathode Ray Oscilloscope screen. These spikes indicated the temporal bone plates on each side of the skull. If the pineal gland was calcified, it also produced a spike midway between the other two spikes. While this method was no more accurate than a x-ray of the skull, its advantage was that it could be performed by the examining physician, and provided a more rapid diagnosis in an emergency situation. A "pineal shift" of one centimeter or more would prompt a call to the neurosurgeon.

Various medical specialties were quick to recognize the diagnostic possibilities that ultrasound could offer their patients. In cardiology it was first used to diagnose aortic aneurysms and pericardial effusions. Later its use evolved to investigate cardiac valve structure and function. In obstetrics a major application of early ultrasound was to determine placental localization as well as fetal size. Later its use expanded to detect fetal anomalies.

Endocrinologists also appreciated the possibilities of this new technology. The first reported use of ultrasound to examine the thyroid gland was by Yamakawa and Naito in 1966 when they proposed a method of applying it to calculate thyroid volume and weight (1). One year later Fujimoto, et al, used ultrasound to describe structural alterations within the gland (2). Soon thyroid ultrasound was being used to differentiate nodules that were solid from nodules that were cystic (3,4,5,6,7,8,9).

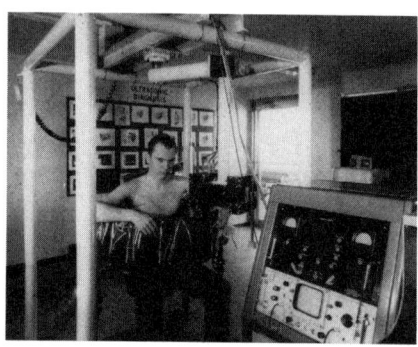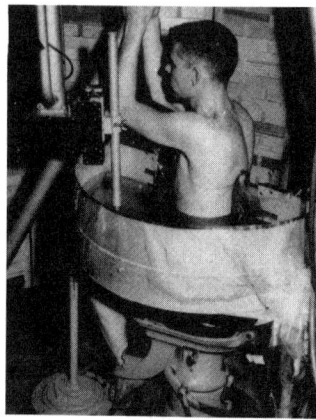

Figures 1.1 and 1.2 Originally diagnostic ultrasound studies required a fluid medium to transmit the sound waves. Submersion in tubs of water was used in some of the early tests. (Courtesy Acuson)

Using A-Mode ultrasound, solid nodules produced multiple spikes throughout the nodule while cysts within the thyroid showed only a spike at the walls of the cyst with an echo-free space in the center of the nodule indicating fluid (Figures 1.4 and 1.5). Initially, it was hoped that finding a cystic nodule indicated it was benign; however as the technique improved it was soon appreciated that very few nodules were entirely cystic while many "solid" nodules contained cystic areas (10,11).

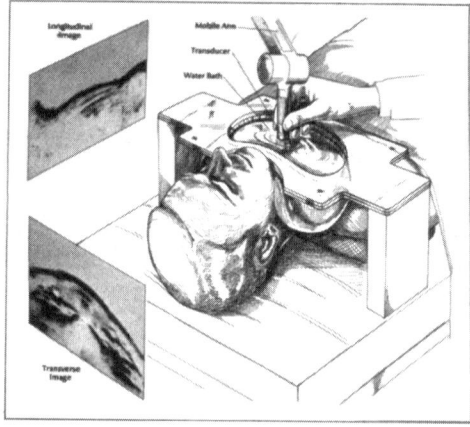

Figure 1.3 A modified water bath was used to perform ultrasound of the thyroid gland. Today an acoustic gel is used to seal the area between the transducer and the skin; this eliminates air which transmits high frequency sound waves poorly. (Courtesy Manfred Blum, M.D.)

The hope that ultrasound would provide a means to easily differentiate benign from malignant tissue, and thus separate nodules in the thyroid that required surgery from those that did not was not realized. Ultrasound could not tell if a nodule was benign or malignant.

B-MODE ULTRASONOGRAPHY

"B-Mode" (brightness mode) ultrasound was developed in the 1970's. Instead of visualizing the echoes as vertical spikes along the horizontal axis, the information was displayed as bright dots of light on the cathode ray tube. This two-dimensional ultrasound made it easier to conceptualize the data by electronically constructing an image of the thyroid gland using the reflected (echo) sound waves. Later, gray-scale imaging using varying shades of gray to depict different echo signals that represented a change in the acoustic impedance of different tissues allowed more detail of the internal structure of the gland. Because acoustic impedance is a product of sound wave velocity and tissue density, gray scale imaging depicted the density of nodules in comparison to the surrounding thyroid tissue. It also demonstrated the presence of a "halo" around some nodules. Originally, eight shades of gray were available, but this has now increased to 256 shades of gray, approximately the same number of shades the human eye can contrast sense. B-Mode ultrasound with gray-scale imaging provided more information than the old A-Mode ultrasound and introduced the capability of accurately and precisely measuring the dimensions and volume of the thyroid and of thyroid nodules, but it still could not reliably differentiate between benign and malignant nodules (12,13,14,15,16,17,18).

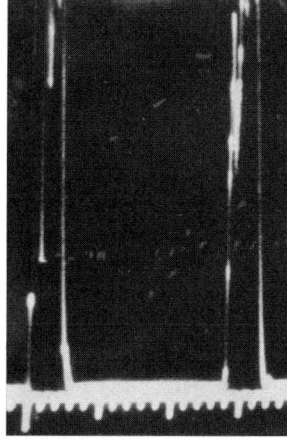

Figure 1.4 A-Mode Ultrasound of a Cyst. The ultrasound tracing shows spikes at the wall of the cyst with an echo-free space between denoting fluid. (Courtesy Manfred Blum, M.D.)

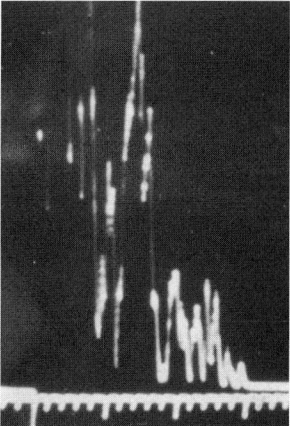

Figure 1.5 A-Mode Ultrasound of a Solid Nodule. Ultrasound tracing shows irregular echoes throughout the nodule indicating it is solid. Courtesy Manfred Blum, M.D.)

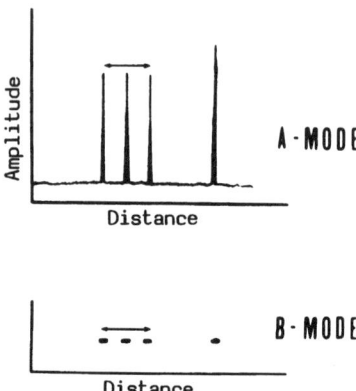

Figure 1.6 Comparison of A-Mode and B-Mode Ultrasound. The same information is depicted in amplitude and brightness mode. (Courtesy Manfred Blum, M.D.)

M-MODE ULTRASONOGRAPHY

In the early 1980's, "M-Mode" (motion mode) ultrasound was introduced and allowed real-time imaging similar to fluoroscopy. This ability to image in real-time permitted the easy recognition of moving structures such as the esophagus, arteries and veins. It also greatly decreased the time it took to do an ultrasound of the thyroid. Much more detail could be seen since views were not limited to one-centimeter "cuts" through the gland. The greatest advantage that real-time imaging provided was allowing guided needle biopsy under direct visualization.

TRANSDUCERS

Improvements were being made in engineering and electronic technology that increased the sensitivity of ultrasound. Simultaneously, the technology of transducers was also being improved. High frequency (7.5 - 10 MHz), hand-held, small parts transducers were developed that were ideal for imaging the thyroid gland. Mechanical, vibrating transducers were replaced by electronically focused, phased-array digital transducers made of a thin wafer of piezoelectric material such as lead zirconate or lead titanate. In addition to drastically improving the resolution of the image, this allowed the transducer to be placed directly on the skin without an intervening water bath greatly facilitating the ease with which ultrasound is done. These digital transducers also allowed focusing the acoustic beam in the near field to permit easy guidance of needles for biopsing the thyroid.

COST-EFFECTIVENESS OF ULTRASOUND

In February, 1982, a widely read and discussed article was published in the Annals of Internal Medicine comparing ultrasound, isotope scanning, and Fine Needle Aspiration (FNA) biopsy in the evaluation of thyroid nodules (19). The article demonstrated that FNA biopsy was the most cost-effective method to evaluate a patient who presents with a thyroid nodule. While this was instrumental in helping FNA achieve widespread use among endocrinologists, it had a dampening effect on endocrinologists' use of ultrasound.

The recent and rapid advances in electronic technology over the past few years have led to the remarkable decrease in the price of extremely sophisticated equipment. Ultrasound machines that are excellent for thyroid ultrasound and ultrasound-guided needle biopsy have decreased from $70,000 - 100,000 down to $20,000. This affordability justifies an endocrinologist having an ultrasound machine dedicated to examining the thyroid. Access to high-resolution ultrasound at the bedside allows endocrinologists to perform ultrasound on their own patients when they are examined rather than referring them to a radiologist. The reduction in equipment cost and the elimination of another level of specialty consultation have made thyroid ultrasound much more cost-effective.

"BEDSIDE ULTRASOUND"

Ultrasound performed by a clinician as part of the examination of the thyroid is not the same as an ultrasound done in a radiology department. Thyroid ultrasound requested in the radiology department of a hospital is almost always performed by a sonographer. When a sonographer performs the thyroid ultrasound and the physician sees only the final images, it is the sonographer who performs *diagnosis* during the study. This is in contrast to gastrointestinal fluoroscopy for example when the physician -not the technologist- decides where to take the spot films. Real-time ultrasound provides vast amounts of information - much of which is discarded. When thyroid ultrasound is performed by the physician as part of the thyroid exam, this information is not lost. In addition, the physician has access to the history and physical examination and has anticipated what pathology may be present. The clinician also has access to other data such as laboratory tests, nuclear scans, and FNA biopsy data and is able to integrate all of this with the ultrasound images to better make the correct diagnosis and provide the correct treatment. This is a vast improvement over static images taken by a sonographer and read by a radiologist who may never even see the patient.

Ultrasound done by the examining physician in the office rather than by a sonographer in the hospital has already been well established by other specialists such as obstetricians and urologists. In Europe, it is common to see an ultrasound machine in the emergency room of most hospitals where it is readily available for use by the general medicine physician or surgeon. Ultrasound should be considered part of the examination of a patient with a thyroid nodule as well as a patient who is being examined post-operatively for thyroid cancer. The sublities sought with a thyroid ultrasound examination are analogous to listening to a heart murmur. The cardiologist does not ask the nurse to auscultate the heart of a patient and describe the patient's pathology! Ultrasound is an extension of the endocrinologist's fingers just as a stethoscope is an extension of the cardiologist's ears. For this reason the endocrinologist must perform the ultrasound and not delegate this important procedure to anyone else.

The importance of the endocrinologist doing the ultrasound becomes even more apparent when this procedure is incorporated into performing ultrasound-guided FNA biopsy. Ultrasound-guided FNA biopsy is now required in biopsing small, non-palpable, or cystic thyroid nodules or if repeat biopsy is required because of insufficient material. In addition, ultrasound guidance is always necessary to biopsy suspicious lymph nodes of patients who have undergone surgery for thyroid cancer.

As will be seen throughout this book, high-resolution real-time ultrasound allows excellent imaging of the thyroid gland and its contiguous soft-tissue structures with dynamic clarity. The procedure has many advantages including being noninvasive, painless, quick, and involving no contrast material or radiation exposure. In addition, it is less expensive than other forms of imaging. Unlike an isotope scan, thyroid ultrasound can be done during pregnancy, in patients who are taking l-thyroxin, and in patients who have been given or ingested large doses of exogenous iodine. Currently there are no licensing requirements for a physician to perform ultrasound.

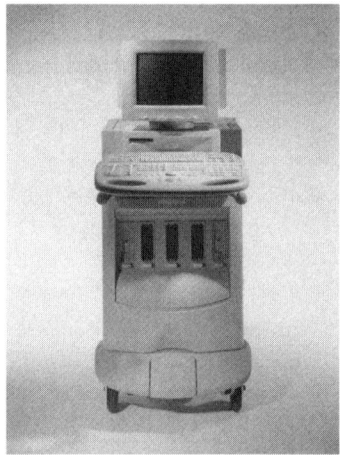

Figure 1.7 Modern Ultrasound equipment. Today's real-time, high-resolution ultrasound equipment is "user-friendly", compact, and portable. (Courtesy Acuson)

Ultrasound continues to be improved. The data can be acquired, stored, and processed to rapidly produce a three-dimensional image with better resolution of the thyroid gland than computerized tomography or magnetic resonance imaging. Nodules as small as three millimeters and cysts as small as two millimeters can be easily seen. The addition of Color Flow Doppler adds another dimension to demonstrate the vasculature and blood flow to the thyroid and will be discussed later in this book.

REFERENCES

1. Yamakawa K, Naito S. (1966) *Diagnostic Ultrasound.* Proceedings of the First International Congress, University of Pittsburgh (Edited by Grossman CH, Holmes JH, Joyner CL, Purnell EW. Plenum Press and Plenum Publishing Corporation, New York. 27-41.
2. Fugimoto Y, Oka A, Omoto R, Hirose M. (1967) Ultrasound scanning of the thyroid gland as a new diagnostic approach. *Ultrasonics* 5:177-180.
3. Damascelli B, Cascinelli N, Livarghi T, Veronesi U (1968) Preoperative approach to thyroid tumours by a two-dimensional pulse echo technique. *Ultrasonics* 6:242-243.
4. Rasmussen SN, Christiansen NJB, Jorgensen JS, Holm HH. (1971) Differentiation between cystic and solid nodules by thyroid ultrasonic examination. *Acta Chir Scand* 37:331-333.
5. Blum M, Weiss B, Hernberg J. (1971) Evaluation of thyroid nodules by A-Mode echography. *Radiology* 101:651-656.
6. Miskin M, Rosen IB, Walfish PG. (1973) B-Mode ultrasonography in assessment of thyroid gland lesions. *Ann Int Med* 79:505-510.
7. Miskin M, Rosen IB, Walfish PG. (1975) Ultrasonography of the thyroid gland. *Radiol Clinics North Am* 8:479-492.
8. Spencer R, Brown MC, Annis D. (1977) Ultrasonic scanning of the thyroid gland as a guide to the treatment of the clinically solitary nodule. *Br J Surg* 64:841-846.
9. Lees WR, Vahl SP, Watson LR, Russell RCO. (1978) The role of ultrasound scanning in the diagnosis of thyroid swellings. *Br J Surg* 65:681-684.
10. Thijs LG. (1971) Diagnostic ultrasound in clinical thyroid investigation. *J Clin Endocrinol* 32:709-716.
11. Rosen IB, Walfish PG, Miskin M. (1979) The ultrasound of thyroid masses. *Surg Clin North Am* 59:19-33.
12. Crocker EF, McLaughlin AF, Kossoff G, Jellins J. (1974) The gray scale appearance of thyroid malignancy. *J Clin Ultrasound* 2: 305-306.
13. Taylor KJW, Carpenter DA, Barrett JJ. (1974) Gray scale ultrasonography in the diagnosis of thyroid swellings. *J Clin Ultrasound* 2:327-330.
14. Chilcote WS. (1976) Gray-scale ultrasonography of the thyroid. *Radiology* 120:381-383.
15. Sackler JP, Passalaqua AM, Blum M, Amorocho RT. (1977) A spectrum of diseases of the thyroid gland as imaged by gray scale water bath sonography. *Radiology* 125:467-472.
16. Crocker EF, Jellins J. (1978) Grey scale ultrasonic examination of the thyroid gland. *Med J Aust* 2:244-250.
17. Allen FH, Krook PM, DeGroot WPH. (1979) Ultrasound demonstration of a thyroid carcinoma within a benign cyst. *AJR* 132:136-137.
18. Scheible W, Leopold GR, Woo VL, Goskink BB. (1979) High-resolution real-time ultrasonography of thyroid nodules. *Radiology* 133:413-417.
19. Van Herle AJ, Rich P, Ljung BE, Ashcraft MW, Solomon DH, Keeler EB. (1982) The thyroid nodule. *Ann Int Med* 96:221-232.

2

PRINCIPLES OF ULTRASOUND TECHNIQUE

Dara R. Treadwell, B.S., R.D.M.S.
President, Innomed Systems, Inc.
100 North Park Avenue
Apopka, FL 32703-4146 USA

INTRODUCTION

With current ultrasound technology, the image that appears on the ultrasound monitor represents some biological structure or structures obtained during the scanning procedure. Upon closer evaluation, however, one recognizes that this image is actually a display of dots or pixels in an arrangement of 256 gray shade levels from white to black, depicting the actual differences in tissue density of the internal body structures and displaying their anatomic relationship to one another. It is essential that one understand the principles of ultrasound propagation and echo generation as they relate to the resultant image if proper procedural and image interpretation skills are to be mastered. This chapter is designed as an introduction to the basic tenets of ultrasound physics affording foundational information for those who desire better knowledge of good ultrasound technique.

PRINCIPLES OF SOUND

Propagation of sound

Understanding the physical characteristics of an ultrasound beam, requires first exploring the properties of audible sound. Sound, by general definition, is the transfer and propagation of kinetic energy through a medium in a series of mechanical waves. The nature of any mechanical wave is to disturb particles in the medium through which it travels. Sound waves are created then, when pressure is applied by a defined source causing a back and forth vibration of molecules and a continual transference of this vibrational energy as the wave moves forward through the medium. The rhythmic pulling and tugging effect on the molecules creates systematic phases of high and low density. Where molecules are pushed closely together, the wave is *compressed* creating a region of density. Conversely, as the wave front passes, the molecules return to their original position and the region assumes a lower density referred to as *rarefaction*. (Figure 2.1) This pattern of molecular compression and rarefaction constitutes a *cycle*, expressed scientifically

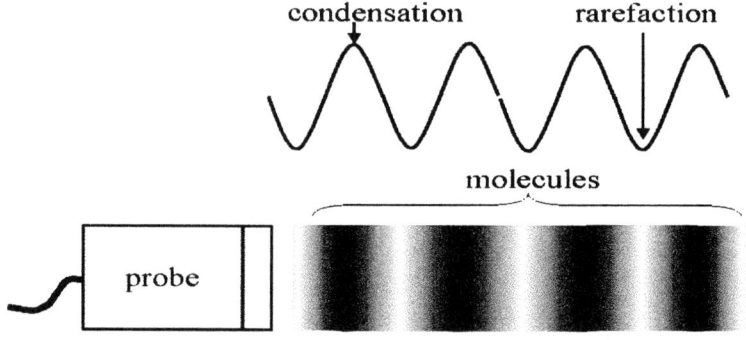

Figure 2.1 Propagation of sound. Sound waves are created when pressure is applied causing a transference of vibrational energy between molecules.

as a sine wave. The amplitude, or positive phase of the wave, signifies the amount of pressure applied for each compressive state and the negative phase of the wave as each point of rarefaction. The number of times this pattern is repeated per second characterizes the *frequency* of the sound wave, and the distance between the "peaks" of compression or "valleys of rarefaction of the repetitive cycles defines the *wavelength*. Frequency and wavelength are inversely related; the higher the frequency, the shorter the wavelength. Frequency is expressed in hertz (Hz), representing *complete cycles per second*. The audible range of sound is approximately 20 Hz to 20,000 Hz (20 KHz). Sound with a resonating frequency below 20 Hz is considered *infrasonic* sound, while above 20 KHz is *ultrasonic*.

Speed of sound
The speed of sound is not determined by the source producing the sound, but by the medium through which it is traveling. The more dense the molecular composition of the medium, and the more rigid or "stiff" its nature, the faster the vibrations between molecules will occur, increasing the rate at which the sound wave is propagated. For example, a metal object, like a tuning fork, will actually transfer sound energy at a faster rate than the air through which we hear its effect. In a biological application, the speed of sound will therefore be faster through bone as compared to a fluid filled structure like a cyst, and the same is true when comparing a cyst to gas in the stomach or intestines; the sound speed through the cyst will be faster. (Figure 2.2)

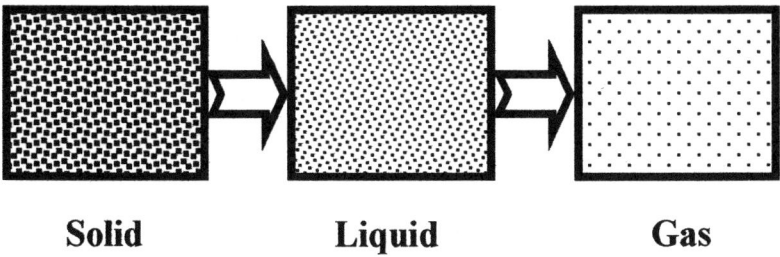

Figure 2.2 Speed of sound. The speed of sound is dependent upon the molecular density and stiffness of a medium. Sound propagates faster through bone than through a cyst.

PRINCIPLES OF ULTRASOUND

Propagation of ultrasound

Ultrasound waves have vibrations of the same physical nature as audible sound, but because they vibrate at frequencies above the human hearing range, they are inaudible to the human ear. For diagnostic imaging purposes, the useful range of ultrasound frequencies is between 1 MHz and 20 MHz, depending upon the application. Like any sound wave, ultrasound propagation depends upon two things: (1) a source of energy and, (2) a medium through which the sound wave will travel.

Ultrasound imaging begins with the transducer, a device that converts energy from one form to another. (Figure 2.3) An ultrasound transducer serves a dual purpose as both a transmitter and receiver of sound waves by converting an electrical signal to sound, or acoustical energy, and acoustical energy back to an electrical signal.

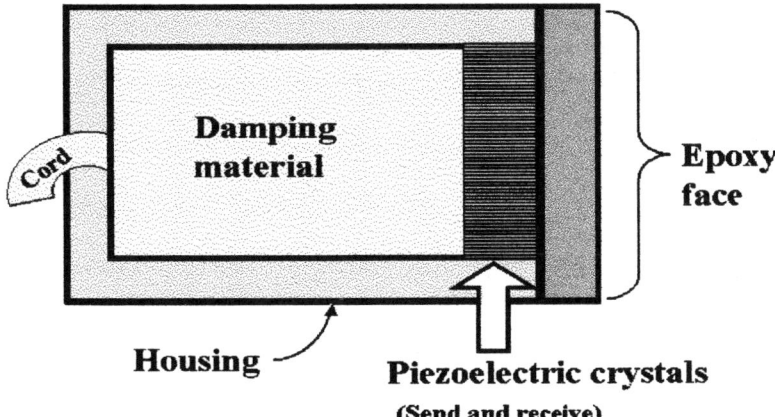

Figure 2.3 Transducer construction. The transducer is a device that converts electrical energy to sound, or acoustical energy, and acoustical energy back to an electrical signal.

Transducers in medical ultrasound employ the *piezoelectric* effect to generate sound waves. Built into the face of the transducer, or probe as it is commonly called, is an arrangement of piezoelectric crystals, which, by their nature, have a unique ability to change shape when a force is introduced. An ultrasound wave is created when a sudden voltage strikes the crystals causing them to first expand, then to vibrate continuously at a stable resonating frequency, much like the tuning fork. Conversely, when squeezed by the high-pressure phase of an incoming, return echo, the crystals contract, producing a small electrical potential. (Figure 2.4) Thus the name *piezoelectric* from the Greek word, "piezo" meaning "pressure". There are naturally-occurring piezoelectric elements such as quartz, but synthetically manufactured ceramic crystals, like lead zirconate titanate, are mainly used for today's diagnostic ultrasound transducers.

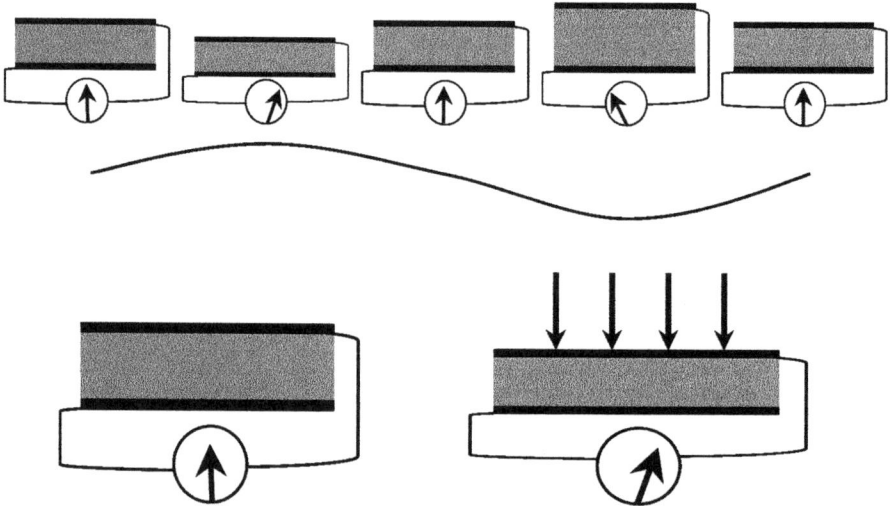

Figure 2.4 The Piezoelectric effect. When squeezed by the high-pressure phase of an incoming, return echo, the crystals contract producing a small electrical potential.

The number of crystal elements will vary depending upon the probe type, size of the probe face or "footprint", and the electronic specifications of the ultrasound system. Probes may have just one element or as many as 250 or more crystals imbedded in the face of the transducer.

Behind the row of crystals is a heavy backing layer. The backing layer dampens the vibration of the transducer elements after each electrical excitation to assure that only short bursts of energy are introduced in the transmission phase of the ultrasound cycle. Another function of the backing layer is to absorb any sound energy that may be propagated in a reverse direction posing a threat of potential damage to the electrical power source of the transducer.

Immediately in front of the crystals are matching layers, designed to optimize the transmission of sound between the piezoelectric elements and the skin of the patient. The acoustic properties of the crystals and human soft tissue are so different that without matching layers to balance the transition, most of the initial energy would be reflected back to the elements with little, if any, transmission occurring. This is called *acoustic mismatch* and will be discussed in more detail later.

The entire transducer is encased in a plastic housing for lightweight handling and ease of cleaning. An electrical power cable extends from the back of the transducer encasing the wires that internally extend to all of the elements. Each individual crystal has two wires attached to it. This enables each element to be excited individually or pulsed in groups for the production of ultrasound scan lines. Additionally, returning echoes are detected by each element, and amplified separately before combining to form one signal per reflector.

Probe types

The two basic probe types available are categorized by whether they are mechanically operated or electronically controlled. Mechanical probes are motor driven creating a cross-sectional image by sweeping the element or elements across the area of interest with each stimulating pulse. There are three types: single crystal (wobbler), rotating wheel, and oscillating mirror. The wobbler has a single piezoelectric element that rocks back and forth over the region to be scanned. In the rotating wheel type, three or four crystals are spun across the area to produce the cross-sectional display. The oscillating mirror operates differently from the other two by having a fixed element with an oscillating mirror sweeping across the body surface. The resulting image display for mechanically operated probes is triangular in shape with a point source in the near field and a broadening beam width in the far field. (Figure 2.5) With only one crystal, the scan head is considerably small making it an ideal choice for scanning between ribs, but discriminating tissues at shorter depths is sacrificed.

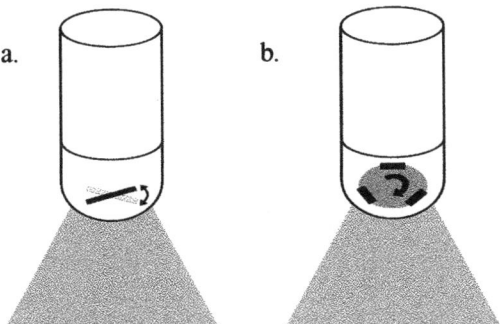

Figure 2.5 Mechanical probe operation. a. single element "wobbler" b. rotating wheel

The majority of ultrasound instruments today use transducer arrays rather than single element transducers. An array assembly consists of rectangular-shaped piezoelectric elements arranged closely together. There are four types of arrays: annular, linear, curved, and phased.

Annular array probes consist of a circular target and "bulls eye" arrangement of concentrically arranged elements. (Figure 2.6) Like sector probes, the beam line of an annular array probe is mechanically swept across the region to be imaged, producing a similar display with a wider footprint. Being mechanically driven, however, annular array probes are subject to breakage and are subsequently more costly to repair.

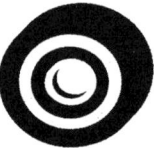

Figure 2.6 Annular array probe

Electronically powered phased, linear, and curved array probes are more widely accepted. The term *linear array* refers to the probe's design, having multiple piezoelectric elements arranged in a linear fashion along the surface of the transducer face. Linear probes will vary in width according the number of crystal elements, ranging from approximately 64 to as many as 250. To produce an ultrasound image, linear array-type probes employ sequential firing of groups of elements rather than sweeping the crystals like sector technology. The resulting display is rectangular shaped, affording the best delineation of near field anatomy.

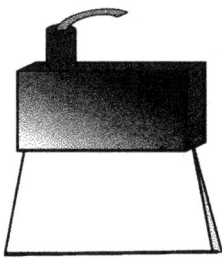 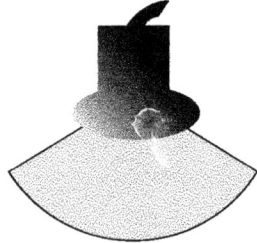

Figure 2.7. Linear array probe   **Figure 2.8** Curved array probe

Curved or *convex array* probes offer the benefits of both sector and linear array transducers. The crystals in the face of convex probes are arranged in the same manner as in linear arrays, but the curvature of the probe face produces a broadening beam width in the far field like mechanical sectors. (Figure 2.8) Curved probes produce good near to far field imaging and are generally used wherever image depth display is desired as in abdominal or pelvic imaging.

A *phased array* transducer also produces a sector display, but has a smaller footprint than a curved array probe. (Figure 2.9) Phased array probes generally have 128 separate elements that are smaller in size than those used for linear or convex array probes. Individual pulses of ultrasound energy are created by activating all 128 elements at the same time. A unique engineering design feature of a phased array probe enables steerage of the ultrasound beam by introducing small time differences (phases) between the pulsation of crystal groups. Although helpful for scanning between the ribs, the skin contact area of a phased array probe is much smaller, producing a limited view beneath the skin surface.

The remainder of this chapter will focus on linear and convex array imaging technique.

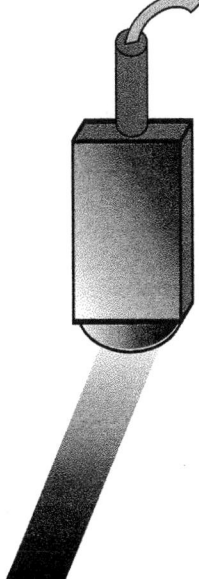

Figure 2.9 Phased array probe

Pulse-Echo Technique
If ultrasound energy were continually transmitted, it would be extremely difficult to recognize any returning echoes. More "noise" would be created than would useful echo information. Ultrasound systems employ a technique; therefore, whereby the piezoelectric crystals are subjected to short bursts of electrical energy, or pulses, during the transmission phase of the ultrasound wave cycle with a longer duration

reserved for "listening" or receiving the reflected echo signals. This is referred to as the *pulse-echo technique,* or *pulse-echo principle.*

A pulse is a group of cycles having both a beginning and an end. To ensure a very short emission time compared to a much longer period of reception, the crystals are initially "shocked" by several hundred volts of electricity, but then quickly dampened so that each transmitted sound pulse consists of only a few cycles.

The frequency of the pulse is dependent upon the *thickness* of the piezoelectric elements. Thin elements have higher frequencies; thick elements produce lower-pitched frequencies. Each transducer has a resonant frequency at which it is the most efficient, but a pulse actually contains a spectrum of frequencies called the *frequency bandwidth*. For this reason, some ultrasound systems afford the operator a selection of frequencies to choose from for each transducer.

An ultrasound wave begins with the "firing" or excitation of ceramic elements. With each sudden pulse of electricity, the piezoelectric crystals vibrate producing a corresponding pulse of ultrasound energy. But, not all of the elements are excited at the same time. To produce a tighter, more efficient ultrasound beam, groups of crystals are "fired", or pulsed, in a sequence with each pulsation creating just one line of ultrasound energy. (Figure 2.10) The number of crystals involved for each firing sequence will vary from system to system. Usually an even number of crystals, like 8 or 16 will be used, even up to 30 at one time. Each resulting acoustic line will be parallel to the next in the sequence, ultimately creating an efficient beam of ultrasound energy. Some systems even have the capability of firing both even *and* odd sequences thereby producing a *double line density* effect. When an even number of crystals are fired, the ultrasound line occurs between the middle two crystals; when an odd number are subsequently excited, the acoustic line emerges from the center crystal creating twice as many lines of information in closer proximity to one another. Basically, the more lines of acoustic energy in an ultrasound beam, the better appearing the image quality will be on the ultrasound monitor.

One complete firing sequence, both the transmission and receiving phases, will be completed in just 1/30 of a second. The transmission phase occurs in 0.5 to 3 *milli*seconds with the remainder of the time devoted to detecting the returning echoes while the next group of crystals is fired, continuing the sequential firing process across the entire array of crystals. The resulting parallel acoustic lines create one frame of an ultrasound image. Since 30 lines can be produced by each group of crystals in one second, the image is displayed as "real time" on the system's monitor.

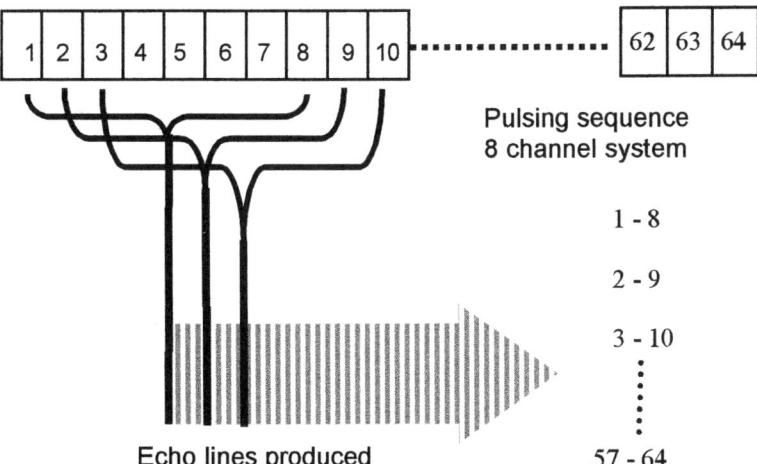

Figure 2.10 Pulse echo technique. Groups of crystals are pulsed in a sequence to create one acoustic scan line.

Huygen's principle

A pulse of ultrasound emitted by the transducer travels in a well-defined beam. Conceptually, the beam is described as a collection of point sources, emanating from the piezoelectric elements, called *Huygen sources.* (Figure 2.11) With each expansion and contraction of a piezoelectric crystal, the corresponding condensation and rarefaction of the molecules produces an individual diverging wave called a *Huygen wavelet.* As multiple elements are fired, the combined wavelets form a wave front. The resulting sound wave continues to move in a longitudinal direction by the back and forth motion of the molecules in the medium.

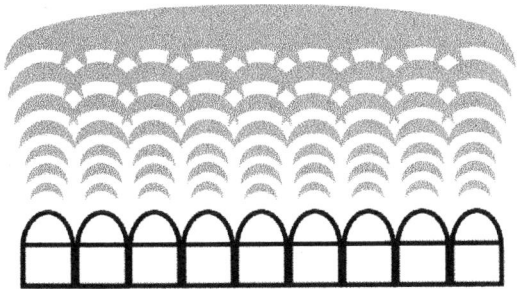

Figure 2.11 Huygen's principle. Each crystal produces a wavelet of condensation and rarefaction. As multiple elements are fired, the combined wavelets form a wave front.

Beam Focusing

All beams have a natural point of focus, the converging point at which the best quality of the beam occurs. (Figure 2.12) The ultrasound beam is divided into three parts: the *Fresnal zone* refers to that area of the beam closest to the source; the *focal zone*, the middle region of the beam encompassing the focal point; and the *Fraunhofer zone*, which defines the distal, diverging section of the beam. Structures lying in the focal zone are displayed on the ultrasound monitor as having the sharpest clarity or *resolution*. This would be fine if everything we wanted to visualize was positioned at a corresponding depth to the focal zone, but clear delineation of structures close to the surface or deep within the body tissues would be sacrificed. Since every probe frequency has its own focal zone, one solution would be to change transducers, (something that earlier generation scanners required), but modern technology offers a better solution.

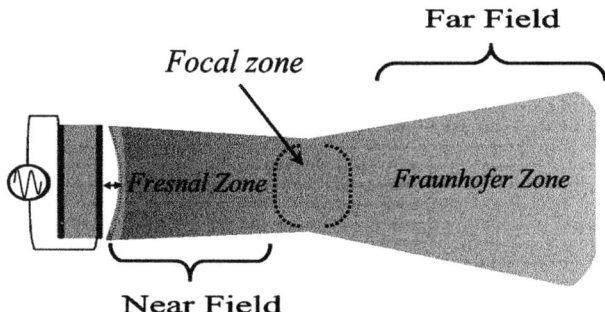

Figure 2.12 Ultrasound beam

By simply varying the time at which individual crystals within a group are fired, the focal zone can be repositioned electronically to coincide with the area of interest. Short delay times are introduced between the firing of elements to alter the focal length. The longer the delay, the shorter the focal point distance will be from the face of the probe. (Figure 2.13)

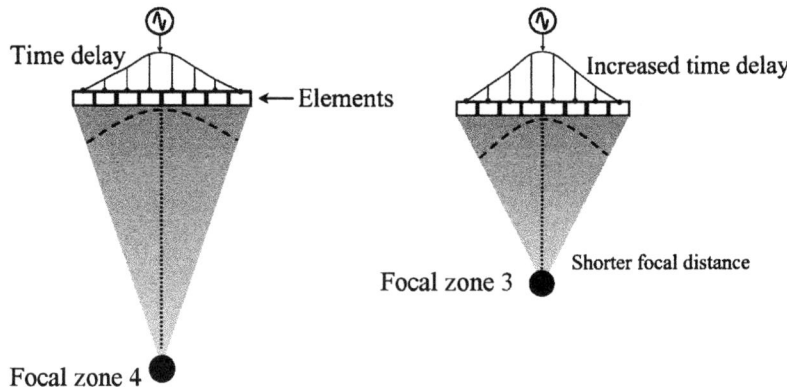

Figure 2.13 Electronic beam focusing. By varying the time at which individual crystals within a group are fired, the focal zone can be repositioned electronically to coincide with the area of interest.

Multiple focal zones may also be simultaneously selected electronically, but with an effect on frame rate. Since one pulse of information is required to form one focused beam, the addition of focal zones will decrease the overall acquisition frame rate. Therefore, for visualizing real time movement, as in echocardiography, just one focal zone is suggested.

Thus far we have discussed the focusing of the beam's width in its propagation plane, but this does not take into consideration the *slice thickness* perpendicular to the image plane. The collection of ultrasound data occurs in three planes, producing a volume of information from which the resultant image is being constructed. Slice thickness represents the width of tissue not visible on the monitor screen. Just as focusing is required to assure the sharpest detail of structures in the two-dimensional scan plane, focusing in the thickness dimension is necessary to achieve optimum focusing capability in the overall image. This is accomplished by introducing a fixed focal lens to the entire array of crystals in the face of the transducer. (Figure 2.14)

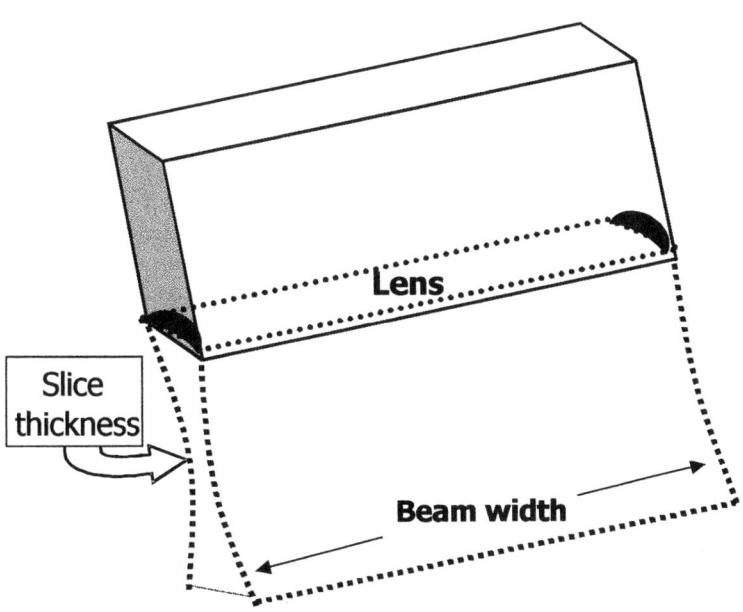

Figure 2.14 Slice thickness. There are three dimensions of tissue but only two appear on the ultrasound display. Slice thickness represents the width of the tissue not visible.

PROPERTIES OF ULTRASOUND

Tissue interaction

Acoustic energy is never stronger than when it emerges from the transducer, before it strikes the skin surface. This is often called the "main bang" of the ultrasound beam. Further transmission of the wave front through the body is dependent upon the *acoustical impedance* (intermolecular stiffness) of each tissue in its propagation path. If two tissues are similar in impedance values, the pulse continues largely unchanged, but if the interface between the tissues is significantly different, reflection of the sound beam will occur with further transmission dependent upon the measure of impedance differences. (Figure 2.15) The acoustic impedance factor is overcome between the transducer and the skin by the introduction of a coupling agent, or gel, thereby assuring the transfer of the initial "main bang" of ultrasound energy between the two surfaces.

Acoustic Impedance
rayls = $g/cm^2 sec \times 10^{-5}$

air	0.004 (rayls)
fat	1.38
water	1.54
blood	1.61
muscle	1.70
piezoelectric polymers	4.0
bone	7.8

Figure 2.15 Acoustic impedance. Reflection of sound is dependent upon the difference in acoustical impedance between tissue interfaces.

Reflection

For an echo to be produced, reflection of the ultrasound beam must occur. As the beam encounters a tissue of differing acoustic impedance, reflection will result, producing an echo signal. The greater the degree of difference, the more intense the reflected echo will be.

The number of returning echo signals received for display is dependent upon the angle at which the reflection occurs and the size of the reflector. If the incident sound beam strikes a surface at a 90° angle to the direction of propagation, optimum direct reflection will be realized. (Figure 2.16) If the primary pulse encounters a surface at any other angle, however, the reflected echoes will be scattered. Any transmitted energy will be refracted at a slight angle to the original vector causing distortion of the image. If the angle difference is significant, echoes will be totally deflected with no transducer reception at all.

The surface of the reflector will also determine the degree of reflection. A large, smooth interface will produce direct or *specular* reflectors. Specular reflectors will determine the contour or shape of a structure as viewed on the ultrasound monitor.

If the surface of the reflector is smaller than the incoming sound beam or has a rough interface, the reflectors will scatter. The scattering effect of these *nonspecular* reflectors determines the echo pattern or texture of the ultrasound image.

Attenuation

As sound interacts with structures of differing molecular density and stiffness, some of the energy will be reflected, but as the signal continues to interact with biological tissue, propagation loss, or *attenuation* will also occur. The more compact the molecular structure, the more scattering of acoustic energy and subsequent energy loss due to attenuation and absorption.

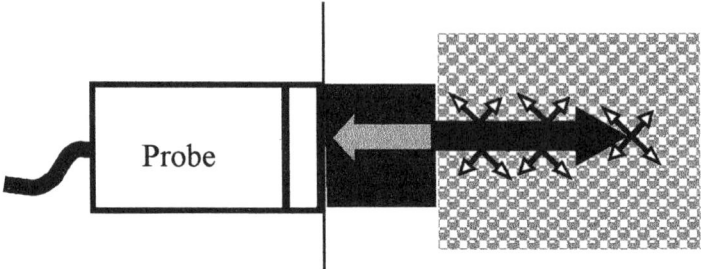

Perpendicular interface = optimum reflection

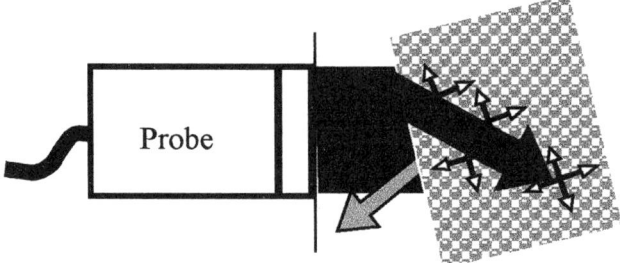

Angled interface = partial reflection and image distortion

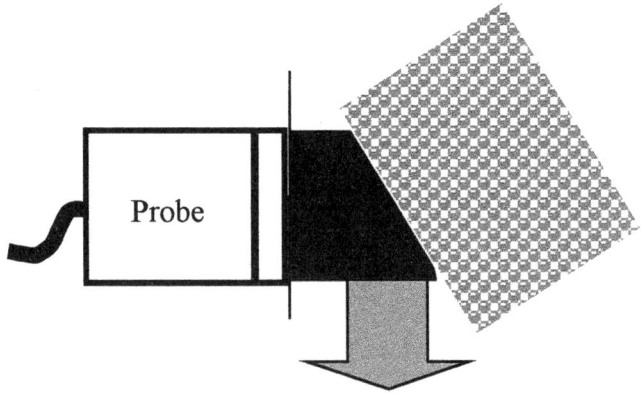

Steeply angled interface = total reflection without transducer reception

Figure 2.16 Reflection. If the incident sound beam strikes a surface at a 90 degree angle to the direction of propagation, optimum direct reflection will be realized.

Resolution

The sharpness or *resolution* of the visual image characterizes the ability of the ultrasound beam to recognize two points as being separate. The closer in proximity the two structures being discriminated are, the better the resolution capability of the system.

There are five types of resolution to be considered in the production of an efficient ultrasound beam.

Temporal resolution is the number of times per second the ultrasound system scans. This is displayed as frames per second. An action can be *temporally resolved* if it is scanned at twice the rate of occurrence.

Gray scale resolution is the maximum number of gray shades available in a system, broken into steps from white to black. The greatest number of shades possible in an ultrasound system is 256

The remaining three parameters are referred to as *spacial resolution*. These are: axial, lateral, and azimuthal resolution.

Axial or *depth resolution* defines the ability of the ultrasound transducer to detect two closely spaced reflectors along the direction of sound travel and is directly proportional to the pulse length. The higher the frequency of the transducer, the shorter the incoming pulse and subsequently, the shorter the wavelength, yielding improved axial resolution. (Figure 2.17). For example, a 7.5MHz transducer, having a shorter wavelength than a 3.5MHz one, will produce a pulse of corresponding short duration.

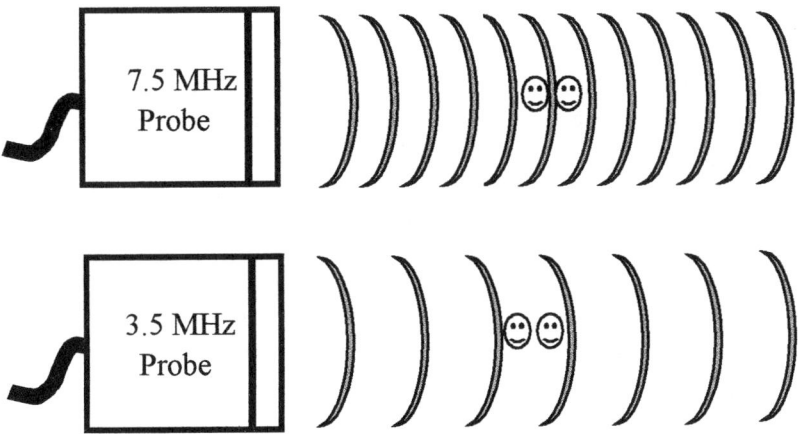

Figure 2.17 Axial resolution. The ability of the ultrasound transducer to detect two closely spaced reflectors along the direction of sound travel.

Lateral resolution is the ability to discern two points perpendicular to the direction of propagation, affecting the horizontal image plane. Since the natural divergence of an unfocused ultrasound beam causes distortion of the image, the beam is electronically focused to minimize the effects of beam width, extending the better lateral resolution properties of the near field. (Figure 2.18).

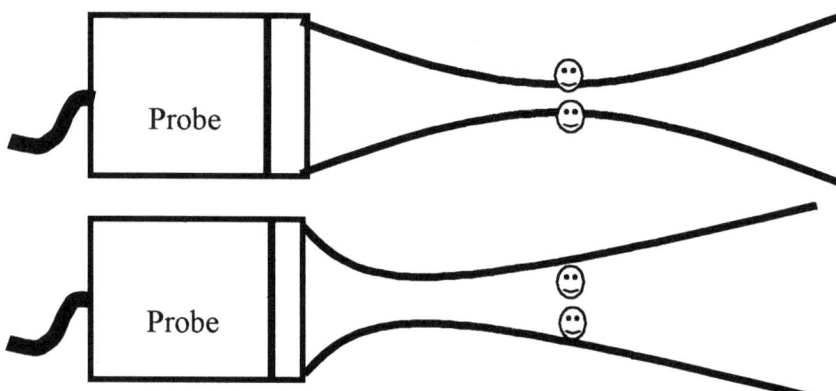

Figure 2.18 Lateral resolution. The ability to discern two points perpendicular to the direction of propagation.

Azimuthal resolution refers to the sharpness of the image in the third dimension, perpendicular to the anatomic scan plane, or slice thickness. The fixed lens in the face of the probe focuses the beam at a specific depth. When axial and lateral resolution have been optimized, structures within the focal zone of the azimuthal plane will be sharpest. There may not be an obvious visual impact, but azimuthal focusing will directly influence the guidance of a needle for FNA biopsy technique.

Beam penetration

The particular physical characteristics of each probe frequency determine its application. Higher frequency probes afford better image resolution, but as the frequency is increased, the beam is also attenuated more quickly resulting in poorer penetration capability. Standard probe frequencies in the high range are between 7.5 MHz and 10 MHz. These are used for viewing small anatomic structures that are relatively close to the surface at imaging depths up to about 7 centimeters. There are even higher frequency probes for certain applications, such as ocular imaging, where penetration limitations are not a factor.

The longer wavelength produced by lower frequency probes affords better tissue penetration to depths as great as 24 centimeters, but conversely, near field resolution is compromised. However, the increased incident energy of the frequency's beam and the subsequent increased scattering effect within the tissues, compensates for any perceived deterioration of the image. Lower frequency probes from 2.5 MHz to 3.5 MHz are best used for abdominal, pelvic, or cardiac imaging.

There are several midrange probe frequencies that overlap the parameters of the other two. Selecting the right probe frequency will depend upon such criteria as the size of the patient and the depth of the structure being examined.

The average speed of sound through human tissue is 1540 m/s. Most ultrasound systems are calibrated on this basis. The time it takes for a signal to be returned by a reflector is calculated and the distance is then plotted from the surface. Each returning echo is constructed in this manner and displayed on the monitor screen.

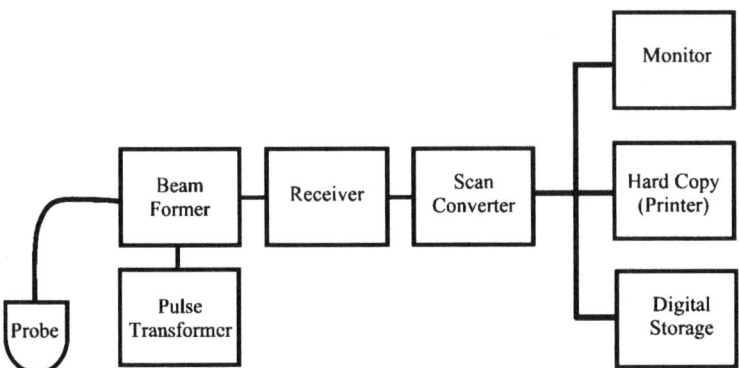

Figure 2.19 Components of an ultrasound system

UNDERSTANDING THE FORMED IMAGE

Instrumentation
(Figure 2.19) is a schematic diagram of the components of the ultrasound system.

The function of the transducer is to convert electrical energy into the mechanical or acoustical energy transmitted through the patient's anatomy, and to convert the ultrasound energy back into electrical energy for processing to the image display.

The *pulser* supplies the electrical shock to the piezoelectric element. It communicates with the receiver and memory that an electrical pulse has been initiated.

The *beam former* provides the pulse-delay sequences applied to the individual elements in order to: focus the beam in the transmission phase; control the beam direction; and control the dynamic focusing of the received echoes. During transmission, beam focusing and direction are controlled by the manner in which the elements are fired, but without some method of focusing the beam in the receiving phase, the returning signals from a particular reflector will arrive at slightly different times to each of the crystals in the group. To produce one signal for each reflector, the beam is *dynamically focused* whereby time delays of different durations are electronically applied to the individual returning signals.

The number of channels activated by the beam former to produce a beam line dictates the number of array elements that can be simultaneously excited to transmit a pulse and receive echo signals. The term, *channel* refers to the transducer element in the array and the pulser-receiver circuit to which it is connected to the system. In theory, the more operating channels a system employs, the better, ("bigger ears hear better", so to speak), but in practical application, certain physical limitations of the ultrasound system will affect the number of elements that can be activated. Systems with as many as 128 channels are presently available with progress being made to develop beam formers with higher channel counts.

The *receiver* provides the initial processing of the received information. There are two principle functions of the receiver: time *gain compensation* (TGC), and *dynamic range*.

> *TGC*
>
> A natural occurrence of sound transmission is a loss of echo strength as the energy of the beam is attenuated. Without some way to correct for this, signal amplitudes would appear brighter in the near field, gradually fading out with depth. A *time-gain-compensation device* is introduced, allowing the operator to independently alter the signal strength in each area of the image, so that the transducer "hears" the sound at the same pitch regardless of the reflector's position. A ramp of sound is thus created by suppressing the intensity of near field echoes and amplifying the signals from reflectors in the far field. The entire ramp, or TGC curve, can also be altered by activating the *overall* gain control. (Figure 2.20)

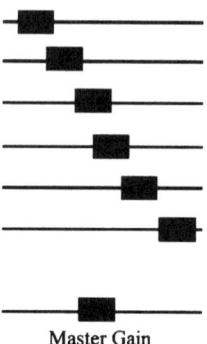

Figure 2.20 TGC (Time Gain Compensation)

Master Gain

Dynamic range

Dynamic range, expressed in decibels (dB), is the ratio of the largest signal to the smallest signal that an electronic device is capable of processing. Different components of the ultrasound scanner have different dynamic range capabilities. The dot brightness, or gray scale of an ultrasound image, is related to the echo signal amplitudes and clinically will be displayed for variations up to 60dB. However, the display monitor has a more limited dB range capability, usually 20 to 30dB. Since the echo amplitudes exceed the display device, the larger signals are "compressed" within the receiver while the lower amplitudes are "boosted". A dynamic range control on the ultrasound system allows the operator to control the effective range of echo signals appearing as shades of gray on the monitor. The wider the dynamic range, the wider the range of displayed gray shades with a maximum display capability of 256 shades.

Most ultrasound units write image data to a memory device called a *scan converter*. Scan conversion is necessary because the times for image acquisition and display to the video monitor occur at different intervals. The scan converter accepts echo image data, converts it to memory and reads out of the memory for viewing. Current ultrasound instruments use digital technology for storage and manipulation of data.

Video display modes

A-mode or *amplitude* mode, registers each signal as a spike along a baseline according to the strength of the returning echo. (Figure 2.21) The higher the spike, the greater the echo intensity. The high acoustic impedance of bone, for instance, will result in a higher amplitude than a fluid filled cyst would demonstrate. The distance from the reference spike or "main bang" to other spikes along the baseline is an indication of the relative distances to other reflectors.

B-mode, or *brightness* mode, plots the returning signals as dots, forming an image representation of the anatomic structure being evaluated. Each dot is assigned a particular gray value in a 256-shade range from white to black according to the strength of the reflected echo. The higher the intensity, the whiter the dot; the weaker the signal, the darker the gray shade.

M-mode, or *motion* mode, utilizes B-mode to display reflector motion plotted over time as in cardiac imaging.

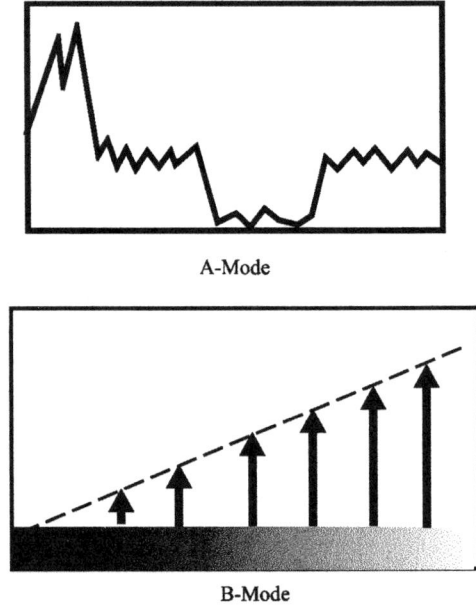

Figure 2.21 Amplitude and Brightness modes

Image display
When viewing the image on a display monitor, the area nearest the transducer is at the top of the screen. By convention, the transverse scan is presented so that the right side of the patient is on the left side of the screen, and for longitudinal or sagittal orientation, cephlad presentation is depicted to the left. All ultrasound transducers have a reference dot or depression on the side of the probe for proper orientation of the transducer during the scanning procedure.

Since an ultrasound image is a two-dimensional display of three dimensional structures, two planes of information must always be acquired for accurate delineation of a structure. A cyst, for example, could appear small in the transverse image, but have a much longer measurement when viewed in the longitudinal plane. (Figure 2.22)

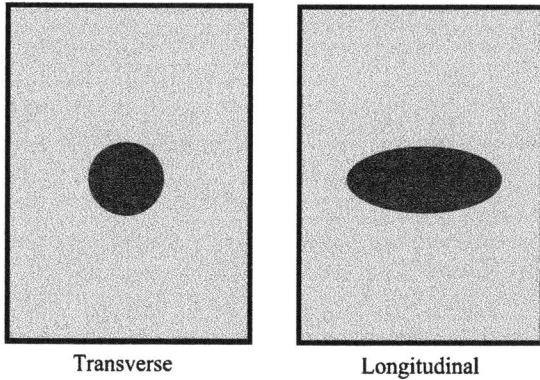

Figure 2.22 Two planes of information must always be acquired for accurate delineation of a structure.

The gain adjustment can dramatically affect the displayed image. Like structures should look alike regardless of location depth. Normal thyroid tissue will have an even or *homogeneous* echo texture from near field to far field with proper gain adjustment.

The amount of gray scale assigned to a returning signal is determined by the molecular composition of the medium and the acoustic mismatch between interfaces. An object with a high acoustic impedance value that will reflect virtually all of the sound waves back to the transducer is depicted as *white*. Such structures are said to be *hyperechoic* or *sonodense*, generating many echoes from the intermolecular interactions with the sound beam. Calcifications will demonstrate this effect. The beam from such hyperechoic structures is highly attenuated so no transmission occurs. This creates an *acoustic shadow* or *sonic tail* posterior to the structure.

The opposite extreme, a fluid-filled cyst, for example, transmits all the ultrasound impulses through it and is therefore considered to be *sonolucent* or *anechoic*, appearing black on the image. Posteriorly, echoes will appear brighter or *enhanced* relative to the surrounding tissue.

Structures with slight differences in acoustic impedance will demonstrate both the ability to transmit and reflect the sound beam, but each structure will have a different gray scale appearance. Recognition of abnormal pathology becomes more apparent as one becomes accustomed to the sonographic depiction of normal anatomic architecture. Thyroid nodules can demonstrate varying sonographic characteristics depending upon their composition. In comparison, lymph nodes will be more echophenic, displaying very few echoes.

The high acoustic impedance value and widely spaced intermolecular composition of a gaseous interface prohibits any transmission of sound from occurring. Air in the trachea, lungs, stomach, etc., will deflect the sound beam and no usable information will be obtained as a result.

Sonographic analysis of an image

There are six phenomena that must be considered in analyzing an image for sonographic interpretation:

1. *Are the margins smooth or rough surfaced?*
   Cysts, adenomas, and vessel walls will display rounded borders while some malignant tumors may have more jagged edges.

2. *What is the retrotumoral acoustic phenomena?*
   Cysts will produce sound *enhancement* while calcifications will demonstrate *acoustic shadowing*.

3. *What is the internal echo pattern?*
   The parenchyma of normal tissue will have a homogeneous or *isoechoic* echo pattern. Sudden changes in echo texture could represent pathology.

3. *What is the echogenicity of the structure being evaluated?*
   Echogenicity is classified according to the following sonographic characteristics: (Figure 2.23)

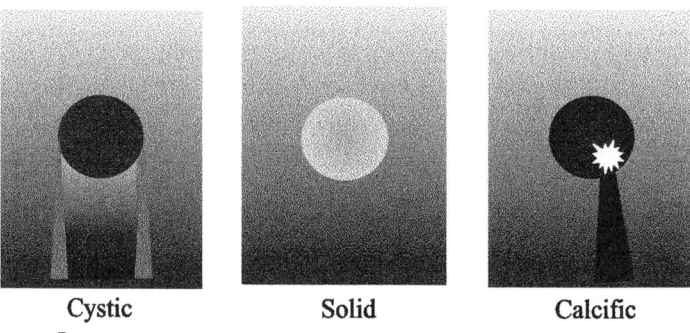

Cystic　　　　Solid　　　　Calcific

Figure 2.23 Sonographic characteristics of a structure.

- *Fluid-filled (cystic)* *Anechoic*
  Smooth, round borders
  Posterior enhancement
- *Solid* *Internal echo pattern*
  Little or no posterior enhancement
- *Calcific* *Hyperechoic*
  Posterior acoustic shadowing

A structure that shows evidence of two or all three of the sonographic patterns is said to be *complex*. An abscess is good example of this, demonstrating both fluid-filled and solid components of varying echogenicity.

4. *What is the effect of compression on the shape of the structure?*
    Thin walled structures are easily compressed. The jugular vein, for example, "winks" when pressure is applied in comparison to the more rigid-walled-carotid artery. Cysts are also compressible, assuming the shape of the anatomic space in which they occur.

5. *What is the effect of compression on the internal echoes?*
    Solid, benign structures, such as fibroadenomas, will become more echo dense when compressed. However, unchanged echogenicity may be indicative of a malignancy.

Artifacts
Artifacts can often cause the obliteration or deterioration of ultrasound information. There are several that have been identified. These are just a few that may be apparent during thyroid scanning.

Contact artifacts
Insufficient contact between the transducer face and the skin will cause intermittent loss of sound through the image. This could be a result of poor operator technique or a lack of transmission gel between the two surfaces.

Gain artifacts
Inappropriate adjustments of TGC or overall gain can cause loss of detail. Not enough amplification could result in the missed diagnosis of pathology. Too much can conversely cause excessive reverberation, filling in cystic structures.

"Halo" effect
Some nodular densities in the thyroid have a sonolucent or echophenic rim. Why this occurs is not clearly explained though speculated causes include edema from the inflammation of capsular tissue, or high vascularity within the capsular rim.

Linear blind spot
The field of view of a linear probe often causes one echo representation to obscure another. The tracheal "ring down", or *comet tail* artifact, will often hamper

visualization of the esophagus, although physically it is in its correct anatomic position.

Refraction
When a sound beam encounters a smooth, round interface, reflection will occur and the beam will be *refracted* at an angle equal to the incident beam. This is the principle defined as Snell's Law and is demonstrated sonographically as edge shadowing.

Reverberation
When sound energy is trapped between two strong reflectors, multiple reflections occur producing a "ring down" effect. This is clearly evidenced by the effect of tracheal cartilaginous rings on a thyroid image.

Side lobes
A *side lobe* is energy in the far field or focal region of an ultrasound transducer that is not part of the main beam. If side lobes are strong, they can degrade the image. A common side lobe artifact is demonstrated when imaging the gallbladder, giving it a sludge effect. The different frequencies in the spectrum of a pulsed transducer however, usually cancel the side lobe effects of one another, making them inconsequential on the image.

BIOLOGIC EFFECTS

Any harmful biologic effects associated with ultrasound imaging remain neither proven nor disproven, but since every ultrasound device transmits energy into the medium at which it is directed, the fact remains that this energy is capable of disrupting biologic systems as evidenced by the therapeutic application called lithotripsy. The major difference between the *diagnostic* and *therapeutic* purposes is in the power of the incident energy.

The FDA (Food and Drug Administration) has established guidelines for acceptable power requirements of an ultrasound system in order to maintain the performance of medically diagnostic ultrasound without apparent incident. The manufacturers of ultrasound equipment must comply with these regulatory standards for such equipment to be used in a clinical environment.

The American Institute of Ultrasound in Medicine (A.I.U.M.) having studied the effects of diagnostic levels of ultrasound, particularly to the fetus in utero, have taken the following official position: "no confirmed biologic effects on patients or instrument operators caused by exposure at intensities typical of present diagnostic U/S instruments have ever been reported. Although the possibility exists that such biological effects may be identified in the future, current data indicates that the benefits of the prudent use of ultrasound outweigh the risks, if any, that may be present."

GLOSSARY OF TERMS

Acoustic impedance Product of density and velocity of sound in a particular material. The amount of reflection of a sound beam is determined by the difference in the impedances of the two tissues.

Acoustic shadow Posterior loss of sound, also called a *sonic tail*.

Amplitude Strength or height of the wave, measured in decibels (dB).

Anechoic Used to refer to a structure which returns no echoes. This could be a simple cyst or cystic structure such as the gall bladder or urinary bladder.

Attenuation Reduction in amplitude and intensity as sound travels due to scatter, reflection and absorption.

Axial resolution Depth resolution; ability to separate two objects lying in tandem along the axis of the beam.

Azimuthal resolution Ability to recognize two distinct reflectors in the plane perpendicular to the anatomic scan plane or slice thickness.

Complex echo pattern Refers to a structure that is heterogeneous and may contain both cystic and solid components.

Dynamic range A log compression value, demonstrating the range of intensity from the largest to the smallest echo that a system can display.

Echo An indication on the monitor of an anatomic structure

Echogenic Refers to any structure capable of returning echoes.

Echophenic Refers to a structure very low in returned echoes.

Echolucent No echoes; anechoic

Heterogeneous Refers to structures with uneven distribution of echo patterns.

Homgeneous Refers to structures with even distribution of echoes.

Hyperechoic	A relative term defining echoes that are returned from a structure. Hyperechoic may mean more echogenic than expected or simply more echogenic than another organ in the same region.
Hypoechoic	A relative term defining echoes that are returned from a structure. Hypoechoic may mean fewer echoes than the surrounding tissue, or fewer echoes than expected.
Interface	Occurs whenever two tissues of different acoustic impedances are in contact.
Isoechoic	A structure in which all of the echoes are of the same intensity.
Lateral resolution	Ability to separate two adjacent objects in the horizontal plane perpendicular to the direction of ultrasound propagation
Piezoelectric	Defines the unique property of the crystals to contract and expand when an electrical current is applied. From the Greek word, "piezo" meaning "pressure".
Reverberation	The phenomenon of multiple reflections within a closed system which causes the echoes to be misplaced in the display thereby representing a false image.
Specular reflection	Reflection from a smooth surface at right angles to the sound beam
Time-gain compensation	Control that compensates for the attenuation of the sound beam as it passes through tissue.

References

1. Curry AC, Tempkin BB: Ultrasonography: An Introduction to Normal Structure and Functional Anatomy. Philadelphia: W.B. Saunders, 1995
2. Heller M, Jehle, D: Ultrasound in Emergency Medicine. Philadelphia: W.B. Saunders, 1995
3. Reynolds, T: Ultrasound Physics: A Registry Exam Preparation Guide. Phoenix: Arizona Heart Institute Foundation, 1996
4. Sanders RC: Clinical Sonography: A Practical Guide, 2nd ed. Boston: Little, Brown and Company, 1991
5. Seeds JW, Chescheir NC, Wade RV: Practical Sonograph in Obstetrics and Gynecology. Philadelphia: Lippincott-Raven Publishers, 1996
6. Zagzebski JA: Essentials of Ultrasound Physics. St. Louis: Mosby-Year Book, 1996

3

METHOD OF PERFORMING ULTRASONOGRAPHY OF THE NECK

Manfred Blum, M.D., F.A.C.E.
Professor of Clinical Medicine and Radiology
Director, Nuclear Endocrine Laboratory

Joseph Yee, M.D.
Clinical Associate Professor of Radiology
New York University School of Medicine
New York, NY 10016 USA

The focus in this chapter is on the technical performance of thyroid ultrasonography, a noninvasive procedure that produces diagnostic and reproducible images. When properly performed, an ultrasound examination answers a clinical question:

- Defines the shape, size and extent of a palpable nodule

- Clarifies controversies about palpation

- Detects a nonpalpable nodule

- Monitors therapeutic goals

- Facilitates aspiration biopsy

- Provides screening for the patient with a high risk of thyroid carcinoma

- Identifies early recurrence of tumor

Overview
There are five interdependent requirements for an excellent thyroid sonogram: 1) the clinician's recognition and expression of the patient's diagnostic problem so that the ultasonographer knows the purpose of the test, 2) the quality of the equipment, 3) the sonographer's technical ability, 4) the interpreting physician's analysis of the images in response to the diagnostic conundrum and the transmission of the information to the clinician, and 5) the clinician applying the results to the patient. The loop starts and ends with the patient. It matters not if

the study is performed by a sonologist, a radiologist, or the clinician, providing there is expertise in technique. Enthusiasm is not enough; quality comes with practice. But even the most experienced operator cannot excel using inferior or archaic equipment. A proper examination requires state of the art technology, that includes hardware, software, and readable images on a screen or film. In some facilities the ultrasound exam, also referred to as a sonogram, is performed in a special laboratory with dedicated personnel or it may be done in an office by the responsible clinician. However, in either setting the essential elements must prevail for a cost-effective and useful study.

Sonography requires science and artistry. In distinction to other procedures that image the thyroid region, such as computerized tomography (CT) or magnetic resonance imaging (MRI) which display anatomy and pathology objectively, ultrasonography requires selectivity by the sonographer to photograph appropriate images that document anatomy and delineate pathology. Not only is knowledge of the anatomy a prerequisite, but an awareness of the clinical problem and the specific question being asked are essential. The operator must attempt to answer the clinical question that has been posed and not merely record the routine anatomy. A standard protocol is essential but must be modified as required by the clinical situation. A team effort is needed to achieve technical excellence, consistency, clinical relevance, and cost-effectiveness.

TECHNICAL

The Equipment
There are basic elements that are similar in all modern commercial ultrasound scanners. Key components include: 1) a transmitter to activate the transducer 2) the transducer itself which generates the sound waves and receives the reflected signal, which are called echoes, 3) a processor, 4) a display of the pictorial data, and 5) a recording of the data. In conventional units the image is displayed in numerous shades of gray whose range, contrast, and brightness are adjusted manually. More sophisticated units will have color and spectral Doppler capability, to detect vascularity and blood flow. This concept will be discussed below. Some technical options are specific for certain manufacturers or "high-end" machines and are not available on all models. Some of these features will be mentioned below when we discuss enhancing the image.

Ultrasound Frequency; Selection of Transducer
The feature that distinguishes sonography is the capability of imaging superficial small parts, such as the thyroid with ultra-high frequency sound waves to produce exquisite resolution (in the order of 1 – 2 mm.) without using ionizing radiation (1). The energy level employed is in the megahertz range (million cycles per second), which is both inaudible and safe.

High frequency transducers that have a linear or curvilinear configuration are used because of their great resolution and their ability to minimize distortion. Currently employed clinical equipment uses a mean frequency between 7 and 13 MHz for nodules and goiters that are less than 6cm in maximal dimension. Large thyroid goiters may require a lower frequency both to include the entire gland for measurement and also to image at depths greater than 5cm. The transducers that are clinically most useful are a curvilinear 5 MHz, curvilinear 7 MHz, and linear 7 MHz, each with multifrequency capabilities. (Figure 3.1)

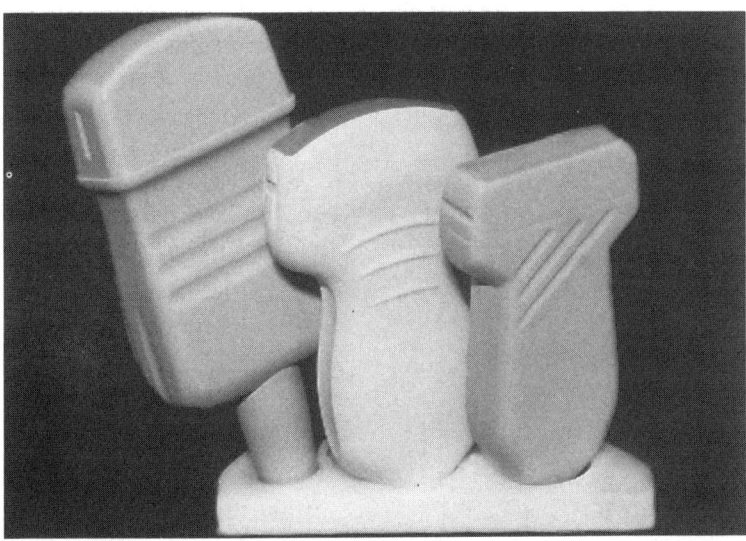

Figure 3.1 Commonly used high frequency transducers are pictured from left to right: Curvilinear 5 MHz, Curvilinear 7 MHz, and Linear 7 MHz. Note that the higher frequency probes have smaller "scanheads" or "footprints."

Doppler Imaging

Doppler imaging is a useful and widely available adjunct to gray scale imaging of the thyroid gland that demonstrates specific blood vessels in tissue and the overall vascularity of organ parenchyma. In the gray scale mode, the Doppler signal is depicted as a very bright region. Color Doppler imaging (2) uses frequency shifts to depict flow with regard to direction (phase shift) and velocity (frequency shift). With color imaging, directional information can be encoded according to convention. Red signifies flow in one direction and blue in the opposite direction. Color Doppler can be modified by increasing its sensitivity at the expense of losing the directional information, which is called Power Doppler. Power Doppler is an angle-independent property, whereas mean frequency shift Doppler is highly dependent on the angle of insonation. Power Doppler draws its greater sensitivity to blood flow by incorporating rather than filtering, baseline noise data. A drawback to this greater sensitivity is the problem of color "flashes" which detect the slightest motion, either by the operator or the patient, including breathing or swallowing. An arbitrary electronic assignment of color, to denote direction, in Power Doppler, has been achieved by one manufacturer, which they call "convergent color". Since each manufacturer has a certain uniqueness in the color

Doppler display, it is important to consult with them as to the most effective way of incorporating color Doppler data in routine practice. As a general rule, it is most important to have color Doppler settings that are appropriate for slow flow; that is, lowest velocity scale, lowest wall filter setting and the most sensitive priority setting. (Figure 3.2) Figure 3.2 also demonstrates that color flow obtained in real-time is oftentimes recorded in the black and white format (3). The higher frequency transducers will also enhance color Doppler sensitivity. In Power Doppler, the highest log compression scale without significant flash artifacts is most desirable.

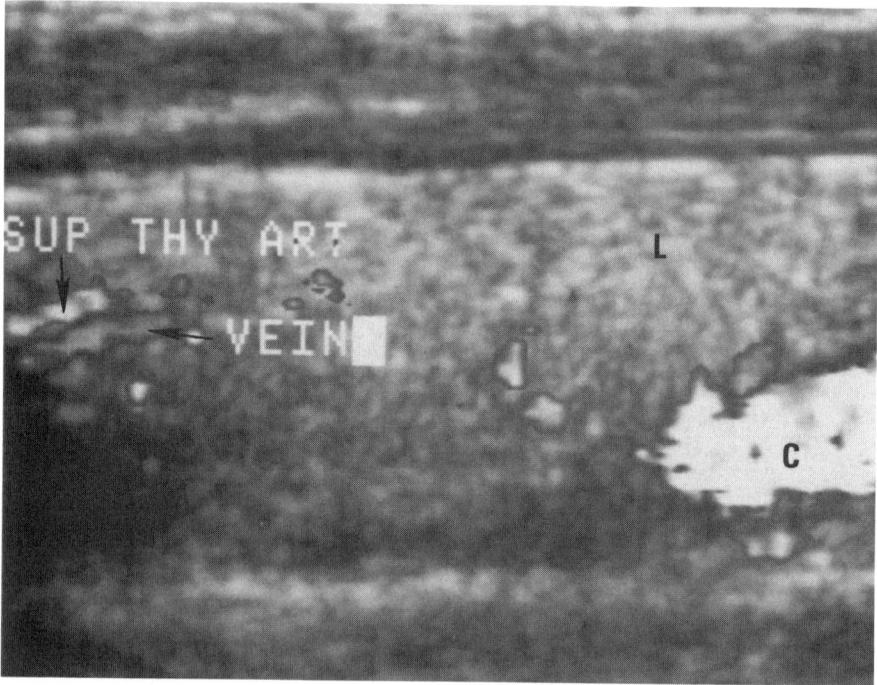

Figure 3.2 Sagittal view of the right thyroid lobe (L). The bright areas are color Doppler flow data, photographed in shades of gray, which show normal vascularity. The superior thyroid artery and vein are seen (arrows). The bright area below and deep to the lower pole of the lobe (C) is an oblique portion of the common carotid artery.

Color Doppler can assess the overall glandular or focal vascularity in a nodule. Diffuse hypervascularity is seen in Graves' disease that has been called, "thyroid inferno" (4), an ultrasound equivalent of a thyroid bruit. Hypervascularity may also be seen in inflammatory conditions such as Hashimoto's thyroiditis (Figure 3.3). In focal lesions, color Doppler may help to delineate a thyroid nodule that is not otherwise defined by distinctive echogenicity when compared with the rest of the lobe. This feature is useful when a thyroid nodule almost replaces the entire lobe. Furthermore, a very hypoechoic nodule on gray scale echography may be incorrectly considered cystic but can be distinguished from a cystic nodule by demonstrating vascularity within the lesion (Figure 3.4). Occasionally, a blood vessel can also simulate a cystic nodule and Doppler examination can identify it properly. Finally, Doppler imaging can demonstrate a vascular halo to reveal an isoechoic nodule (Figure 3.5A and 3.5B)

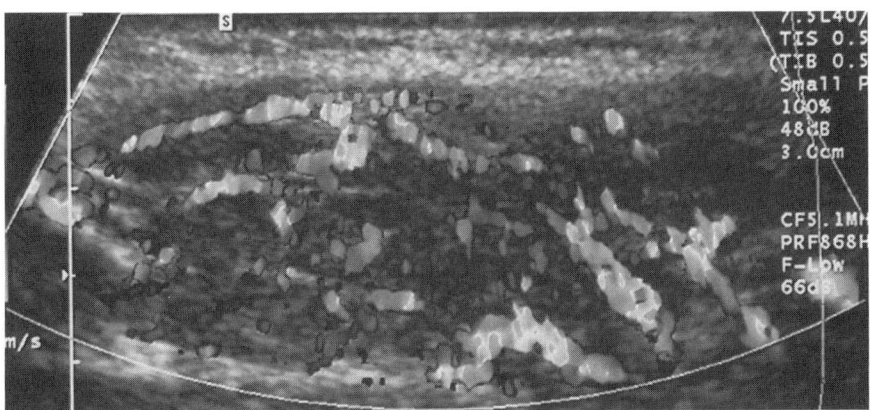

Figure 3. 3 Color Doppler image in the sagittal plane of a lobe, photographed in shades of gray with parenchymal hyperemia (the two toned bright areas) in a patient with Hashimoto's thyroiditis.

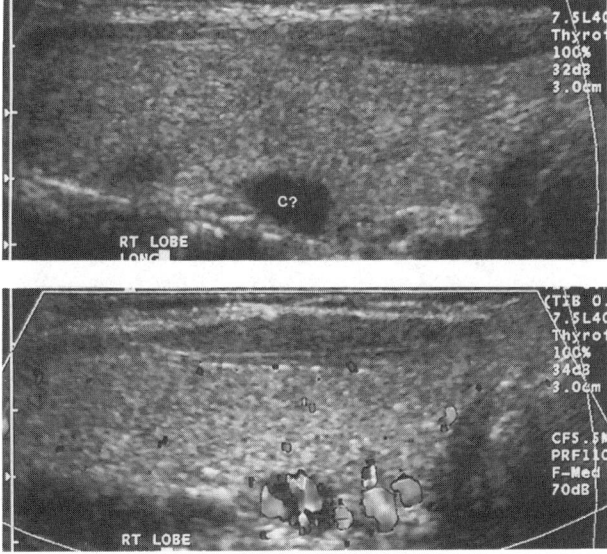

Figure 3. 4 Panel A shows a gray scale image in the sagittal plane of an anechoic structure that was initially considered cystic (C?). Panel B shows Doppler imaging and demonstrates that the structure is vascular and not a cyst.

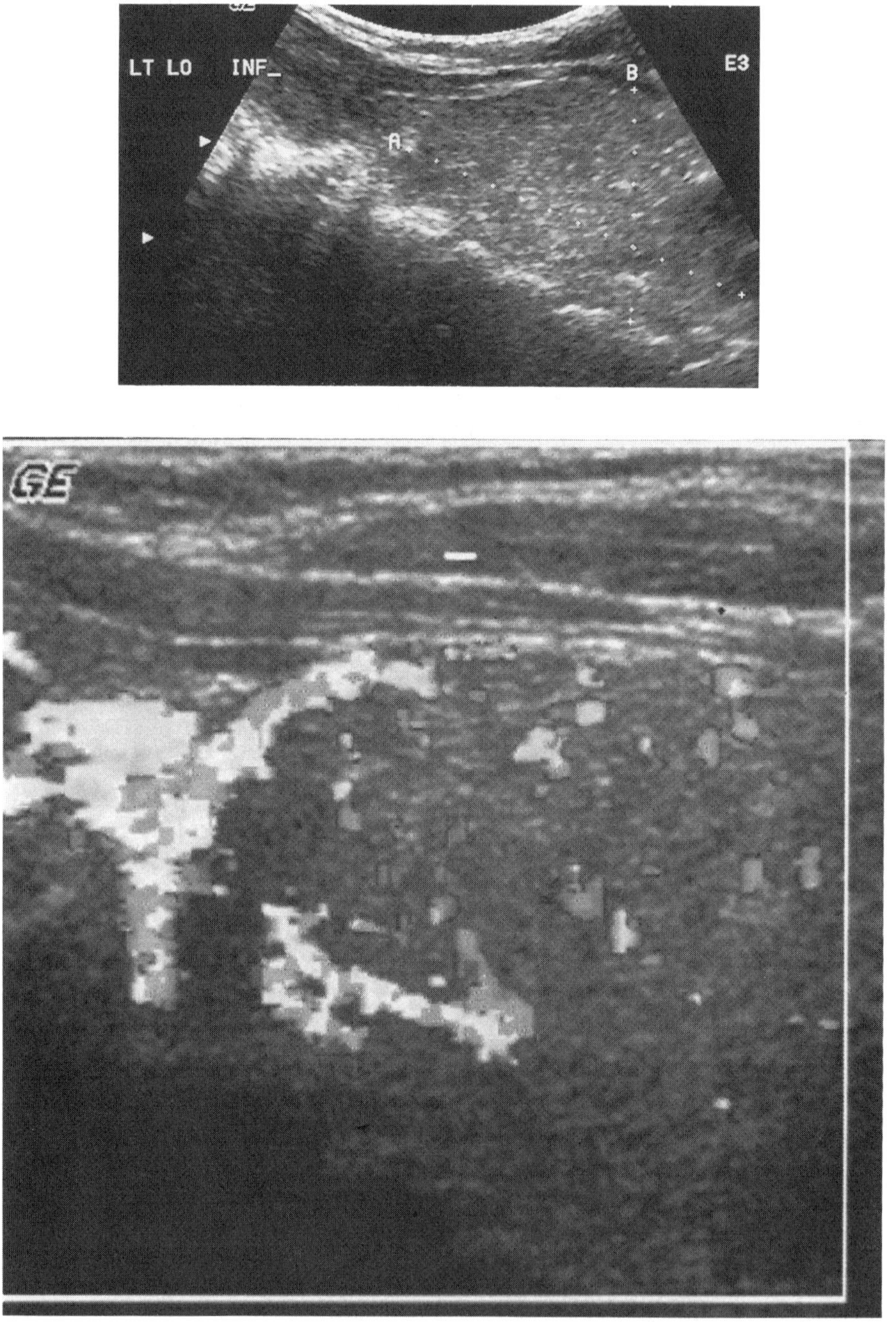

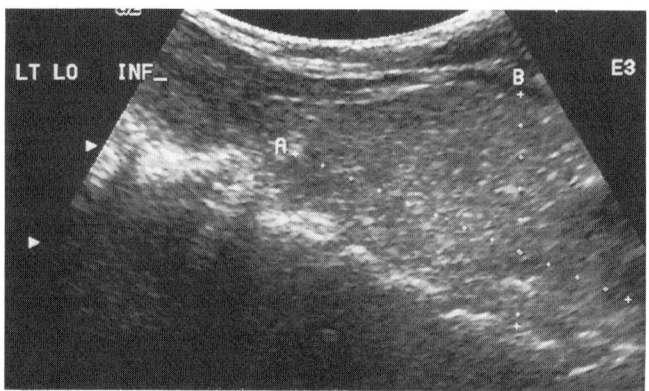

Figure 3. 5 Panel A shows a sagittal view of a palpable solid nodule (A-B) that is isoechoic and is not "seen". Panel B shows the Doppler signal added, demonstrating a vascular halo that makes the nodule more obvious.

Color Doppler has not been successful in distinguishing benign from malignant nodules. However, Clarke et al. (5) has reported that "hot" nodules on scintigraphy have been shown to have more central vascularity and cold nodules, more peripheral vascularity.

Improving the Conventional Image
There have been several recent innovations that probably will be widely used because of their greater sophistication leading to enhanced diagnostic accuracy.

"Extended Field of View" instrumentation allows high resolution real-time scanning with a linear probe as well as demonstrating an anatomic area that is considerably larger than the conventional images. Thus, an entire gland whose dimensions exceed the width of the probe can be visualized. This is accomplished by electronically storing and assembling images from adjacent fields to produce a composite picture (Figure 3.6). In this mode, the high-resolution images are continuously summated to form one large image. A modification of this approach is the electronic transformation of the usual linear field of view into a trapezoidal field, so that the region examined is expanded at two margins. Most commercial units allow for a dual summation of only 2 linear images, thus providing a limited extended field of view.

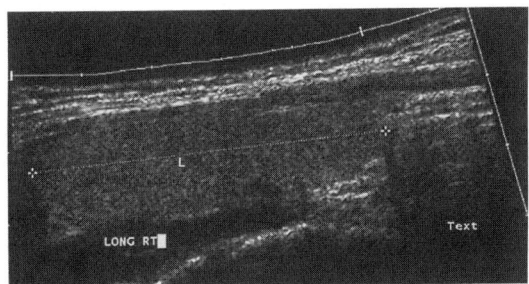

Figure 3.6 Shows a sonographic image of an enlarged right lobe of the thyroid gland (L) in the sagittal plane using extended field of view imaging that shows the entire lobe. This lobe has normal texture and no nodule.

More sophisticated units are also available to assemble, modify and reformat multiple images in depth to produce 3-dimensional imaging. Such data can be acquired in color Doppler to show global vascularity or in gray scale for relationship anatomy. When 3rd dimensional images are examined in real time, the study is referred to as 4th dimensional imaging.

An innovative way of improving image resolution by decreasing the noise clutter that is inherent in all images is called native tissue harmonics. In simplest terms, with harmonic imaging, digital filters select harmonics of the fundamental ultrasound frequency. The resultant higher frequency echo is a weaker signal than the fundamental one and requires amplification but yields better resolution. While this approach was initially introduced for deep abdominal imaging, newer applications are now available for small parts imaging.

PERFORMING THE EXAMINATION

Patient Positioning

The patient is typically scanned in the supine position with mild hyperextension of the neck. Support for the shoulders is provided in the form of a foam wedge or a "oatmeal" pillow, consistent with comfort. Patients with cervical spine disease such as degenerative arthritis may require some modification in the degree of hyperextension. The operator (sonographer) may stand at the head of the examining table, as one might do for carotid examinations (Figure 3.7), or from the right side of the patient, as one might do for abdominal studies (Figure 3.8). A slight tilt of the transducer, to conform to the skin surface, facilitates a high quality image. For the right-handed sonographer, the ultrasound equipment is set up such that the right hand does the actual scanning and the left hand adjusts the scanning features of the machine. At the outset of the test, it is important to establish on the equipment the superior and inferior margins in the cephalo-caudad plane and the medial or lateral margins in the axial or transverse plane. To confirm correct orientation of the system relative to the patient, the sonographer touches either end of the gel-coated transducer in the plane of scanning to demonstrate that the orientation is correct in the right/left or cephalo/caudad planes.

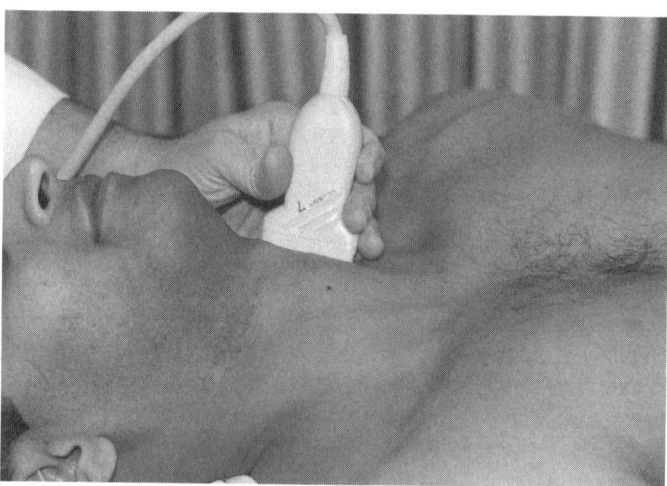

Figure 3.7. Scanning the left side of the neck in the sagittal plane. The sonographer is at the head of the table, using the "carotid" approach.

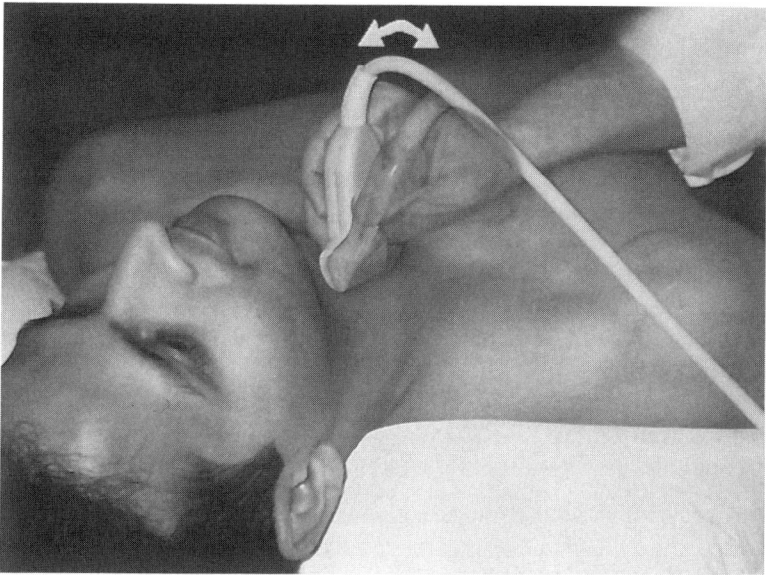

Figure 3.8 Scanning the right side of the neck in the sagittal plane, where the sonographer stands at right side of the patient using the "abdominal" approach. Note that a slight tilt of the transducer (arrow) may be advantageous to conform to the surface of the neck. However, excessive tilt must be avoided to prevent imaging in the coronal, rather than the sagittal plane.

Problem Oriented Scanning Protocol

The sonographer must be aware of the clinical question and be certain that the scope of the study will address this issue. The thyroid gland is initially scanned in real-time, in both the sagittal and axial planes for general orientation. Especially when the thyroid gland is atrophic, surgically absent, or ectopic, it is important to identify the submandibular glands and the strap muscles to avoid a false impression that they are thyroid tissue.

Next, the entire region is systematically explored with static images in the sagittal plane starting in the midline (for the isthmus and pyramidal lobe), and then laterally on each side, to view the medial, central, and lateral aspect of each lobe and the regions peripheral to the thyroid. Each sagittal scan is done from the sternal notch to the submandibular region. The common carotid artery and the jugular vein are the vascular landmarks used to define the most lateral or outer border of the thyroid gland. Using a Valsalva maneuver, the jugular vein becomes distended and forms a useful landmark for the lateral border of the gland. The superior and inferior boundaries are also demonstrated in the sagittal plane. At times, swallowing is a useful maneuver to demonstrate the inferior border, because the entire thyroid gland is drawn superiorly when swallowing takes place. However, because swallowing may be a rapid process, the "frozen" image may not depict the lower pole of the gland on its upward position. In that case, the cine function of most modern units allows the operator to recall the last series of images for a sharp undistorted view of the inferior margin of the gland. This technique is particularly useful for some substernal goiters. Still in the sagittal plane, scanning superiorly beyond the level of the thyroid cartilage depicts craniad structures such as the pyramidal lobe or thyroglossal duct cysts.

The axial plane is studied next. Representative images are taken in the upper, middle, and lower portions of each lobe and also in regions where pathology has been demonstrated on the sagittal views.

Finally, attention is re-focused on the clinical question to be certain that a correct and pertinent response has been obtained. Correlation of the images with other studies, when available, especially a radionuclide study of the thyroid gland is helpful to that end.

ANATOMY AND PATHOLOGY
Anatomy
The normal thyroid gland is homogeneous and has the appearance of ground glass and is more echogenic than the strap or sternocleidomastoid muscles. The thyroid gland is superficial to the anterior and lateral aspect of the larynx and trachea. The thyroid in the female is located higher in the neck when compared with the male. In women, the upper poles may be located lateral to the lower part of the thyroid cartilage. The gland consists of right and left lobes that are joined by a bridge of tissue, the isthmus. The pyramidal lobe, which is a remnant of the thyroglossal duct, is demonstrated to extend upward from the thyroid isthmus. It can be seen in 10 – 40% of normal patients, especially in younger patients (6) (Figure 3.9). It is similar in echo-density to the thyroid gland and is more definable and prominent in those patients who have a goiter or Graves' disease. It is important not to confuse a prominent pyramidal lobe with an isthmus nodule (Figure 3.10) or pretracheal lymph node. Anterior to the thyroid gland are the strap muscles, namely, the sternothyroid and sternohyoid muscles. (Figure 3.11) The sternohyoid muscle is medial in location compared to the sternothyroid muscle. Lateral to the strap muscles is the much larger sternocleidomastoid muscle (SCM), which is used to classify the neck into the anterior and posterior triangles. The various triangles in the anterior and posterior neck is summarized in a review by Harnsberger et al. (7). The insertion of the SCM is readily apparent near the base of the neck, especially when the head is turned laterally. Posterior to the trachea and thyroid, and usually to the left of the midline, is a hypoechoic structure, the esophagus, which should not be mistaken for a thyroid nodule, parathyroid lesion or a lymph node. It can be shown in the sagittal plane as a tubular structure that is distended when the patient drinks water. The longus colli muscles define the posterior border of the thyroid gland and frame the deepest useful penetration of conventional transducers.

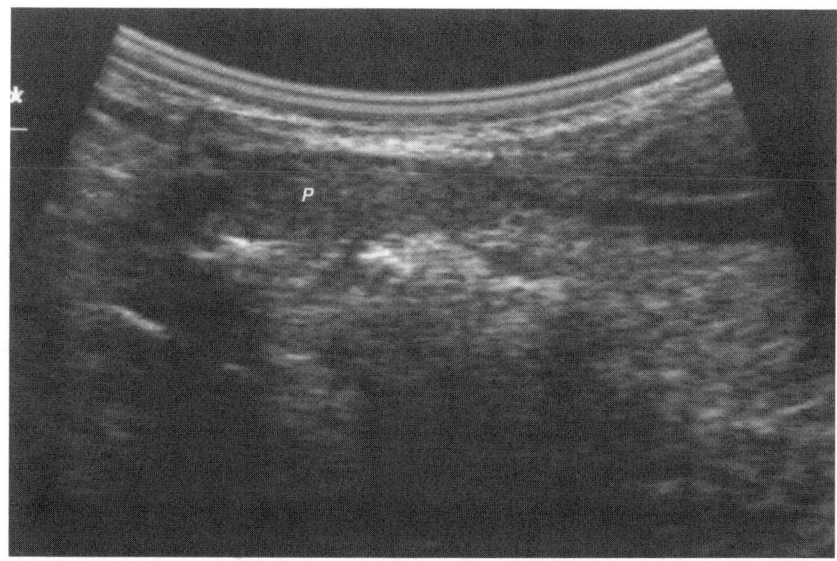

Figure 3.9 Sonogram of the sagittal view of an enlarged pyramidal lobe (P), containing no nodule.

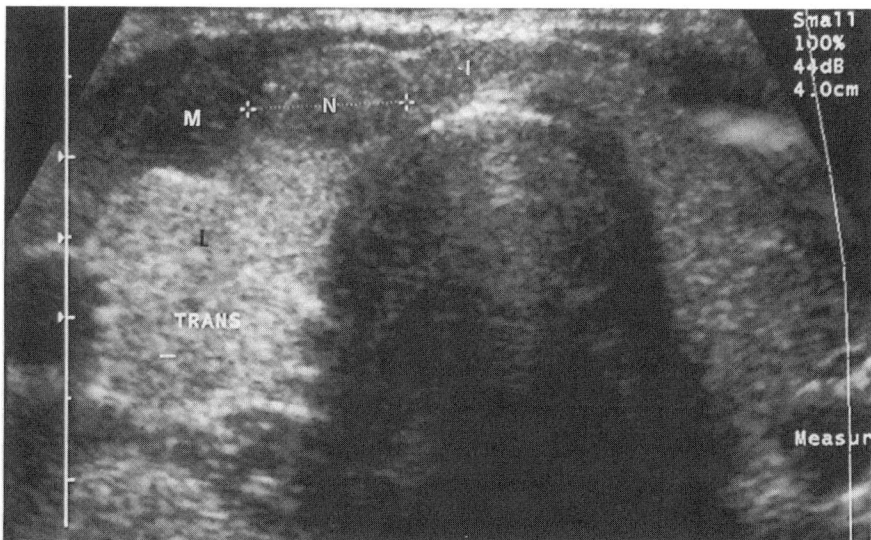

Figure 3.10 Sonogram of the transverse view of a palpable solid hypoechoic nodule (N), that was located at the intersection of the isthmus (I) and the right lobe (L). Because of the location and it is hypoechoic, the nodule, it may be confused with the strap muscle (M). The brightness of the right lobe compared with the left lobe is an artifact due to greater probe to skin contact.

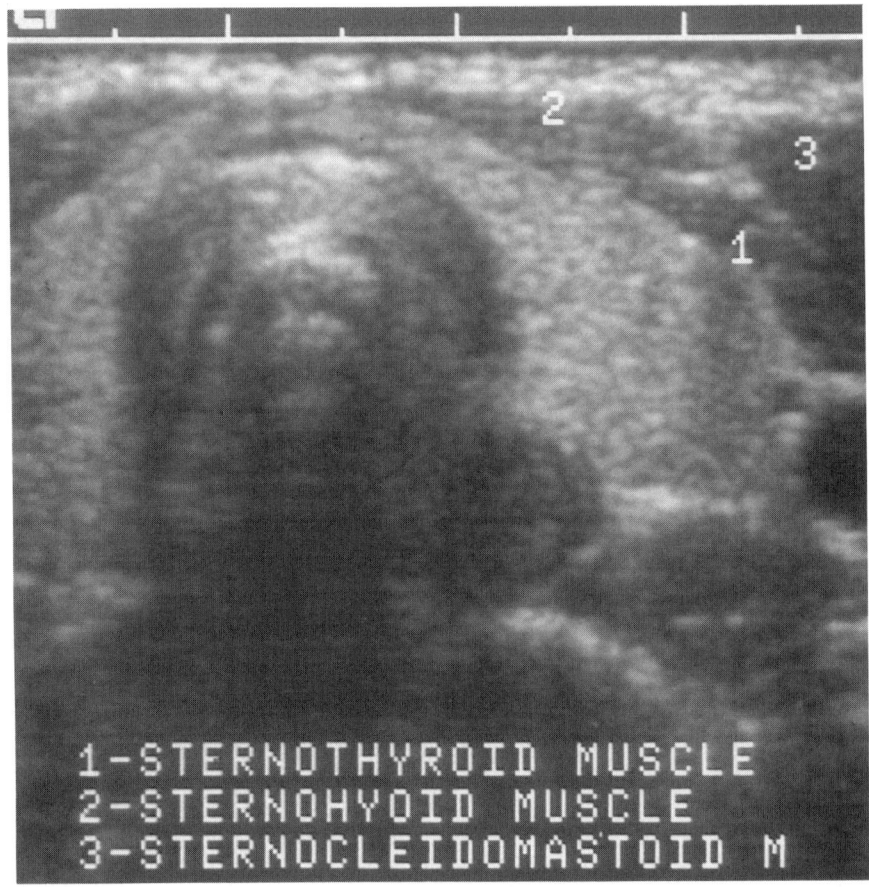

Figure 3.11 Sonogram of the transverse view of the thyroid gland with delineation of the three major regional muscles: (1) sternothyroid, (2) sternohyoid, and (3) sternocleidomastoid muscles.

The skin and subcutaneous tissue including the platysma may also be demonstrated using higher frequency transducers, (10-13MHz.). Their image is enhanced by displacing the transducer from the skin to reduce the "near field" artifact, using extra gel or a disposable silicon pad "offset" (8) (Figure 3.12 and 3.13).

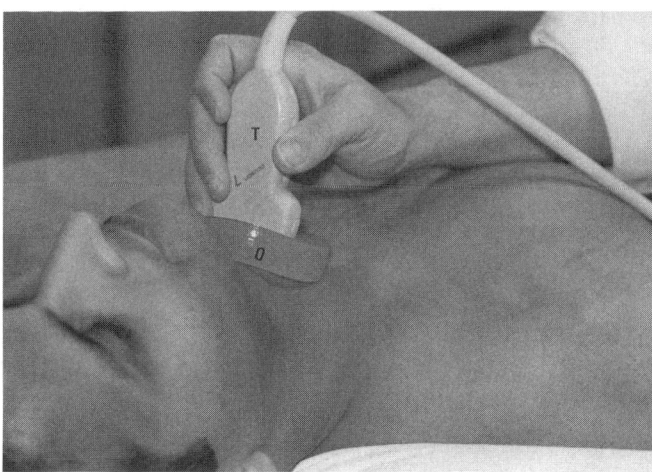

Figure 3.12 Superficial structures that are in the near field may be best imaged with a silicon offset (O), so that the skin surface is not at the surface of the transducer (T). Both sides of the offset must be moistened or gel-coated to allow optimal probe contact. Overall receiver gain settings should be increased to allow greater depth penetration. Increased gel volume on the skin with "light touch" scanning may be a useful alternative.

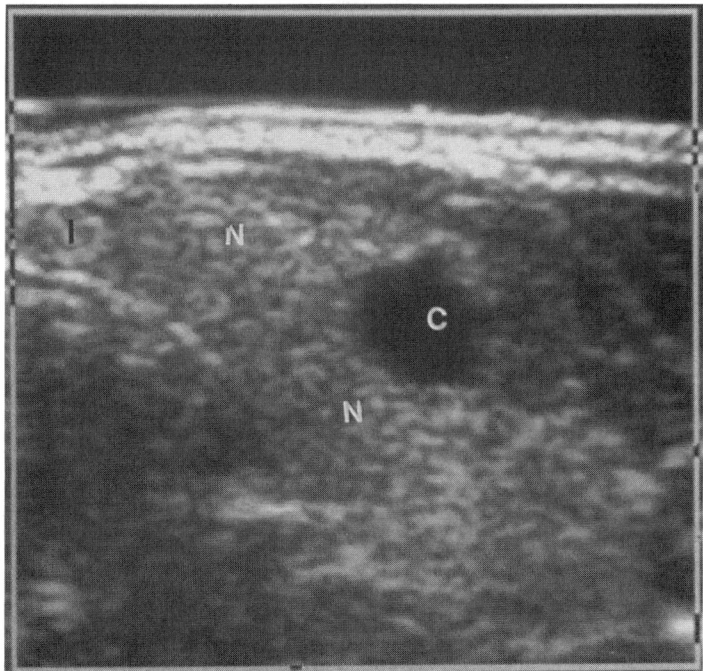

Figure 3.13 Transverse image of a superficial thyroid nodule (N) near the isthmus (I), using an offset, to allow enhanced resolution. The nodule contains an area of cystic degeneration (C).

Thyroid Size

The size of each lobe is measured in the mid-sagittal plane to obtain the length (L) and anterior-posterior (AP) dimension. The transverse plane (Figure 3.14) is taken to estimate its cross sectional width (W), usually taken at mid-portion.(Figure 3.15) Each lobe is an ellipsoid that is usually 4 X 1 - 1.5 X 1 cm. in length, width, and depth (AP), respectively. Volume is estimated using the formula for a prollate ellipse, Volume = 0.5 (L x AP x W). The isthmus of the gland in the transverse plane forms a bridge between the two lobes in the midline and usually is less than 5 mm in height and 3mm in depth. The average volume of a thyroid lobe in normal subjects is 12-40 cc.(9)

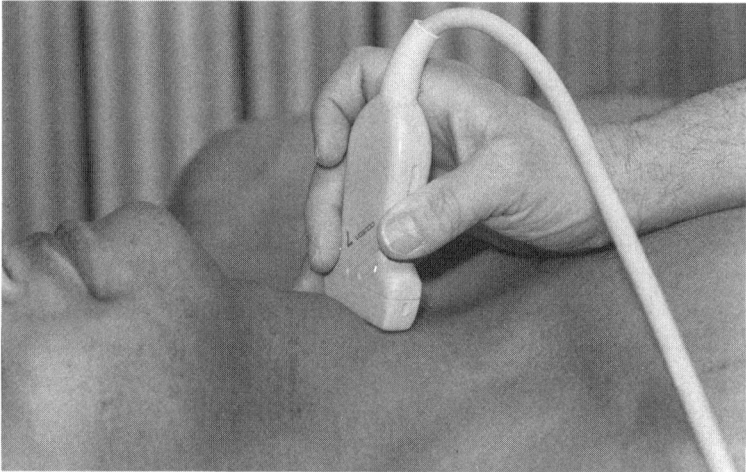

Figure 3.14 Scanning the thyroid gland below the level of thyroid cartilage in the transverse plane to image the isthmus of gland and to obtain the axial (transverse)views of each lobe.

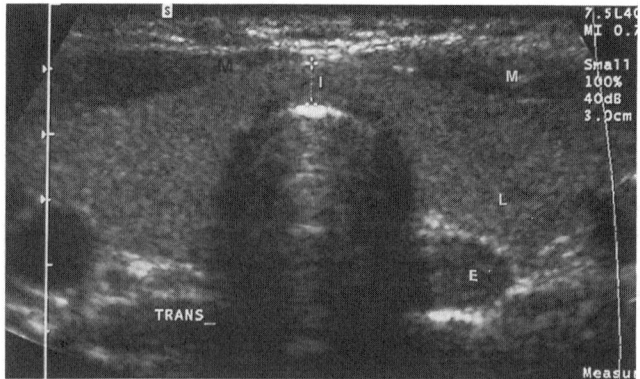

Figure 3.15 Sonographic image of the anterior part of the neck in the transverse plane. The isthmus (I) is 3 mm. in depth, which is normal. The lobes (L) are uniform, without nodules. Note the hypoechoic strap muscles (M), anteriorly, and the esophagus (E) on the left side, posteriorly.

Pathology
Abnormalities of the gland are described as either focal or diffuse. Although these changes are non-specific, they may offer clues that are useful or even essential in clinical management, and must be revealed by the sonographer.

Nodules
Focal, discrete areas are called nodules, whose echo-density may be greater (hyperechoic), lower (hypoechoic), or equal (isoechoic) than the rest of the gland. Figure 3.16 illustrates both an isoechoic thyroid nodule and a hypoechoic solid parathyroid nodule in the same person. Hyperechoic or hypoechoic nodules are seen as distinct by virtue of their relative echogenicity. Isoechoic nodules are not identified by their echogenicity but rather by a defined rim or halo, calcification or altered blood flow. Hyperechoic or hypoechoic nodules may also have these features. Furthermore, nodules may be entirely solid, fluid-containing (cystic), or complex, having a mixture of solid and cystic regions. Complex nodules may appear to be cystic on one image but additional views will demonstrate a small solid component, septae, or calcifications (Figure 3.17). Nodules may be large, and when greater than 1 - 1.5 cm in diameter, may correlate with palpation. West and associates (10) reported what many have long suspected that high frequency ultrasound at 7.5 MHz is more sensitive in the detection of nodules when compared with clinical palpation. However, sonography may detect nodules as small a 2-3 mm which are not palpable and are called "incidentalomas" because of their uncertain clinical meaning. It is the sonographer's role to identify the nodules and define their location and characteristics. The clinician has the responsibility to decide if further diagnosis and management are required.

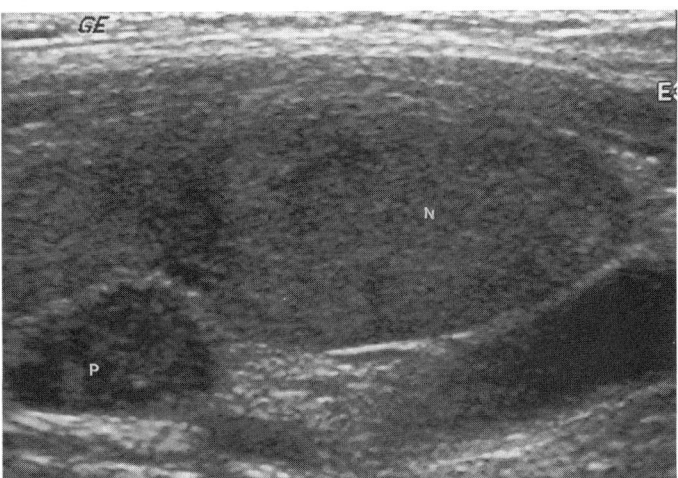

Figure 3.16 Sagittal view of a large solid thyroid nodule (N) that is nearly isoechoic with adjacent tissue. There is a smaller parathyroid mass (P) which is more hypoechoic. The parathryoid mass was confirmed with a Technetium sestamibi nuclear scan.

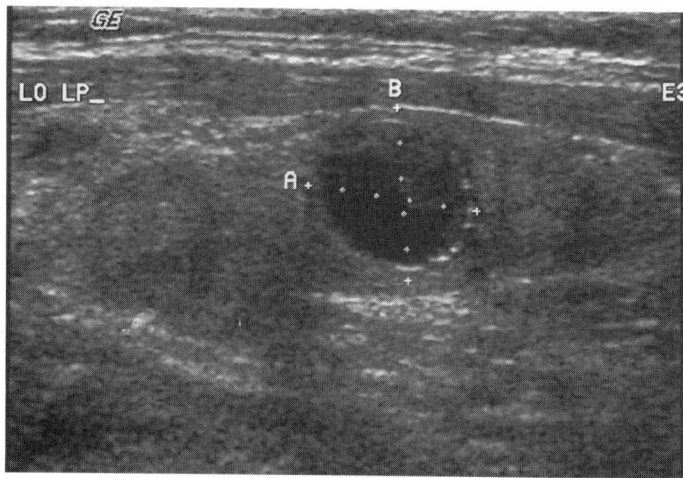

Figure 3.17 Sagittal view of a nodule (A-B) that has undergone cystic degeneration. Note that the periphery of the nodule has bright spots due to small calcifications in the rim.

When there are multiple nodules, it is useful for the sonographer to make a map of the anterior neck (5). This diagram depicts the gland in the coronal plane to indicate the number and location of defined nodules in a simplified format. It helps to transmit anatomic data to the clinician and to facilitate follow-up examinations by subsequent sonographers (Figure 3.18).

Goiters
Diffuse thyroid abnormalities involve size, and/or the texture and intensity of the echo pattern. (Figure 3.19) Glands that are larger than defined above are called goiters. They may be uniform or heterogeneous in echo-texture, in which case they are called, multinodular. The goiter or nodularity may be hyper or hypo echo-dense, solid, cystic, or complex, or have areas of calcification. All of these attributes need to be documented for clinical interpretation.

Dominant nodule in a goiter
There may also be a dominant nodule within a multinodular or a uniform goiter. The sonographer must call attention to such a nodule, its location, its echo characteristics, and whether it corresponds to a palpable mass or tender region. Occasionally, a posterior nodule may be confused with a parathyroid nodule. See Figure 3.16. The sonographic texture may help to distinguish a thyroid nodule from a parathyroid nodule.

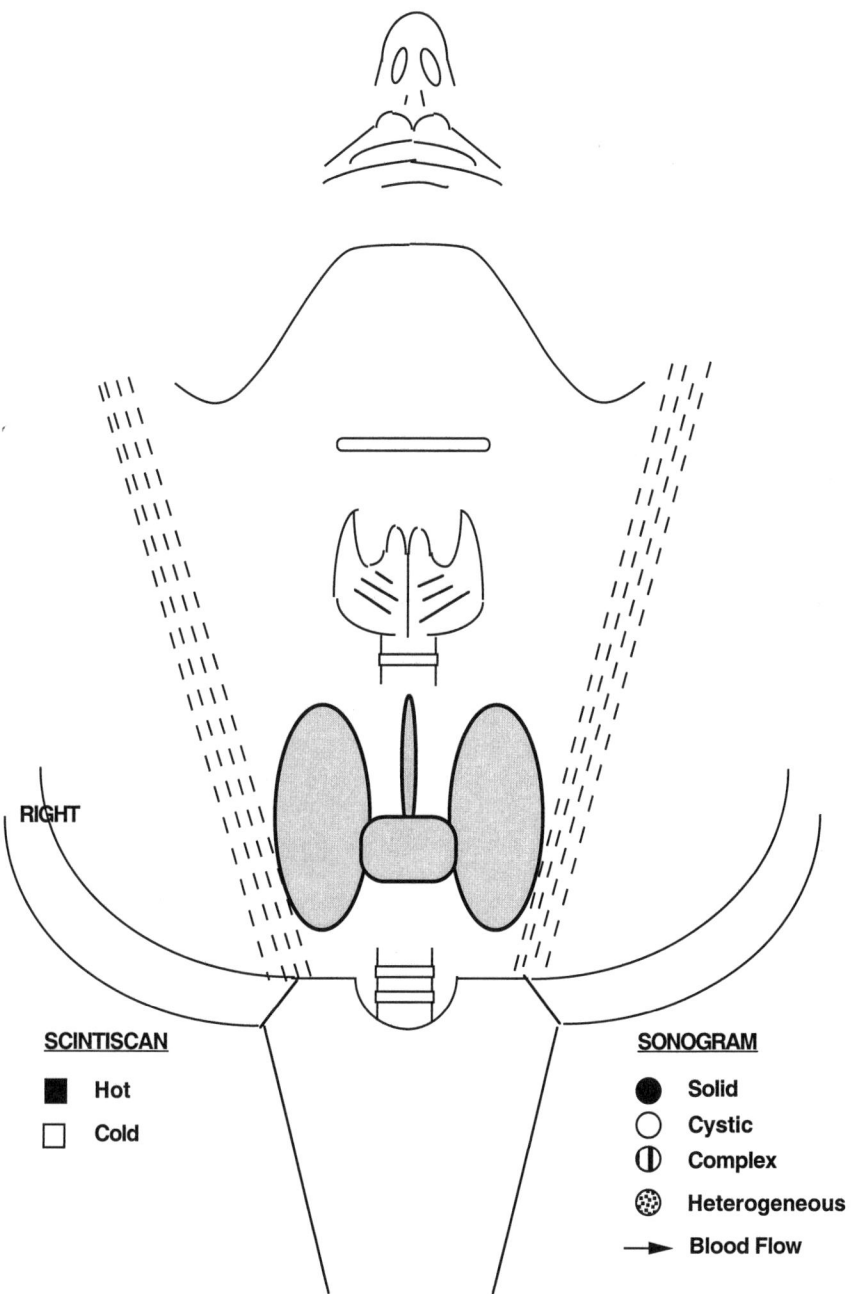

Figure 3.18 Mapping thyroid nodules can be accomplished with a diagram portraying the gland in the coronal plane.

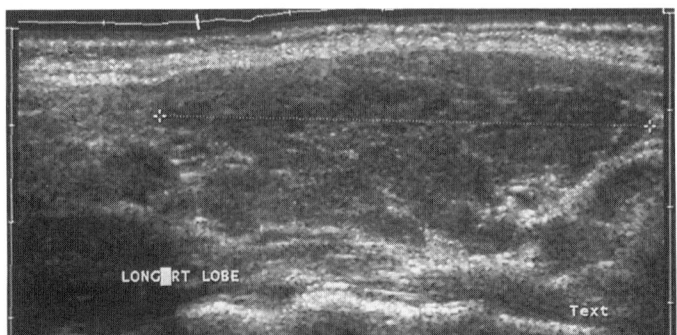

Figure 3.19 Sagittal view of an enlarged diffusely multinodular lobe (*---*) in a patient with Hashimoto's thyroiditis. Extended field of view imaging, at 7 MHz, was used to include the entire length of the lobe.

Cervical Nodes

A normal node is elliptical or bean-shaped and has an echo-dense hilum. (Figure 3.20 A and 3.20B) The ratio of the length to width of a node that is not involved with tumor is usually greater than 2 (Length divided by anterior-posterior thickness >2) (11). If the node is smaller than 1 cm. in maximal dimension, this criterion may not be valid. However, fortunately, such small nodes are usually not clinically significant unless they enlarge or change shape.

To identify adenopathy, which is essential information that is sometimes not clinically apparent, the sonographer must evaluate the regions where lymph nodes are usually situated. The examination is extended laterally beyond the common carotid artery and jugular vein to identify the jugular chain of lymph nodes. (Figure 3.21) The simplest approach is to scan these regions in the transverse plane from the base of the neck to the carotid bifurcation to locate the groove between the carotid artery and the jugular vein. Other nodes may be seen inferior to the thyroid gland (Figure 3.22) above the isthmus in the midline, (the Delphian node), and in the submental and submandibular regions.

Extrathyroidial Lesions

The need to identify an extrathyroidial mass sonographically is usually occasioned by the discovery of a mass by palpation, radiologically, or by an abnormal blood test like hypercalcemia. In any case, the clinical clue must be recognized and understood and the clinical concern communicated to the sonographer. It helps for the sonographer to know that that there is something ectopic suspected, and where it may be located. Sometimes an accomplished sonographer may see an unsuspected ectopic mass and alert the clinician to a problem.

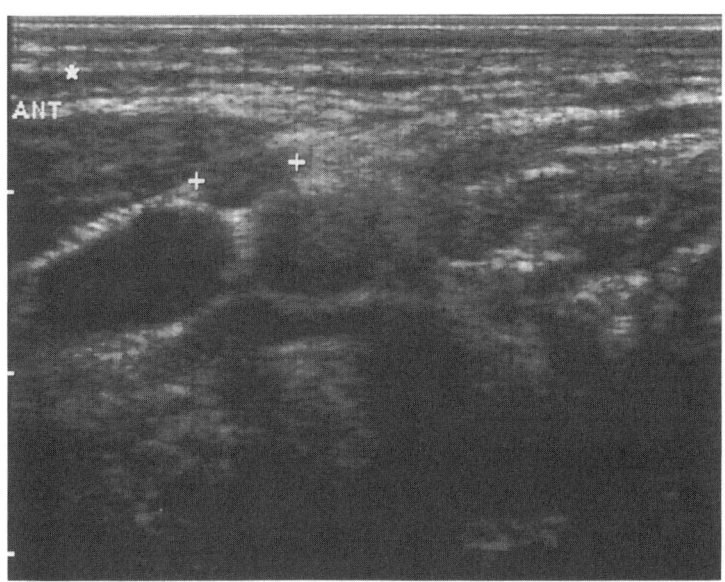

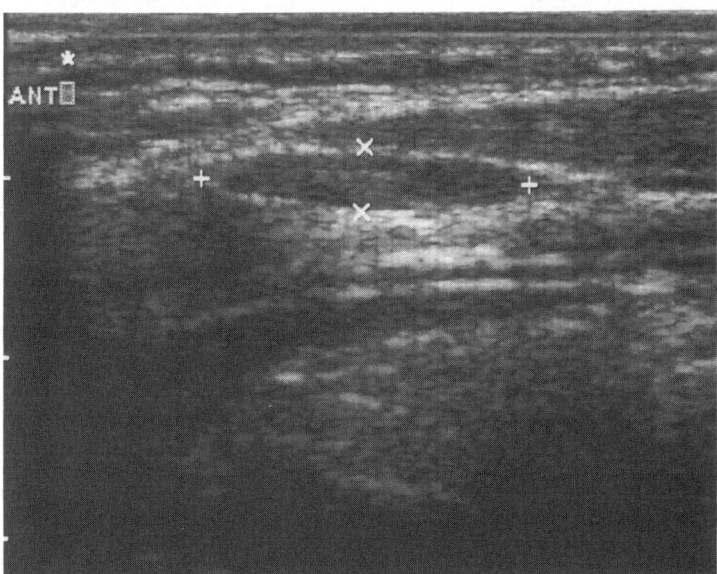

Figure 3.20 Panel **A** shows the transverse image of an anterior cervical node (+ --- +) in the jugular chain in the sulcus between the right jugular vein and common carotid artery. Panel **B** shows a sagittal view of the anterior cervical node previously identified (+ --+, x – x). It was obtained by rotating the probe 90 degrees, clockwise. This node has a slender elliptical shape and a thin echogenic hilum.

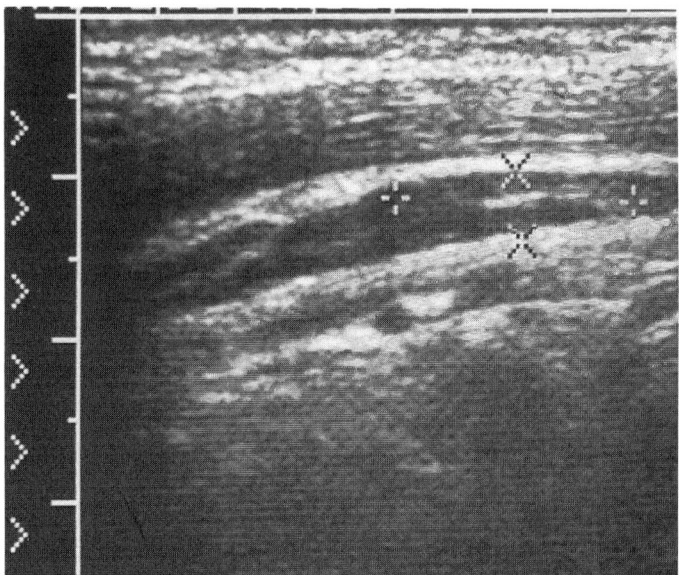

Figure 3.21 Sagittal view of jugular chain lymph nodes. Portions of the sternocleidomastoid muscle is imaged anterior to the jugular nodes, all of which are normal.

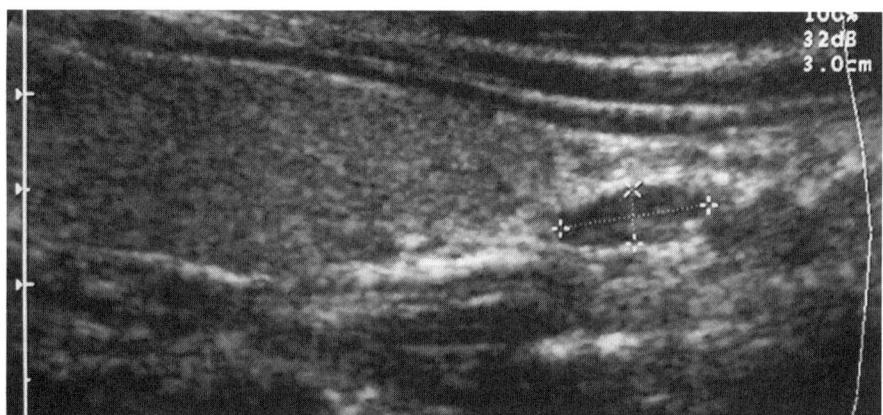

Figure 3.22 Sagittal view of a small lymph node (+ --+, x – x) inferior to the thyroid lobe. An echogenic hilum may help to distinguish it from a parathyroid lesion.

A frequently encountered extrathyroidial lesion in the anterior, infrahyoid neck is a parathyroid mass. Adenopathy, either reactive or malignant is another frequent cause of neck masses. Less commonly seen are thyroglossal duct cysts (usually midline), branchial cleft cysts (usually para-median or laterally located), cystic hygromas, arteriovenous malformations, ectopic thyroid tissue, and subcutaneous lesions such as lipomas, sebaceous cysts or other mesenchymal lesions. The most common pulsatile neck mass is a buckled innominate artery, although a common carotid artery aneurysm may also pulsate. Certain extrathyroid masses are probably better evaluated by spiral CT and MR imaging than sonography, especially for deep lesions like those involving the brachial plexus (12).

Parathyroid

In our experience, the normal parathyroid glands are not generally visualized using current state of the art commercial scanners with high frequency imaging up to 13MHz. Reading and colleagues (13) however, claims that occasionally normal parathyroid glands, with typical measurements of 5 x 3 x 1 mm, may be visualized in young adults.. A normal parathyroid gland is 20 – 40 mg in weight, and is less than 6 mm in its greatest dimension. While lymph nodes of this size can be visualized sonographically when they are adjacent to muscle or a blood vessel, normal parathyroid glands are poorly imaged because their echogenicity is not significantly different from the contiguous thyroid gland. However, an enlarged parathyroid gland may be quite distinctive. The usual parathyroid adenoma is identified as a hypoechoic ovoid mass that has a definable cleavage plane with the posterior margin of the thyroid gland. There may be one enlarged gland when the lesion is an adenoma, or there may be multiple adenomas, or four enlarged glands in the case of parathyroid hyperplasia.

Areas that are difficult, if not impossible, to evaluate for a parathyroid lesion include the retrotracheal, retroesophageal, retropharyngeal regions, and the superior mediastinum. Similarly, an intrathyroid parathyroid mass will usually be obscure. However, if there is a non-nodular thyroid gland, a hypoechogenic parathyroid lesion may be identified as the cause for hypercalcemia and elevated parathyroid hormone levels. This diagnosis is much more difficult when there is a multinodular gland as seen in Figure 3.16. It is noteworthy that a peripheral or exophytic thyroid nodule or a cervical lymph node can mimic a parathyroid mass. The importance of correlating the ultrasound image with a technetium 99M sestamibi parathyroid nuclear scan using cannot be overemphasized. Color Doppler has shown parathyroid lesions to be vascular, usually with a feeding artery and a draining vein. However, neither the Doppler pattern of the adenoma nor the spectral analysis of these vessels seem to reliably differentiate a parathyroid mass, a thyroid mass, or an abnormal lymph node.

It is best to scan the parathyroid glands by first doing a thorough thyroid ultrasound examination of the neck using the protocol previously discussed. The general approach to scanning for patients who are at risk for parathyroid lesions is to extend the area scanned superiorly from the base of the jaw, above the hyoid bone to include the area inferiorly to the sternal notch. Most cervical ectopic parathyroid glands will be included in this survey. When the inferior regions are scanned the patient should be asked to swallow to raise the lower poles of the thyroid gland.

Sonographically, there is no distinguishing characteristic between a parathyroid adenoma and the very rare parathyroid carcinoma, except by size or presence of metastases.

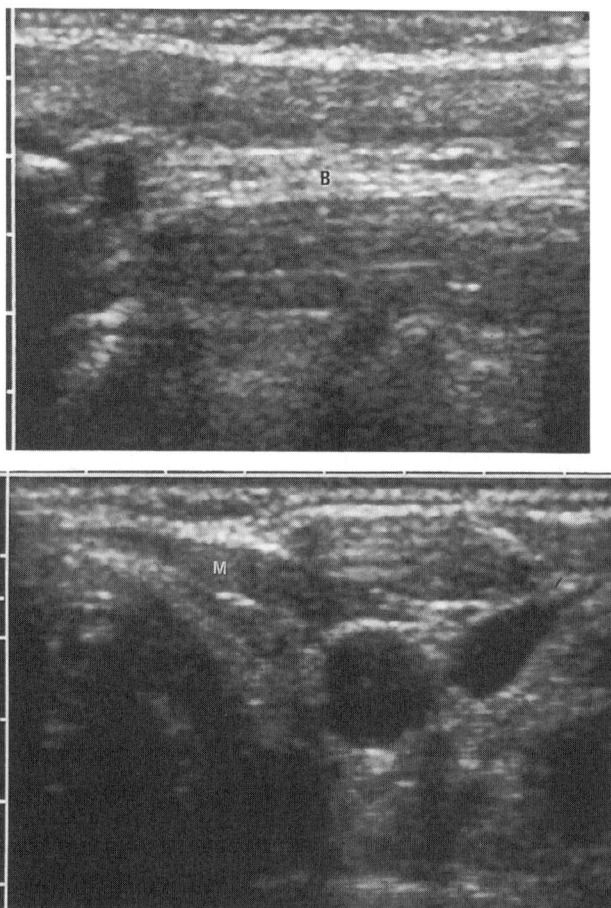

Figure 3.23 Panel **A** shows that the postoperative thyroid bed (B) in the sagittal plane is hyperechoic and there is no residual thyroid tissue. Anterior to this area is a strap muscle and posteriorly is the longus colli muscle. Panel **B** shows the postoperative thyroid bed in the axial /transverse plane. The strap muscle (M) should not be confused with residual tissue or mass. Muscle tends not to round in shape in either plane.

Post-operative Neck

One of the most important functions of thyroid sonography is to examine the thyroid carcinoma patient after total thyroidectomy. The most common finding is an empty thyroid bed that is demonstrated sonographically as hyperechoic fibrous tissue. (Figure 3.23A and 3.23B) Residual or recurrent tumor can be identified before it becomes palpable, which is the goal. In the postoperative patient, the strap muscles can be mistaken for tumor that is a source of confusion. Differential features include a lack of mass effect in 2 projections and a tapered, fibrillar appearance typical for strap muscles.

UNDERSTANDING THE PITFALLS OF THYROID ULTRASOUND

There are numerous potential pitfalls in performing thyroid sonography. The entire team, including the sonographer, interpreting physician, and clinician, must strive to avoid technical problems that are easily forgotten.

A frequent trap is related to diversity of equipment even within a single department. When sequential studies are done with machines of different manufacturers or transducers with different characteristics, a nodule that is seemingly new or altered in size may not really be a significant change. When dissimilar equipment is unavoidable, direct comparison the images is important to reveal subtleties, especially when there is a question of a new finding. It is paradoxical that opposing technical goals of objectivity, inventiveness, responsiveness to clinical need, and artistry are necessary. Standardization should be as impartial as possible. However, while consistency is a major requirement in every study, the operator must also customize the examination to answer the question that has been posed and not merely to record the routine anatomy. This is particularly true in the post-operative patient where it is important to know the extent of the surgery and the pathology. For example, after cancer surgery, as mentioned above, the strap muscles may be mistaken for residual disease (which can clarified in the orthogonal plane), and meticulous evaluation of cervical lymph nodes is essential.

Certain technical problems are frequently encountered. The size of the gland should be consistently measured in the sagittal and axial planes. The axial, transverse dimension is generally best measured using a high-resolution transducer that is 7.5 MHz or higher. However, the sagittal length is frequently "under-measured" using this transducer. As a rule, a 5Mhz transducer, with a larger "footprint" than a 7.5 MHz instrument, can better image the entire length of the gland. The pitfall in measuring the length of the thyroid gland with a conventional 7.5 MHz linear transducer is that it will erroneously "measure" the length transducer rather than the gland. A frequent source of error is a tendency to foreshorten the gland to fit the probe's field of view. Advanced transducers that allow extended field of view imaging or that can elecctronically transform a linear into a trapezoidal field tend to minimize these sources of error.

Interpeting the films also has a major pitfall. Pertinent clinical information is needed to interpret a sonogram properly. It is the responsibility of both the clinician and the sonologist to share this knowledge. Thyroid ultrasound testing performed by sonographers or sonologists who do not have a full understanding of the clinical problem provide an inferior report.

References

1. Mittelstaedt, CA. (ed.) General Ultrasound. Chap. 3, pp. 105-142, Churchill Livingstone Inc. 1992.
2. Blum M and Yee J. Advances in Thyroid Imaging: Thyroid Sonography : When and How should it be used? Vol. XX, No. 3 1997
3. Tempkin, BB. Ultrasound Scanning: Principles and Protocols. Chapter 16. pp. 205-215. W.B. Saunders, Philadelphia, 1993.
4. Ralls PW, Mayekawa DS, Lee K, Colletti PM, Radin DR, Boswell WD, Halls JM: Color flow Doppler sonography in Graves' disease: "thyroid inferno," AJ Roentgen 150: 781 – 784, 1988.
5. Clarke DK, Cronan J, Scola F. Color Doppler sonography: Anatomic and physiologic assessment of the thryroid. *J. Clin. Ultrasound* 23 (4): 215-223, 1995.
6. Rumack C, Wilson S, Charboneau JW. Diagnostic Ultrasound. Ch. 21 – 22, pp 703 – 750. Mosby, New York. 1998
7. Harnsberger HR. Handbook of head and neck imaging. Ch. 9 pp. 150 – 198. Mosby, New York, 1995.
8. McGahan JP, Goldberg BB. Diagnostic Ultrasound – A logical approach. Ch 35 pp. 74-75 Lippincott-Raven, Philadelphia. 1998
9. Bruneton JN. Ultrasonography of the Neck. Chapters 1 – 3. pp. 1 –63. Springer Verlag, Berlin, 1987..
10. West PW, Hartsborne MF, Inskip PD, et. al. Thyroid palpation versus high resolution thyroid ultrasonography in the detection of nodules, *J Ultrasound. Med.* 17:487-496,1998
11. Vassallo P, Wernecke K, Roos N, Peters PE. Differentiation of benign from malignant superficial lymphadenopathy:, the role of high resolution *US. Rad.* 183: 215 – 220 , 1992.
12. Sigal R., Infrahyoid neck in Radiologic Clinics of north America 36: 5, pp.781 799, 1988.
13. Reading CC. Palpable Neck Masses in RSNA Special Course in Ultrasound . pp. 351 - 361 , 1996

4

COMPARISON OF ULTRASOUND WITH OTHER TYPES OF THYROID IMAGING

H. Jack Baskin, M.D.,F.A.C.E.
Florida Thyroid and Endocrine Clinic
Orlando, FL 32804 USA

INTRODUCTION

Imaging of the thyroid gland began in 1951 when the first scanner was developed at the University of California, Los Angeles, by Cassen and Curtis (1). Thyroid scintigraphy using a radioactive isotope remained the primary method of imaging the thyroid for over a quarter of a century. It provided both an *anatomical* and *functional* image of the thyroid gland. The development of high-resolution real-time ultrasound, computed tomography (CT), and magnetic resonance imaging (MRI) now offers alternative means to visualize thyroid anatomy. While the recent development of single photon emission computed tomography (SPECT) and positron emission tomography (PET) have the potential to measure tissue function as well as anatomy, the use for that purpose remains experimental and is not widely available. Although ultrasound demonstrates only thyroid anatomy and not thyroid function, it has emerged as the most widely used method of thyroid imaging. This chapter will concentrate on comparing the advantages and disadvantages of ultrasound with isotope scans, CT, and MRI.

THYROID SCINTIGRAPHY

Choice of Isotope

Initially, radioiodine-131 (^{131}I) was the standard isotope used in performing thyroid scans. It could be given orally and was long lasting, inexpensive, and readily available. However, ^{131}I emits not only gamma radiation, which is used for imaging, but also particle or beta radiation, which can damage tissue. Although this property is an advantage in treating patients with Graves' disease or thyroid cancer, it is a distinct disadvantage when this isotope is used for imaging. In addition, ^{131}I has a high-energy emission of 364 keV (Table 4.1). This high-energy peak penetrates tissue well and can be an advantage in the search for metastatic thyroid cancer involvement, which remains the primary use for ^{131}I scanning today. When scanning is done in the follow-up of patients with thyroid cancer, ^{131}I should always be used.

Table 4.1-Radiopharmaceutiacl Agents Used for Thyroid Scanning

Isotope	Dose Given	Route	Dose Absorbed	Half-life	Energy
^{131}I	100uCi	Oral	75 rad	8.1 days	364 KeV
^{99m}Tc	10mCi	IV	1.3 rad	6 hours	140KeV
^{123}I	100uCi	Oral	0.75 rad	13 hours	159KeV

With the widespread use of the gamma camera in the 1970's, technetium pertechnetate (^{99m}Tc) became more readily available and began to replace ^{131}I for thyroid scanning. ^{99m}Tc is inexpensive, with an energy emission at 140keV, it imposes a low radiation dose and produces a sharp image. These advantages notwithstanding, no effective method is known for measuring ^{99m}Tc uptake that will replace the radioiodine uptake data. The major problem with using ^{99m}Tc to image the thyroid gland, however, is that ^{99m}Tc, while taken up by thyroid tissue is not organified. ^{99m}Tc is not metabolized the same as iodine, and it does not represent the true function of thyroid tissue. In the 1970's, many published reports described malignant nodules that were hot with the use of ^{99m}Tc but were cold with the use of radioiodine (2-7). Such results make the test unreliable for the evaluation of the function of thyroid nodules, and ^{99m}Tc scans are no longer recommended for this purpose.

By the late 1980's, radioiodine-123 (^{123}I) became available throughout the continental United States and has now replaced both ^{131}I and ^{99m}Tc as the isotope of choice for imaging the thyroid gland. It emits pure gamma radiation with an ideal energy peak of 159 keV which produces a sharp image and provides a very low dose of radiation, approximately 1% of that received from an equivalent amount of ^{131}I. Thus radiation exposure is a nonissue except in pregnant women or nursing mothers. If ^{123}I is available, it should be the only isotope used to image the thyroid gland.

^{131}I remains the primary isotope used to scan patients after they have had surgery for thyroid cancer. While ^{123}I has been suggested as an alternative to avoid stunning the tissue with beta radiation, it would significantly increase the cost (8). The low energy peak of ^{123}I also might not be as effective in penetrating tissue and miss bone metastasis (9). Thallium-201 (^{201}Tl) and other isotopes have also been suggested when ^{131}I scans are negative, but have generally been less sensitive, less specific, and less accurate than ^{131}I scans (10). More recently technetium-99m methoxyisobutyl isonitrile (Tc-MIBI) has been proposed as a scanning agent for patients with thyroid cancer, but this agent is not approved for use in the United States (11). Scanning with such agents would provide little clinically useful information because treatment still depends upon iodine uptake by the tissue. An exception is the use of Indium-111 Pentetreotide (octreotide), which is used for scanning neuroendocrine tumors and is about 70% successful in identifying medullary cancer metastasis (12,13).

A radioiodine scan will identify thyroid nodules greater than one centimeter in size, but it is much less sensitive if the nodule is less than one centimeter. Nodules less than 0.5 centimeter will not be seen; therefore ultrasound is a much more sensitive test for detecting nodules. The single big advantage of a radioiodine scan over ultrasound is the ability to observe thyroid *function* as well as thyroid *anatomy*. Neither CT nor MRI has this ability. If radioiodine uptake is high, thyroid scans often detect a pyramidal lobe appearing as a finger-like projection of activity attached to the right or left lobe or the isthmus, or as activity near the midline above the tips of either lateral lobe (14-16). This is a vestige of the thyroglossal duct tract, and it is often seen in scans of patients with Graves' disease. The pyramidal lobe can usually be seen with ultrasound.

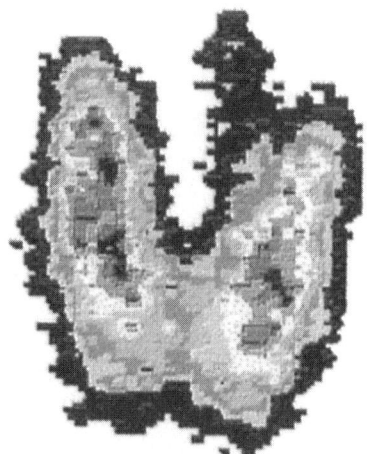

Figure 4.1- Pyramidal Lobe. This represents thyroid tissue in the thyroglossal duct tract attached to the left upper lobe. A pyramidal lobe can be attached to the upper pole of either lobe or to the isthmus. It is most likely, to be seen in patients with Graves' Disease.

Rectilinear Scans
Until the late 1960's, all scans were done using a rectilinear scanner. Although it is more time consuming than a gamma camera, and this is a major obstacle in imaging larger organs such as the lungs or liver, it takes only about fifteen minutes to image a thyroid gland using a rectilinear scanner. The scanner probe on a rectilinear scanner moves back and fourth over the neck producing a 1:1 linear image of the thyroid gland depicting its actual size and shape. Any palpable nodule(s) can be easily marked and the collimator focused to produce a tomogram through the center of a nodule, ignoring the surrounding thyroid tissue above and below the nodule. This makes it easier to determine if a nodule it hot or cold, and eliminates the need to perform oblique views. (Figure 4.2 & Figure 4.3) New rectilinear scanners are now computerized presenting color images that indicate the function of the tissue within the gland and calculate the size of the thyroid and the nodules. Most endocrinologists prefer a rectilinear scan, but the older scanners have disappeared from most nuclear medicine laboratories, and the new computerized rectilinear scanners are not always available.

Figure 4.2-Cold Nodule in Right Lobe A rectilinear scanner takes a planogram through the center of the nodule and visualizes no uptake of the isotope within the nodule. At surgery, this proved to be a papillary carcinoma.

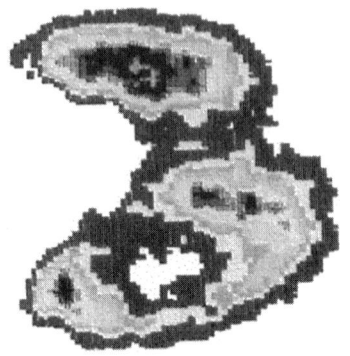

FIGURE 4.3. Hot Nodule in Right Lobe. A planogram through this nodule shows an increased concentration of isotope in the nodule in comparison to the rest of the thyroid gland. It is safe to assume that such a nodule is not malignant.

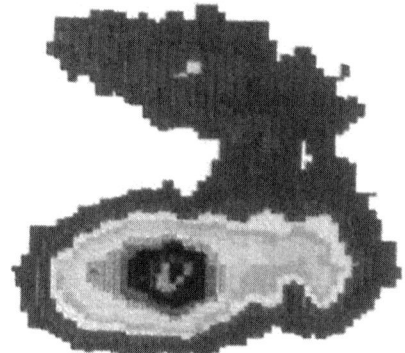

Gamma Camera Scans

Most scans done today are done with a gamma camera since they are readily available in any nuclear medicine facility. When the thyroid gland is scanned, a pinhole collimator is placed over the detector head in order to visualize thyroid nodules; if a pinhole collimator is not used, even large thyroid nodules will not be seen (17,18). The collimator distorts the image much like a fisheye lens on a photographic camera. The size of the image is dependent upon the distance of the thyroid to the pinhole; therefore, the lateral border of the thyroid appears larger than the isthmus and medial border. This sometime leads to the appearance of false nodules along the edge of the thyroid that is just normal "scalloping". In order to avoid "scalloping" and not miss nodules, it is important to do right and left oblique views in addition to an anterior image of the thyroid (19,20). The image is not a linear reproduction of the gland and cannot be used to determine its size as can be done using a rectilinear scan. This makes it difficult to mark nodules, and it is critical that a skilled physician be present to palpate the thyroid at the time of scanning to determine the size and attempt to mark any obvious nodules. Because a gamma camera can scan much quicker than a rectilinear scanner, it is always used to do total body scans on patients being scanned after thyroid cancer surgery.

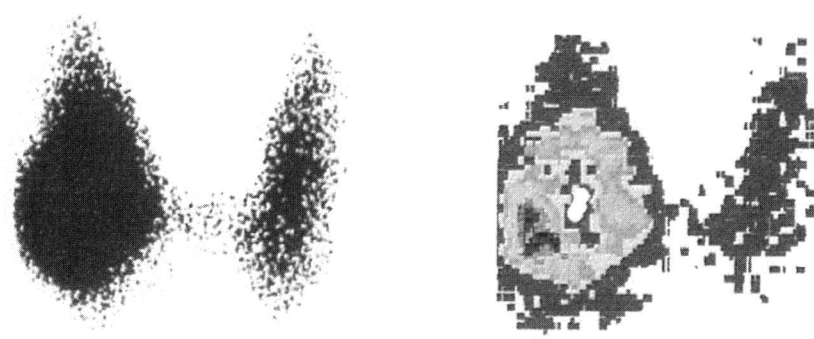

FIGURE 4.4. Comparison of Gamma Camera with a Rectilinear Scanner. The gamma camera scan on the left shows a hot nodule; however the rectilinear scan of the same nodule on the right shows a cold area in the center of the hot nodule that could represent a thyroid cancer. An ultrasound revealed that this was a necrotic cyst inside the hot nodule and did not require surgery.

INDICATIONS FOR THYROID SCANS

Thyroid scans were overused in the past and remain so today. Thyroid scans are virtually useless in the evaluation of hypothyroidism, simple goiter, or to measure thyroid size (unless done with a rectilinear scanner), and most thyroid abnormalities can be adequately diagnosed and treated without the expense and radiation exposure of an isotope scan. Scans done using radioiodine require discontinuation of l-thyroxin for six weeks and triiodothyronine for two weeks. In patients who have had surgery for thyroid cancer, this can result in discomfort to the patient and the potential that the TSH elevation during the pre-scanning period may act as a growth factor allowing the thyroid cancer to progress. Instead of stopping thyroid hormone, we now have the option of the administration of recombinant TSH but this increases the expense further. In addition, one should be certain that the patient has not received iodine contrast material or ingested large doses of iodine for approximately eight weeks before the scan. The performance of a thyroid scan should generally be limited to one of the indications listed in Table 4.2. Even for some of the conditions listed, thyroid scanning can often be avoided by using other simpler or newer tests. In general, there has been a diminishing need to do thyroid scans in recent years.

Table 4.2-Indications for Radioiodine Scan

1.	Identify and Evaluate Nodules
2.	Assess Thyrotoxicosis
3.	Post-op Follow-up of Thyroid Cancer
4.	Localization of Aberrant Thyroid Tissue

Thyroid Nodules

For decades, a thyroid scan was considered the first and most important test to order whenever a patient presented with a thyroid nodule. The rational was that a thyroid scan would identify and avoid surgery in nodules that were "hot" in comparison to the surrounding thyroid tissue or autonomous using the Werner Suppression Test giving triiodothyronine for several days to suppress the normal thyroid tissue. However 'hot" or autonomous nodules account for only 5% of all nodules; therefore, the scan provided little useful information in the great majority of patients with thyroid nodules.

It is well recognized that FNA biopsy is a much more accurate method to approach a thyroid nodule than to do an initial thyroid scan (21,22). A FNA biopsy is less expensive than a thyroid scan, and the procedure is widely available by endocrinologists. Only patients in whom the FNA biopsy is said to show a follicular neoplasm or in whom the TSH is suppressed will require a thyroid scan using ^{123}I.

Thyrotoxicosis

Today some authorities argue that a thyroid scan is not needed in patients who have thyrotoxicosis (23). If all patients with thyrotoxicosis had Graves' disease, perhaps this would be acceptable; however, Graves' disease accounts for only 80% of these patients. Other thyroid conditions often present as Graves' disease, but the elevation of thyroid hormones in the blood is due to another cause (Table 4.3). Patients with subacute and postpartum thyroiditis or those with iodine-induced hyperthyroidism (Jod Basedow) often present with clinical symptoms and thyroid function tests no different than those with Graves' disease. Only after the scan is ordered and the radioiodine uptake is found to be low is the true diagnosis confirmed and the proper treatment prescribed. Patients with toxic nodular goiter are sometimes diagnosed as having Graves' disease, but these patients often do not respond well to antithyroid medication, require larger doses of ^{131}I, and may even need surgery. There are few endocrinologists who have not been occasionally misled initially into thinking a patient has Graves' disease when the radioiodine uptake and scan revealed another problem.

Table 4.3- Causes of Thyrotoxicosis

1.	Toxic Diffuse Goiter (Graves' Disease)
2.	Toxic Nodule(s)
3.	Subacute Thyroiditis (de Quervain's)
4.	Silent and Postpartum Thyroiditis
5.	Iodine-induced Hyperthyroidism (jod Basedow)
6.	Excess T_4 or T_3 Ingestion
7.	Aberrant thyroid Tissue
8.	Secondary to Increased TSH

In the United States most patients with Graves' disease are treated with ^{131}I, and many recommend that a radioiodine uptake be done to evaluate the treatment dose; a scan should definitely be done if the patient is being given a radioactive isotope for an uptake determination. Even if antithyroid medicine is being contemplated, one should be certain of the diagnosis before embarking on a long-term course of potentially fatal medicine. The presence of Graves' disease does not rule out the coexistence of thyroid cancer, and occasionally the pre-treatment scan of a patient with Graves' disease reveals an unexpected thyroid cancer (Figure 4.5). Such a "discovery" will drastically alter the recommended treatment. Most endocrinologists feel that a thyroid scan remains mandatory for all patients diagnosed with Graves' disease regardless of the treatment that is planned.

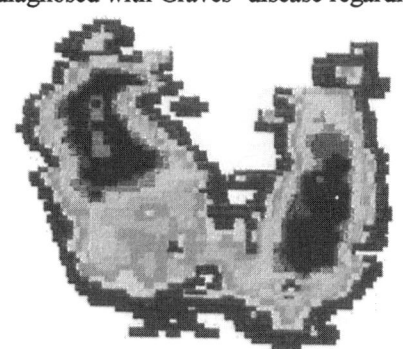

FIGURE 4.5. Graves' Disease with a Nodule. This nine year old female presented with Graves' disease and a small nodule in the right lower lobe. The scan shows the nodule to be "warm" but less active than the surrounding thyroid tissue. A FNA biopsy indicated a neoplasm and a mixed papillary-follicular cancer was found at surgery. Note radioactive saliva in esophagus below thyroid; this disappeared after swallowing water.

Thyroid Cancer

For over four decades, a radioiodine scan using ^{131}I has been the primary method of evaluating patients post-operatively for recurrent disease or metastasis. As will be discussed in Chapter 10, the availability of accurate and sensitive thyroglobulin (Tg) assays and high-resolution, real-time ultrasound in the 1990's has lead to a diminishing need to do routine total body scans. Except for always ordering a total body scan after giving a cancer treatment dose of ^{131}I, thyroid scans are seldom the first or even second test to order in such patients. The sensitivity of scans in detecting recurrent or metastatic cancer is low and is dependent on the dose of ^{131}I used; doses greater than 2-3 mCi have been shown to cause stunning making subsequent treatment with ^{131}I more difficult (24). While the availability of recombinant TSH ($_{rh}$TSH)has reduced the morbidity for patients who must be scanned, it has not increased the sensitivity of the test nor has it eliminated the problem with stunning. Many now feel that a rising Tg level in a post-operative thyroid cancer patient with negative thyroglobulin antibodies, especially when accompanied by a positive ultrasound-guided FNA biopsy of a lymph node, is adequate to treat a patient with ^{131}I without the need for a pretreatment scan. A total body scan is then ordered after treatment and provides much more information (25). Studies show that thyroid scans done after treatment reveal one third more lesions than do pretreatment scans using a tracer dose of ^{131}I; therefore using a post-treatment scan as the "gold Standard", thyroid scanning before treatment has a sensitivity of only 67% - a fact not often appreciated.

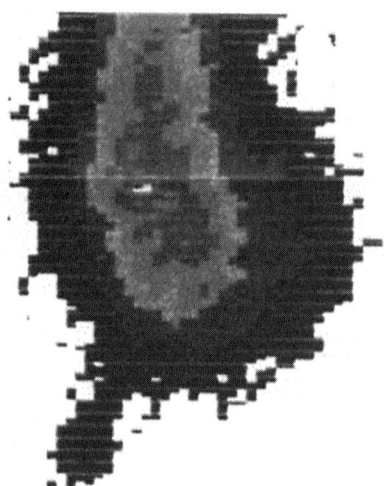

FIGURE 4.6. Pedunculated Mass. This patient presented after having a hemithyroidectomy of the left lobe due to a metastatic lymph node that was removed from the left neck. The left lobe did not reveal a primary thyroid cancer. The pedunculated lesion seen on this scan of the right lobe was the only cancer found. It is unusual for a thyroid cancer to metastasize to the contralateral neck.

Evaluation of a Mediastinal Mass
Aberrant thyroid tissue can occur anywhere from the tongue (lingual thyroid) to the pelvis (strumi ovarii), including intracardiac thyroid tissue (strumi cordis) (26,27). Although localization of aberrant thyroid tissue, such as a mass in the mediastinum, accounts for a small proportion of all thyroid scans performed, no more reliable or less expensive method exists to confirm its presence. ^{99m}Tc should never be used to evaluate a peritracheal mass because the uptake of this isotope by the heart and great vessels is high and can be confused with a substernal goiter. Avoid ordering a CT first since this will not confirm thyroid tissue and will delay doing a radioiodine scan for weeks.

Summary
There continues to be a need in specific circumstances for ordering a thyroid scan, but this need has greatly decreased. This is in part due to the development of newer diagnostic tools such as FNA biopsy and sensitive TSH and Tg assays (28-30). In addition, high-resolution, real-time ultrasound has provided a more sensitive, less expensive, easier and quicker method to fulfil the thyroid imaging requirements without the use of radioactive isotopes. Hopefully, we will see a more judicious use of scans in the future than has existed in the past.

CT AND MRI

The introduction of CT in the 1970's and MRI in the 1980's provided two additional methods for imaging the thyroid gland. While both CT and MRI provide detailed images of the thyroid, neither produces images superior nor detects nodules as well as high-resolution, real-time ultrasound. Both are more expensive than ultrasound, and CT involves radiation exposure. The iodine contrast media used with CT will delay scanning or treatment with radioiodine, and it also exposes the patient to the potential of an allergic reaction. After twenty years, there has been found little clinical use for CT in patients with thyroid disease.

MRI avoids the use of iodine contrast material, and it provides better anatomic definition than CT because of multiplanar imaging (31). However, it is more expensive and takes longer than CT and is not well tolerated by patients with claustrophobia. MRI is affected by motion from breathing, swallowing, and cardiac or vascular pulsation; this deteriorates the images so that they are not as good as the images obtained using high-resolution, real-time ultrasound. A primary use is in the evaluation of a substernal goiter where ultrasound is hampered by the bony structures. MRI is very good for determining the degree of tracheal obstruction caused by such a mass.

The primary use of MRI in thyroid disease is in the evaluation of patients who have been operated on for thyroid cancer. While ultrasound, combined with ultrasound-guided FNA, is preferable for detecting recurrent or metastatic thyroid cancer in the neck, MRI can detect metastatic lymph nodes in the mediastinum. It can detect recurrent cancer in patients with elevated Tg and a negative WBS. However, it is not specific and cannot separate metastatic disease from inflammatory lymph nodes, neuromas, or even a normal thymus (32). An MRI is indicated for the pre-operative evaluation of a patient with known recurrent thyroid cancer in order to determine the extent of the cancer and the involvement of the lymph nodes and surrounding muscles. MRI is good at separating recurrent cancer from fibrosis and scar tissue, and it has been especially helpful in the evaluation of patients with medullary cancer.

Summary
Because of better soft tissue contrast and the elimination of the need to use iodine contrast material, MRI is usually preferred to CT. Both of these imaging methods

should be considered adjunctive to ultrasound and radioiodine scanning in imaging the thyroid gland. They have a very narrow and limited use and neither can be used to perform guided FNA biopsies.

REFERENCES

1. Beierwaltes W.H. (1979) The history of the use of radioactive iodine. *Seminars Nucl. Med.* 9:151-155.
2. Turner J.W., Spencer R.P. (1975) Thyroid carcinoma presenting as a pertechnetate "hot"nodule, but without 131I uptake: case report. *J. Nucl. Med.* 16:22-23.
3. Usher M.S., Arzoumanian A.Y. (1970) Thyroid scans made with pertechnetate and iodine may give inconsistent results. *J. Nucl. Med.* 12:136-137.
4. Steinberg M., Cavalieri R.R., Choy S.H. (1970) Uptake of technetium 99-pertechnetate in a primary thyroid carcinoma: need for caution in evaluating nodules. *J. Clin. Endo.* 31:81-84
5. Shambaugh G.E., Quinn J.L., Oyasu R., Freinkel N. (1974) Disparate thyroid imaging; combined studies with sodium pertechnetate Tc 99m and radioactive iodine. *JAMA* 228:866-869.
6. Erjavec M., Movrin T., Auersperg M., Golouh R. (1977) Comparative accumulation of 99mTc and 131I in thyroid nodules: case report. *J. Nucl. Med.* 18:346-347.
7. Dos Remedios L.V., Weber P.M., Jasko I.A. (1971) Thyroid scintiphotography in 1000 patients: rational use of 99mTc and 131I compounds. *J. Nucl. Med.* 12:673-677.
8. Baskin H.J. (1998) Follow-up of patients with thyroid cancer. *Endocrine Practice* 4:63-64.
9. Baskin H.J. (1998) Thyroid cancer follow-up: editorial. *Endocrine Practice* 4:294.
10. Burman K.D., Anderson J.H., Wartofsky L., Mong D.P., Jelinek J.J. (1990) Management of patients with thyroid carcinoma: application of thallium-201 scintigraphy and magnetic resonance imaging. *J. Nucl. Med.* 31:1958-1964.
11. Alam S., Kasagi K., Misaki T., Miyamoto S., Iwata M, Iida Y., Konishi J. (1998) Diagnostic value of technetium-99m methoxyisobutyl isonitril (99mTc-MIBI) scintigraphy in detecting thyroid cancer metastases: a critical evaluation. *Thyroid* 8:1091-1100.
12. Krenning E.P., Kwekkeboom D.J., Bakker W.H., Breemen W.A.P., Kooij P.P.M., Oei H.Y., van Hagen M., Postema P.T.E., deJong M., Reubi J.C., Visser T.J., Reijs A.E.M Hofland L.J., Koper J.W., Lamberts S.W.J. (1993) Somatostatin receptor scintigraphy with [111In-DTPA-d-Phe1] and [123I-Tyr3]-octreotide: the Rotterdam experience with more than 1000 patients. *Eur. J. Nucl. Med.* 20:716-731.
13. Olsen J.O., Pozderac R.V., Hinkle G., Hill T., O'Dorisio T.M., Schirmer W.J., Ellison E.C., O'Dorisio M.S. (1995) Somatostatin receptor imaging of neuroendocrine tumors with indium-111 penetreotide (octreoscan). *Seminars Nucl. Med.* 25:251-261.
14. Izenstark J.L., Horwitz N.H. (1968) The pyramidal lobe in thyroid imaging. *J. Nucl. Med.* 10:519-524.
15. Levy H.A., Sziklas J.J., Rosenberg R.J., Spencer R.P. (1987) Incidence of a pyramidal lobe on thyroid scans. *Clin. Nucl. Med.* 12:560-561.
16. Siraj Q.H., Aleem N., Inam-ur-rehman A., Qaisar S., Ahmad M. (1989) The pyramidal lobe: a scintigraphic assessment. *Nucl. Med. Communications* 10:685-693.
17. Hurley P.J., Strauss H.W., Pavoni (1989) P., Langan J.K., Wagner H.N. (1971) The scintillation camera with pinhole collimator in thyroid imaging. *Radiology* 101:133-138.
18. Sostre S., Ashare A.B., Quinones J.D., Schieve J.B., Zimmerman J.M. (1978) Thyroid scintigraphy: pinhole images versus rectilinear scans. *Radiology* 129:759-762.
19. Karelitz J.R., Richards J.B. (1974) Necessity of oblique views in evaluating the functional status of a thyroid nodule. *J. Nucl. Med.* 15:782-785.
20. Smith M.L., Wraight E.P. (1989) Oblique views in thyroid imaging. *Clin. Radiology* 40:505-507.

21. Van Herle A.J., Rich P., Ljung B.E., Ashcraft M.W., Soloman D.H., Keeler E.B. (1982) The thyroid nodule. *Ann. Int. Med.* 96:221-232.
22. Baskin H. J., Guarda L.A. (1987) Influence of needle biopsy on management of thyroid nodules: Reasons to expand its use. *South. Med. J.* 80:702-705.
23. Ripley S.D., Freitas J.E., Nagle C.E. (1984) Is thyroid scintigraphy necessary before I-131 therapy for hyperthyroidism? concise communication. *J. Nucl. Med.* 25:664-667.
24. Park H., Perkins O.W., Edmondson J.W., Schnute R.B., Manatunga A. (1994) Influence of diagnostic radioiodines on the uptake of ablative dose of iodine-131. *Thyroid* 4:49-54.
25. Balachandran S., Sayle B.A. (1981) Value of thyroid carcinoma imaging after therapeutic doses of radioiodine. *Clin. Nucl. Med.* 4:162-167.
26. Noyek A.M., Freidberg J. (1981) Thyroglossal duct and ectopic thyroid disorders. *Otolaryngology Clin. N. A.* 14:167-201.
27. Rieser G.D., Ober K.P., Cowan R.J., Cordell A.R. Radioiodine imaging of struma cordis. (1988) Clin. Nucl. Med. 13:421-422.
28. Baskin H.J. (1995) Thyroglobulin: a clinical review. *Endocrine Practice* 1:365-367.
29. Baskin H.J. (1994) Effect of postoperative 131I treatment on thyroglobulin measurements in the follow-up of patients with thyroid cancer. *Thyroid* 4:239-242.
30. Baskin H.J. (1997) Thyroid ultrasonography-a review. *Endocrine Practice* 3:153-157.
31. Higgins C.B., McNamara M.T., Fisher M.R., Clark O.H. (1986) MR imaging of the thyroid. *AJR* 147:1255-1261.
32. Toubert ME., Cyna-Gorse F., Zagdanski AM., Noel-Wekstein S., Cattan P., Billotey C., Sarfati E., Rain JD. (1999) Cervicomediastinal magnetic resonance imaging in persistent or recurrent papillary thyroid carcinoma: clinical use and limits. *Thyroid* 9:591-597.

5

ULTRASOUND OF THYROID NODULES

H. Jack Baskin, M.D., F.A.C.E.
Florida Thyroid & Endocrine Clinic
Orlando, FL 32804 USA

INTRODUCTION

Ultrasound is the most sensitive test available to detect thyroid nodules. It can recognize nodules that have been missed on physical examination, isotope scanning, computer tomography (CT), and magnetic resonance imaging (MRI). High-resolution, real-time ultrasound can readily identify nodules as small as 2-3 millimeters and accurately measure their dimensions and volume. In spite of its high *sensitivity*, its *specificity* in determining whether a nodule is cancer and needs surgery or is benign and does not need surgery is less accurate.

Experience with ultrasound has resulted in scores of articles that have increased our knowledge about thyroid nodules. This knowledge has led to new questions concerning our approach to the evaluation and treatment of nodules. For example, ultrasound has revealed that small nodules are much more common than once realized, questioning the advisability of performing ultrasound on a patient whose thyroid gland is normal to palpation. Ultrasound has also shown that nodules will often disappear with no specific treatment; this makes the necessity of treating all benign nodules with l-thyroxin suppression uncertain.

ULTRASOUND OF NORMAL THYROID

As a general rule, performing ultrasound of a thyroid gland that is normal on physical examination or using ultrasound as a substitute for a physical examination should be avoided. Several studies have shown a high incidence of unsuspected non-palpable nodules when normal people have ultrasound. Brander, et al performed ultrasound on one hundred and one normal adult women and found that thirty-six had at least one nodule (1). It is unlikely that the increased anxiety caused by discovering many benign nodules will be offset by earlier diagnosis of cancer that would result in saving many lives.

However, some exceptions to the rule of avoiding an ultrasound of a normal thyroid gland exist. Patients who received external radiation during childhood or have a history of familial thyroid cancer will benefit from ultrasound screening. Ultrasound of a normal appearing thyroid gland is sometimes indicated in managing patients with thyroid cancer (Table 5.1).

Table 5.1 Indications for Ultrasound of Normal Thyroid

1. External radiation during childhood
2. History of familial thyroid cancer
3. Thyroid cancer with hemithyroidectomy
4. Lymph node metastasis that is Tg positive

Patients who were exposed to external radiation during childhood or teenagers treated with radiation for acne have an increased likelihood of developing nodular abnormalities of the thyroid, both benign and malignant. There is a consensus of opinion to be more aggressive with these patients, and ultrasound provides the easiest means to detect a nodule even before it becomes palpable. Should the nodule be malignant, this allows earlier intervention. A normal ultrasound will also provide an easy method to rule out cancer in these individuals without resorting to more radiation using an isotope scan. A good example of this occurred when ultrasound was used effectively to screen large populations in the USSR and eastern Europe following the 1986 Chernobyl accident where the incidence of thyroid cancer among children from certain high radiation exposure areas increased 100 fold within four years.

Another situation in which an ultrasound of a "normal" thyroid gland may be indicated is in patients who have a family history of medullary thyroid cancer or multiple endocrine neoplasia-type II as well as patients who have a family history of familial papillary cancer. A negative ultrasound study is often reassuring to such patients.

Patients who present after having a hemithyroidectomy for well-differentiated thyroid cancer sometimes present a dilemma as to the need for a completion thyroidectomy. An ultrasound of the remaining lobe that seems normal on physical examination is often helpful in deciding on the course of treatment.

Sometimes patients with a normal thyroid on physical examination present with lymphadenopathy in the neck. After the lymph node is removed, an immunoperioxidase stain is found to be positive for thyroglobulin indicating its thyroid origin. An ultrasound of the "normal" thyroid will reveal the primary carcinoma.

COINCIDENTAL DISCOVERY OF A THYROID NODULE

The increasing use of CT and MRI along with the use of ultrasound for carotid imaging for the evaluation of atherosclerosis has resulted in the accidental discovery of many unsuspected non-palpable nodules of the thyroid gland (2). While some authorities have suggested that these non-palpable nodules, often referred to as "incidentalomas", be treated as normal anatomic variants of thyroid tissue and ignored, it is not altogether certain that this is wise. Several studies have shown that the incidence of malignancy in these non-palpable nodules is the same as that in palpable nodules; therefore ignoring their presence would not be prudent (3-6). While one might assume that a small thyroid cancer is of less concern than a large palpable thyroid cancer; this does not seem to be the case. Rosen, et al reported ninety-nine thyroid cancer patients whose primary neoplasm was less than 1.5 centimeter in size and found that one third metastasized beyond the thyroid gland with two patients having metastasis to the lungs and one to bone (7). Others have reported that patients who present with a metastatic lymph node and a "normal" thyroid by palpation have a more aggressive cancer with a higher recurrence and mortality rate than thyroid carcinoma presenting with a palpable mass in the thyroid gland (8,9).

Clearly, the finding of a small non-palpable nodule with ultrasound cannot be ignored. If the nodule is less then one centimeter in size, it should be re-examined in six months using ultrasound, and an ultrasound guided fine needle aspiration (UG FNA) biopsy should be performed if there is an increase in size. Non-palpable nodules greater than one centimeter in size should undergo FNA biopsy using ultrasound guidance.

ULTRASOUND OF DIFFUSE GOITER

Ultrasound can accurately measure the size of the thyroid gland, and this has some limited clinical application in the evaluation and treatment of patients with diffuse goiter. Usually, the thyroid gland appears hypoechoic in patients with both Hashimoto and Graves' disease (10). Although Color Flow Doppler (CFD) will show increased blood flow in Graves' disease, other tests are more practical for determining the function of the thyroid gland.

By measuring the maximum length (L), width (W), and depth (D) and using the formula for Lobar Mass, one can calculate the weight of the thyroid in grams (11).

$$\text{Lobar Mass} = 4.9D + 0.07L^2W - 2.3$$

This formula gives the weight in grams of one lobe of the thyroid and the adjoining isthmus; each lobe's weight is calculated separately and added to obtain the total weight. This along with the radioiodine uptake, provides an objective method of delivering a predetermined amount of ^{131}I to treat Graves' disease. Doses of 75 to 150 uCi ^{131}I per gram of thyroid tissue yield 5000 – 10,000 rad which will generally stop thyrotoxicosis. The total dose is calculated as follows:

$$\text{Dose in mCi} = \frac{uCi\ ^{131}I/Gm \times \text{weight of gland (Gm)}}{RAI_u \times 10}$$

Ultrasound is also used in epidemiological surveys for endemic goiter in areas outside North America. Measuring the size of the thyroid gland by ultrasound provides an inexpensive and effective method to monitor for iodine deficiency.

Ultrasound is often helpful in defining the anatomy of the neck. It is very useful in differentiating a thyroglossal duct cyst, a brachial cleft cyst or an enlarged lymph node from a thyroid mass (Figure 5.1). It will also readily identify agenesis of a thyroid lobe or other anatomic abnormalities of the thyroid gland (Figures 5.2 and 5.3). Still, the most common use for thyroid ultrasound has been for the evaluation of nodular goiter.

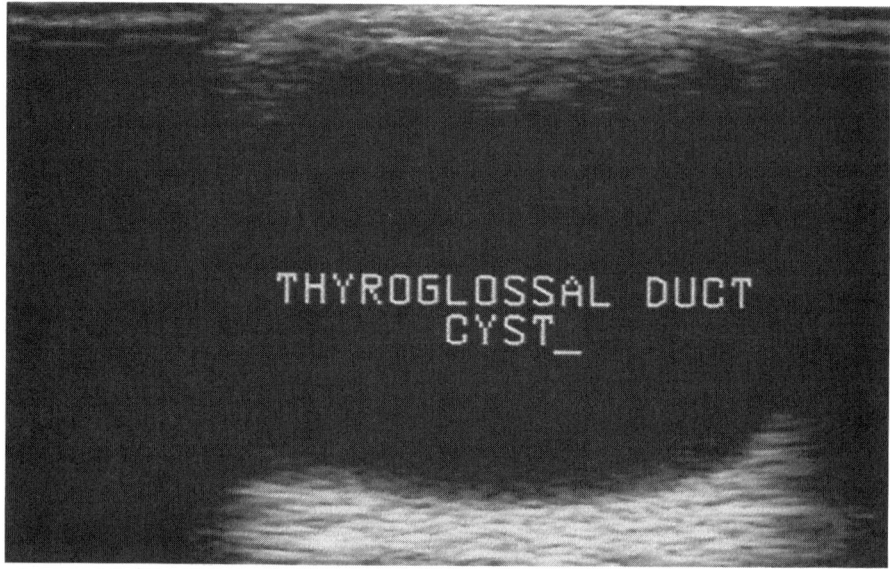

Figure 5.1 Thyroglossal Duct Cyst. These cysts occur in the thyroglossal duct tract above the isthmus and are usually superficial. Note the proximity of the cyst to the skin surface, the absence of echoes in the cyst, and the increased density or *enhancement* below the cyst.

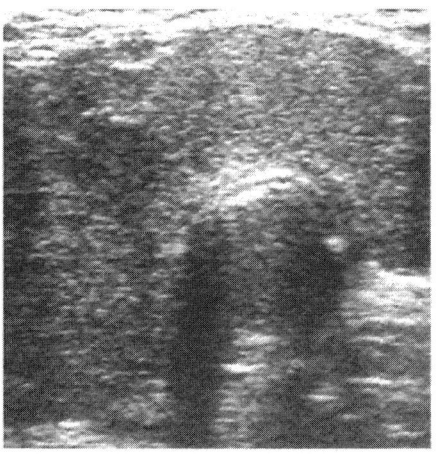
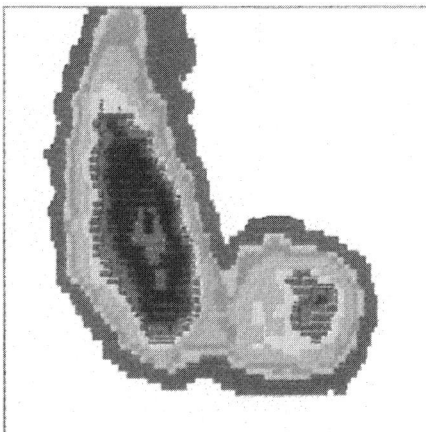

Figure 5.2 Hemiagenesis of Left Lobe in Patient with Graves' Disease. Ultrasound shows the thyroid to be hypoechoic with a thick isthmus (both signs associated with Graves' Disease) with an abrupt end of gland on the left. Scan shows enlargement of the right lobe and isthmus with the "Hockey Stick Sign" typical of hemiagenesis. Hemiagenesis usually involves the left lobe.

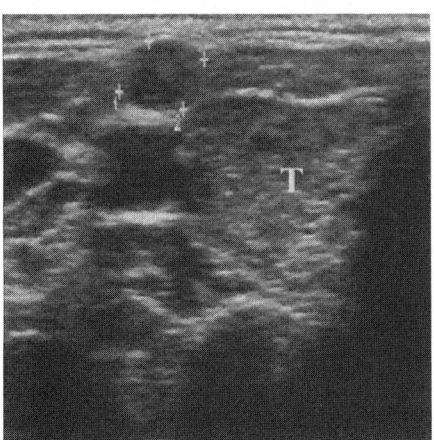
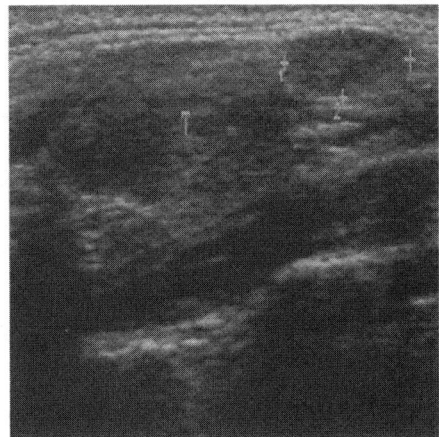

Figure 5.3 Aberrant Thyroid Tissue. Patient presented with a one-centimeter mass located superficially in the lower neck. Transverse and longitudinal ultrasound views show the mass to be attached to the lower lateral right lobe of thyroid gland. An UG FNA biopsy of the mass revealed it to be normal thyroid tissue.

ULTRASOUND CHARACTERISTICS OF NODULES

Unfortunately, there is no single ultrasound finding or combination of findings that will tell whether every nodule is benign or malignant. This led some authorities to minimize the value of ultrasound, compared with FNA biopsy, in the evaluation of thyroid nodules. However, it is important to realize that ultrasound does not replace or compete with FNA biopsy, but the two modalities are complementary (11). As explained in Chapter 1, an ultrasound done by the examining physician is different than one done by a sonographer in a radiologist office. Ultrasound extends the clinician's diagnostic acumen by allowing visualization of the architectural characteristics of thyroid nodules that do have predictive value in deciding if a nodule is benign or malignant. It also allows observation of changes in thyroid nodules over time that often aids in making the decision regarding surgery.

Cystic Nodules
Using A-mode and B-mode ultrasound, nodules were divided into either solid nodules or cysts, but when real-time ultrasound became available, it revealed that most cysts had a thick wall and contained debris indicating that the nodule had been solid and had undergone cystic necrosis or hemorrhage. There were very few purely cystic (thin wall) cysts. Likewise, many solid nodules were found to have some cystic components. The majority of nodules seem to be complex, containing varying amounts of both solid and cystic areas (Figure 5.4). Only if a nodule is a thin wall cyst that can be fully evacuated and not recur, can one assume that it is benign – this accounts for approximately 1% of all thyroid nodules (12). Other cystic nodules should have the fluid aspirated and the solid component biopsied, preferably using ultrasound guidance.

Sometimes it is difficult to tell if a low-density (hypoechoic) nodule is a cyst or is solid by ultrasound. The distinction can be made because ultrasound of a fluid filled cyst causes *enhancement* or reinforcement of the echoes along the posterior wall of the cyst. This bright line along the distal wall is not present with a solid hypoechoic nodule. One should look for *enhancement* in a hypoechoic nodule; when present, it indicates a cyst. However, cysts less than 1.5 centimeters may not show enhancement. When performing a FNA biopsy of a cyst, the fluid may be so viscous that it cannot be aspirated using a small 25-27-gauge needle leading to the false impression that the cyst is solid. If the clinician knows in advance because of *enhancement* that the nodule is cystic, this allows drainage using a larger 21-22-gauge needle. A smaller gauge needle can then be used on the remaining solid component of the nodule.

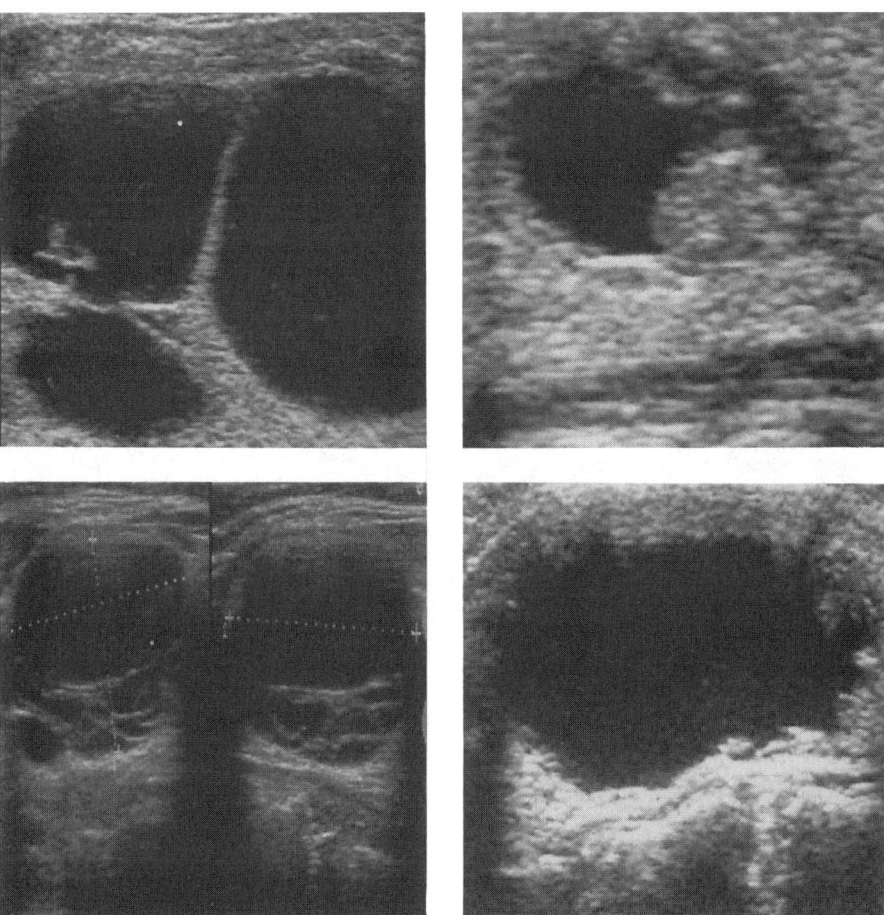

Figure 5.4 Complex Nodules. Many nodules are mixed solid and cystic. They demonstrate a thick wall and the fluid frequently contains debris indicating hemorrhage or necrosis. Septa are common, and occasionally a pedunculated solid mass can be seen growing in the cystic area. If the cystic area is over 1.5 centimeter, *enhancement* of the tissue distal to the cyst may be seen.

The nodule in Figure 5.5 is a thin wall cyst and the bright line of *enhancement* is seen along the posterior wall. The fluid that was aspirated was water-clear and contained a very high concentration of parathromone (PTH) indicating that it was of parathyroid origin (13).

The peripheral PTH and calcium levels in the serum were normal. Although this cyst recurred after drainage, a second drainage was performed several weeks later and there was no recurrence. Malignancy is uncommon in a cyst if there is no palpable residual following aspiration (14).

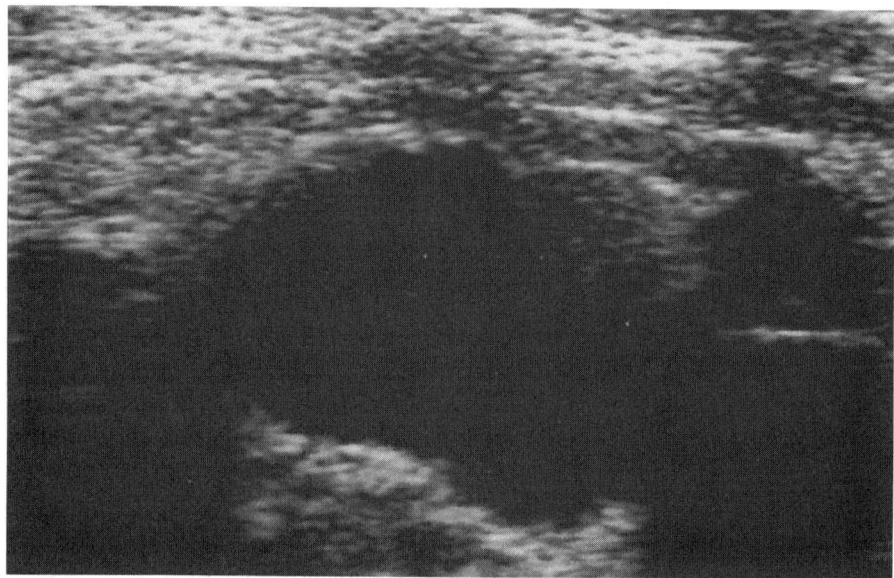

Figure 5.5 Thin Wall Cyst. This cyst has no solid component, and there an *enhancement* of the distal wall. Water-clear fluid was aspirated and contained a high concentration of PTH, indicating it was a parathyroid cyst. After aspiration, the nodule could not be palpated.

Echo Density

A nodule in which the echo pattern is denser than the surrounding thyroid tissue is referred to as being *hyperechoic* (Figure 5.6). Nodules showing a less dense echo pattern are *hypoechoic* (Figure 5.7). Although *isoechoic* nodules do exist, modern high-resolution gray-scale ultrasound generally shows a difference in the density of the nodule compared with the density of the rest of the thyroid gland. Therefore, most nodules can be categorized as either hyperechoic or hypoechoic.

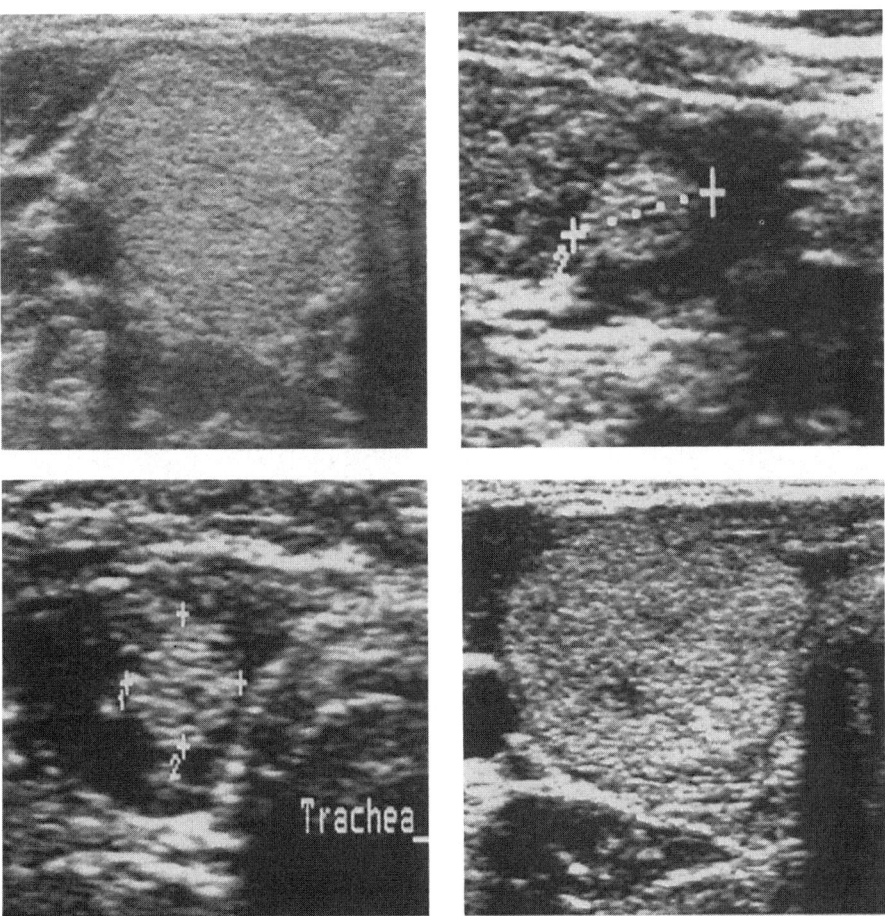

Figure 5.6 Hyperechoic Nodules. These nodules have increased density compared with the surrounding thyroid tissue and appear lighter. Only about 2% of hyperechoic nodules turn out to be malignant.

Thyroid malignancies, regardless of their cell type, are usually hypoechoic. Although malignancy often appears as a hypoechoic nodule, most benign nodules are also hypoechoic. Several large series report a low rate of malignancy if the nodule is hyperechoic (15). Solbiati, et al reported only three of 139 malignancies to be hyperechoic (16). Although a hyperechoic nodule is not likely to be malignant, enough exceptions have occurred that one cannot completely rely on this finding and omit doing a FNA biopsy.

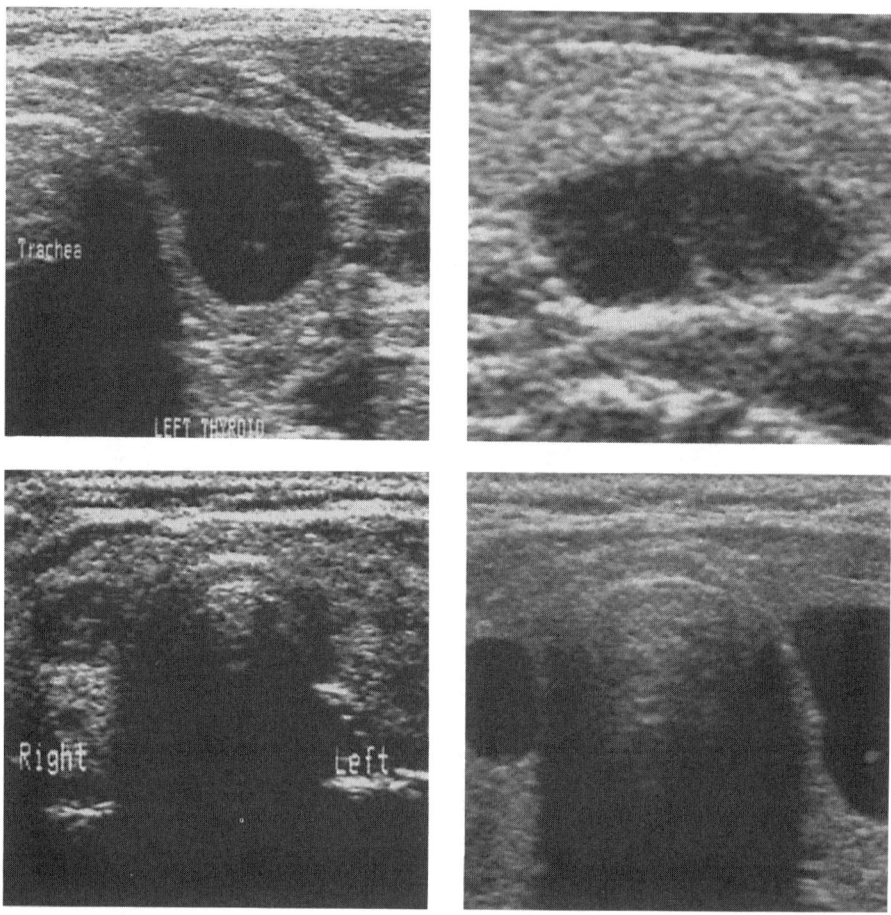

Figure 5.7 Hypoechoic Nodules. These nodules have decreased density compared with the surround thyroid tissue and appear darker. Most malignances of the thyroid gland appear hypoechoic; however, most benign nodules are also hypoechoic.

Margins

The interface between the margins of a nodule and the surrounding thyroid tissue tends to be less well-defined in malignant nodules compared with benign nodules. Cancer frequently has an irregular border rather than a smooth border; and this irregular or obscure margin of a nodule can be an indication of malignancy. Invasive growth of a lesion into the surrounding structures, while rare, is almost a certain indication of cancer.

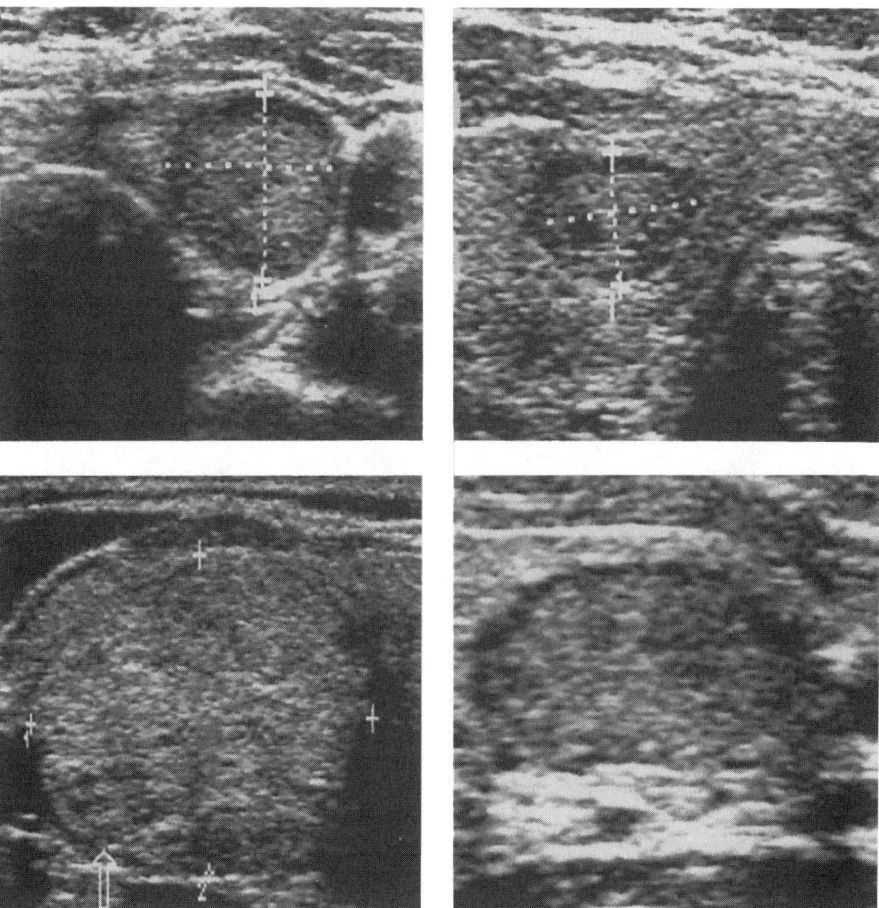

Figure 5.8 Haloes. A sonolucent dark rim around a nodule is referred to as a "halo". While a halo is more common with a benign nodule, it occurs with enough frequency in malignancy that it is not a very helpful in diagnosis. In measuring nodules with haloes, one should be consistent in whether or not the halo is included in the measurement.

Many benign nodules have a sonolucent rim around the nodule referred to as a "halo" (Figure 5.8). While a halo is much more likely to occur with a benign adenoma, it is sometimes seen with malignancy, especially papillary carcinoma, and cannot be used to rule out cancer (17). The cause for a halo is controversial. It is thought to represent inflammation or compression around a nodule rather than a true capsule (18). It needs to be considered when measuring the size or volume of a nodule. It makes no difference if a nodule is measured inside or outside the halo; however, it is critical that the measurement always be done the same way. The inconsistency of different individuals measuring the nodule differently can lead to the false impression that a nodule is growing or shrinking when it is doing neither.

This problem is alleviated if the clinician performs the ultrasound and uses a consistent technique.

Calcifications

Several varieties of calcifications occur with thyroid nodules. The most common types are amorphous dense calcifications that block ultrasound waves and cause *shadowing* distal to the sound wave beam. Although these calcifications can occur anywhere within the nodule, they frequently appear as concentric rings around the rim of a nodule and are referred to as "eggshell" calcifications (Figure 5.9). This type of calcification is associated with chronicity, is common in benign nodules, and is only occasionally seen with malignancy.

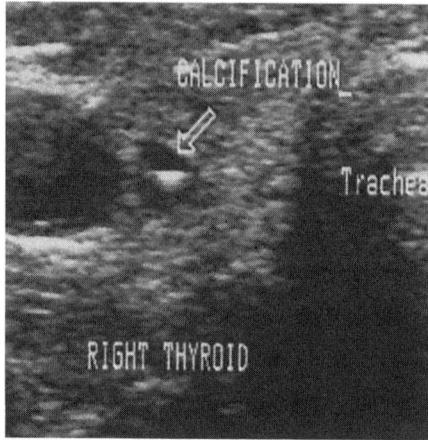 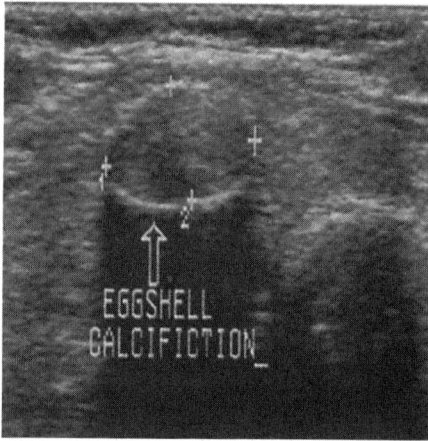

Figure 5.9 Calcifications. Dense amorphous calcifications can occur inside or around the edge of a nodule and cause shadowing or blocking of the sound waves distal to the calcification. They tend to be most common in longstanding benign nodules.

Other types of calcification, referred to as *microcalcifications*, are punctate flecks of calcium within the nodule that are too small to cause acoustic *shadowing* (Figure 5.10). Using high resolution ultrasound, movement of the transducer causes these microcalcifications to appear as bright pinpoints of light that seem to blink or twinkle within the nodule. Pathologically, the fine calcifications are probably due to calcified psammoma bodies, and their presence within the nodule has a high degree of correlation with malignancy approaching 70% (19).

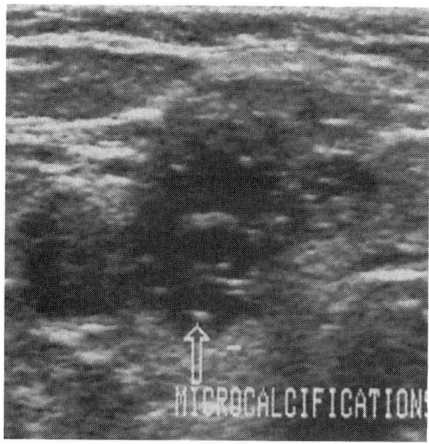
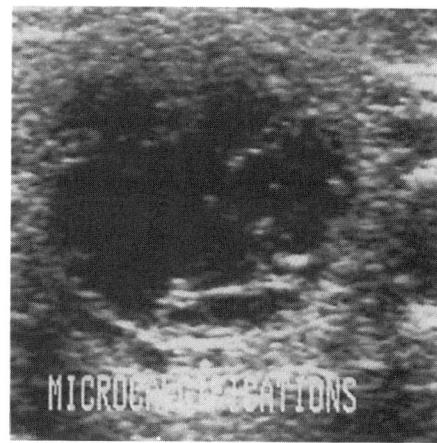

Figure 5.10 Microcalcifications. These tiny flecks of calcium are too small to cause shadowing and are seen within the nodule as pinpoints of light. Using real-time ultrasound, they appear as twinkling stars when the transducer is moved. They have a high correlation with malignancy.

Multinodularity

Ultrasound is the best way to tell if a gland is anatomically normal or has a solitary or multinodular pathology. For years, it was said that the incidence of malignancy was very low in multinodular goiter, ranging from less than 1% to no more than 6% (20,21). This was perhaps a valid assumption when the diagnosis of multinodular goiter was made by physical examination, but ultrasound has shown this to not be true. When ultrasound is performed because of a single nodule, other unsuspected nodules are commonly detected elsewhere in the thyroid gland (22). A small nonpalpable nodule detected by ultrasound does not have the same significance as finding several large palpable nodules on physical examination. Therefore, a dominant nodule in a multinodular goiter should undergo the same evaluation as a solitary nodule.

Change in Size

Although the size of a nodule does not correlate with whether a nodule is benign or malignant, the single best indication that a nodule is benign is its shrinkage or disappearance over time. This can best be determined by using ultrasound that gives an objective measure of a nodule's dimensions and volume. Obviously, a nodule that is decreasing in size is not likely to require surgery. While an estimate of nodule size can be obtained by physical examination, ultrasound provides a much more objective evaluation of what is happening (23). For example, patients taking l-thyroxin suppression may experience a decrease in the surrounding thyroid tissue and it will appear that the nodule is decreasing in size on physical examination. An ultrasound may reveal that the nodule has remained the same or even increased in size. Conversely, a nodule may suddenly increase in size on physical examination, and ultrasound reveals a hemorrhagic cyst occurred that explains the sudden increased size.

In today's mobile society where patients are frequently seen by different physicians in different localities, patients are not always under the care of the same physician for the entire course of their treatment. Ultrasound provides an objective, reproducible, and precise method to measure the size of a nodule that allows different physicians in different geographic locations to follow patients over an extended length of time with continuity of care.

The use of l-thyroxin to induce TSH suppression and cause a decrease in nodule size has been controversial. Although some patient's nodules do seem to decrease while taking l-thyroxin, others may decrease with no treatment at all. Papini, et al followed a random group of patients with thyroid nodules over a five year period with one half taking l-thyroxin and one half taking placebo and found a slight decrease in average volume of nodules in patients taking l-thyroxin (24). However, patients who were taking placebo showed a significant increase in average volume, suggesting that l-thyroxin is beneficial in preventing nodular growth. Just as shrinkage of a nodule is strong evidence that a nodule is benign, a nodule that is increasing in size while TSH is suppressed with l-thyroxin would be a strong signal to re-biopsy the nodule.

Extrathyroidal Extension

As mentioned earlier, ultrasound demonstration of invasion of the anatomical structures around the thyroid is a rare but certain sign of cancer (25). It is most likely to be seen in rapidly growing malignancy such as anaplastic carcinoma. One may see infiltration of the strap muscles or encasement of the jugular vein by metastatic nodes. Ultrasound of a thyroid nodule should always include examination of the lateral neck. Enlargement of cervical lymph nodes, with or without cystic degeneration or microcalcifications, may indicate metastatic spread. Often metastatic lymph nodes in this area may not be palpable and would only be seen with ultrasound.

ULTRASOUND BEFORE FNA BIOPSY?

The majority of thyroid nodules can be easily felt and biopsied without ultrasound. In the past most endocrinologists did not recommend an ultrasound before performing a FNA biopsy. It delayed the biopsy and increased the cost by having to refer the patient to another specialist. However, with office ultrasound there is no delay in doing the biopsy and performing the ultrasound at the time of the biopsy offers certain definite advantages (Table 5.2).

Table 5.2 Advantages of Performing Ultrasound before FNA Biopsy

1. Record the size of the nodule
2. Record the physical characteristics of the nodule
3. Better selection of needle size and length
4. Selection of dominant nodule in multinodular goiter

Because ultrasound provides an objective record of a nodule's size, it can be helpful in the majority of nodules that will be treated medically. It also allows the clinician to record the physical characteristics of the nodule. For example, finding microcalcifications or enlarged cervical lymph nodes is information that would be useful to the cytopathologist. Visualization of the nodule prior to FNA biopsy allows for better selection of needle size (a large gauge for fluid and a small gauge for solid) and needle length. Ultrasound will also reveal other unsuspected nodules and allow FNA biopsy of the dominant nodule(s). Performing ultrasound at the time of the FNA may decrease the number of inadequate specimens and save time and an extra visit.

SUMMARY

Although ultrasound has not yet fulfilled the hope that it could be used to definitely tell if a nodule is benign or malignant, the physical characteristics of nodules are often quite helpful in diagnosis and management of treatment. A hypoechoic nodule with microcalcifications has a higher predictive value of being malignant than a hyperechoic nodule with a sharp halo; however a FNA biopsy is still required of both nodules. Ultrasound does not replace the need to do a FNA biopsy, but the two procedures complement each other. Chapters eight and nine will discuss combining the two procedures into a single procedure, UG FNA biopsy, which many investigators have shown has better predictive value for selecting patients for surgery than either procedure alone (26-30).

REFERENCES

1. Brander A., Viitinkoski F., Nickels J., Kivisarri L. (1989) Thyroid gland: US screening in middle-aged women with no previous thyroid disease. *Radiology* 173:507-510.
2. Carroll B. (1982) Asymptomatic thyroid nodules: incidental sonographic detection. *AJR: 138; 499-501.*
3. Yokozawa T., Miyauchi A., Kuma K., Sugawara M. (1995) Accurate and simple method of diagnosing thyroid nodules by modified technique of ultrasound-guided fine needle aspiration biopsy. *Thyroid* 8; 141-145.
4. Hagag P., Strauss S., Weiss M. (1998) Role of ultrasound-guided fine-needle aspiration biopsy in evaluation of nonpalpable thyroid nodules. *Thyroid* 8; 989-995.
5. Leenhardt L., Hejblum G., Franc B., du Pasquier Fediaevsky L., Delbot T., le Guillouzic C., Menegaux F., Guillausseau C., Hoang C., Turpin G., Aurengo A. (1999) Indications and limits of ultrasound-guided cytology in the management of nonpalpable thyroid nodules. *J Clin Endocrinol Metab* 84; 24-28.
6. Yokozawa T., Fukata S., Kuma K., Matsuzuka F., Kobayashi A., Harai K., Miyauchi A., Sugawara M. (1996) Thyroid cancer detected by ultrasound-guided fine-needle aspiration biopsy. *World J Surg* 20;848-853.
7. Rosen I., Azadian A., Walfish P., Salem S., Lansdown E., Bedard Y. (1993) Ultrasound-guided fine-needle aspiration biopsy in the management of thyroid disease. *Am J Surg* 166;346-349.
8. Takashima S., Matsuzuka F., Nagareta T., Tomiyama N., Kozuka T. (1992) Thyroid nodules associated with hashimoto thyroids: Assessment with ultrasound. *Radiology* 185; 125-130.
9. Nussbaum M., Bukachevsky R. (1990) Thyroid carcinoma presenting as a regional neck mass. *Head & Neck* 12; 114-117.
10. Watters D., Ahuja A., Evans R., Chick W., King W., Metreweli C., Li A. (1992) Role of ultrasound in the management of thyroid nodules. *Am J Surg* 164; 654-657.

11. du Cret R., Choi R., Roe S., Boudreau R., Park H., Loken M. (1987) Improved prediction of thyroid lobar mass from parameters obtained by routine thyroid scintigraphy. *Clin. Nucl. Med.* 12:436-439.
12. Yokozawa T., Matsuzuka F., Kobayashi A., Harai K., Fukata S., Kuma K., Miyauchi A., Katayama S. (1993) 80 Years of Hashimoto Disease ed: Nagataki S., Mori T., Torizuka K. Elsevier Science Publishers
13. Simeone J., Daniels G., Mueller P., Maloof F., vanSonnenberg E., Hall D., O'Connell R., Ferrucci J., Wittenberg J. (1982) High-resolution real-time sonography of the thyroid. *Radiology* 145; 431-435.
14. Ross D. (1992) Evaluation of the thyroid nodule. *J Nucl Med* 32; 2181-2192.
15. Clark O., Okerlund M., Cavalieri R., Greenspan F. (1979) Diagnosis and treatment of thyroid, parathyroid, and thyroglossal duct cysts. *J Clin Endocrinol Metab* 48; 983-988.
16. Solbiati L., Cioffi V., Ballarati E. (1992) Ultrasonography of the neck. *Radiol Clin North Am* 30;941-954.
17. Solbiati L., Volterrani L., Rizzatto G., Bazzocchi M., Busilacchi P., Candiani F., Ferrari F., Giuseppetti G., Maresca G., Mirk P., Rubaltelli L., Zappasodi F. (1985) The thyroid gland with low uptake lesions: Evaluation by ultrasound. *Radiology* 155; 187-191.
18. Propper R., Skolnick L., Weinstein B., Dekker A. (1980) The nonspecificity of the halo sign. *J Clin Ultrasound* 8;129-132.
19. Scheible W., Leopold G., Woo V., Gosink B. (1979) High-resolution real-time ultrasonography of thyroid nodules. *Radiology* 133; 413-417.
20. Takashima S., Fukuda H., Nomura N., Kishimoto H., Kim T., Kobayashi T. (1995) Thyroid nodules: Re-evaluation with ultrasound. *Clin Ultrasound* 23;179-184.
21. Cole-Beuglet C., Goldberg B. (1983) New high-resolution ultrasound evaluation of the diseases of the thyroid gland. *JAMA* 249; 2941-2944.
22. Katz J., Kane R., Reyes G., Clarke M., Hill T. (1984) Thyroid nodules: Sonographic-pathologic correlations. *Radiology* 151; 741-745.
23. Spencer R., Brown M., Annia D. (1977) Ultrasonic scanning of the thyroid gland as a guide to the treatment of the clinically solitary nodule. *Br J Surg* 64; 841-846.
24. Rosen I., Walfish P., Miskin M. (1979) The ultrasound of thyroid masses. *Surg Clin North Am* 59; 19-33.
25. Papini E., Petrucci L., Guglielmi R., Panunzi C., Rinaldi R., Bacci V., Crescenzi A., Nardi F., Fabbrini R., Pacella C. (1998) Long-term changes in nodular goiter: A 5-year prospective randomized trial of levothyroxine suppressive therapy for benign cold thyroid nodules. *J Clin Endocrinol Metab* 83; 780-783.
26. Hayashi N., Tamaki N., Yamamoto K., Senda M., Yonekura Y., Miski T., Iida Y., Kasagi K., Endo K., Konishi J., Torizuka K., Mori T., Makimoto K. (1986) Real-time ultrasonography of thyroid nodules. *Acta Radiologica Diagnosis* 27; 403-408.
27. Takashima S., Fukuda H., Kobayashi T. (1994) Thyroid nodules: Clinical effect of ultrasound-guided fine-needle aspiration biopsy. *Clin Ultrasound* 22; 535-542.
28. Cochand-Priollet B., Guillausseau P., Chagnon S., Hong C., Guillausseau-Scholer C., Chanson P., Dahan H., Warnet A., Tran Ba Huy P., Valleur P. (1994) The diagnostic value of fine-needle aspiration biopsy under ultrasonography in nonfunctional nodules: A prospective study comparing cytologic and histologic findings. *Am J Med* 97; 152-157.
29. Danese D., Sciacchitano S., Farsetti A., Andreoli M., Pontecorvi A. (1998) Diagnostic accuracy of conventional sonography-guided fine-needle aspiration biopsy of thyroid nodules. *Thyroid* 8; 15-21.
30. Khurana K., Richards V., Chopra P., Izquierdo R., Rubens D., Mesonero C. (1998) The role of ultrasonography-guided fine-needle aspiration in the management of nonpalpable and palpable thyroid nodules. *Thyroid* 8; 511-515.
31. Carmeci C., Jefrey B., McDougall R., Nowels K., Weigel R. (1998) Ultrasound-guided fine-needle aspiration biopsy of thyroid masses. *Thyroid* 8; 283-289.

6

NECK ULTRASOUND AND THE ENDOCRINE SURGEON

Edward Paloyan, M.D.
Professor Emeritus
Hinsdale, IL 60521 USA
Regina P. Walker, M.D.
Ann M. Lawrence, M.D., Ph.D.
Loyola University Medical Center
Maywood, IL 60153 USA

PREFACE

During the course of surgical residency training, the young "apprentice" is taught a number of universal principles which s/he transgresses only at the patients' peril and their own risk.

Two such principles were indelibly imprinted on the senior author's cerebral cortex during the first year of residency by two surgical giants, one a thoracic surgeon and the other a general surgeon par excellence.

In sequential fashion this young resident was taught that you perform a lobectomy/pneumonectomy *only* after *you*, the *operating surgeon,* had performed a bronchoscopy personally and had examined and evaluated the bronchial mucosa that you were going to incise and suture and determine whether it was in an optimal condition to heal with minimal risk of a leak or a devastating breakdown of the suture line.

The second principle taught by the premier general surgeon was similar: You perform a colorectal resection/anastomosis only after you personally have performed a sigmoidoproctoscopy to examine the mucosa distal to the lesion you were going to resect.

Those universal principles are applicable in many other fields of health care. In this essay, the authors discuss and illustrate the importance of preoperative and postoperative ultrasonographic examination and evaluation of the thyroid/parathyroids/cervical lymph nodes, *through* the "eyes" of the *operating* surgeon, for preoperative planning and postoperative evaluation/ critique of the operation performed.

The essence of Endocrine Surgery includes specific knowledge in anatomy, endocrinology and endocrine histopathology, a background in laboratory and clinical research and clinical experience (1).

The endocrine surgeon, to be fair to his/her patient, must be able to interpret and be aware of the pitfalls of laboratory endocrine evaluation and imaging. Preoperative evaluation should include specific information in regards to the pathological anatomy, best obtained by physical examination combined with hands-on ultrasonography (US).

Postoperative evaluation, short-term and long-term, includes chemical evaluations and imaging of the neck by US, histopathologic evaluation of the resected tissue, and long-term follow-up to evaluate the long-term consequences of the operation that the operating surgeon performed, sometimes characterized as "agonizing self-appraisal."

It is only since the emergence of ultrasonographic equipment from the domain of "big, black boxes" to manageable and portable equipment, with excellent resolution, that clinicians have been able to add this most important imaging tool to their diagnostic armamentarium.

A number of years ago the editor of this volume urged us to consider in-office, "hands-on" sonographic evaluation of our patients with thyroid and parathyroid pathology: we now wonder how we ever ventured in a thyroidectomy or parathyroidectomy without having evaluated the pathologic anatomy personally. Needless to say, we are highly indebted to the editor, as should be our patients.

An anecdote will epitomize the importance of hands-on US examination by the endocrine surgeon: when we started some years ago, we obtained the assistance of two highly skilled ultrasonographers with a combined experience of 50 years. *They had never* imaged a parathyroid tumor, let alone a normal parathyroid gland. After a few months on the job in our office, they had imaged numerous parathyroid tumors *and* quickly developed the skills to image normal parathyroid glands in most patients examined for parathyroid or thyroid pathology.

The net result is that in a patient evaluated for hypercalcemia and hypophosphatemia the first examination is ultrasonographic. If a parathyroid tumor is noted, the diagnosis is made without any further testing. We believe that such a diagnostic sequence in the evaluation of hypercalcemia is not only very important for the planning of a parathyroidectomy, but is also *cost effective.*

This chapter is comprised of specific illustrations of ultrasonographic items of interest to the endocrine surgeon in the preoperative evaluation of patients with thyroid and parathyroid pathology.

THYROID

Evaluation of Tumors of The Thyroid With Equivocal Fine Needle Aspiration Cytology

In a large number of patients with thyroid nodules, the cytological diagnosis is equivocal and the clinician must rely on a number of other parameters to determine whether a thyroidectomy is indicated.

These parameters include various characteristics of the nodule on physical examination and of the ultrasonographic features in particular, in terms of the size of the tumor, the presence or absence of a halo surrounding the tumor (secondary to significant vascularity in the periphery of the tumor), the presence of concentric or stippled calcifications, and whether the tumor is "solid" through and through, cystic, or "mixed." The presence of other, smaller nodules in the ipsilateral or contralateral lobe is of significance. Finally, of great importance, is the presence of cervical adenopathy, which may be ipsilateral, contralateral, bilateral, and may be related to the tumor in terms of possible metastases or to a coexisting chronic, autoimmune thyroiditis.

In patients where the recommendation for a thyroidectomy is still equivocal, the response to TSH suppressive doses of thyroid hormone may be a deciding factor. The response to TSH is best measured by ultrasonography in terms of changes in the size of the dominant tumor, other coexisting nodules, the remainder of the gland, and the response of coexisting cervical adenopathy, both ipsilateral and contralateral.

When the remainder of the gland shows a significant reduction in size, as do other coexisting nodules, whereas the dominant tumor does not demonstrate any response in terms of size and texture, that fact alone may be the deciding factor in recommending a thyroidectomy.

Preoperative Evaluation

An axiom that has withstood the test of time and logic in surgical philosophy, is that as much information as feasible should be obtained prior to an elective operation. Obviously, other types of information become available during the course of an operation which may modify the original plans. However, the specific information regarding the pathologic anatomy of a thyroid tumor is just as important as the thyroid functional status of a patient about to undergo a major operation under general anesthesia.

Therefore, the importance of ultrasound examination cannot be overstated in terms of location of the tumor, its size, its characteristics, its relationship to the recurrent nerve and the external branch of the superior laryngeal nerve, its vascularity and the vascularity of the surrounding tissue.

The presence/absence of inflammatory changes in the remainder of the thyroid is of great importance to the operating surgeon. The great majority of recurrent nerve problems following thyroidectomies is not due to the primary tumor itself, but to the coexisting chronic thyroiditis which creates a great deal of scarring, edema, and inflammation along the course of the recurrent laryngeal nerves.

Furthermore, the presence and location of cervical adenopathy is important in planning a possible cervical node dissection and the dissection along the recurrent laryngeal nerves, since many of these lymph nodes surround the nerve or may be densely adherent to it.

Finally, it is important to visualize the parathyroids in patients about to undergo a thyroidectomy, since there is a significant occurrence of coexisting parathyroid pathology in many subgroups of patients with thyroid tumors and chronic thyroiditis (2,3,4,5,6,7,8,9,10).

The preliminary decision to perform a lobectomy or a total thyroidectomy is based on a variety of factors, many of which are delineated by detailed ultrasound examination and documentation of the various characteristics described above.

Postoperative Evaluation of Patients with Thyroid Neoplasia
The endocrinologist and endocrine surgeon assume a primary role in the long-term treatment of patients with thyroid neoplasia, whether an adenoma or a carcinoma.

The senior author along with a group of endocrinologists and specialists in nuclear medicine has minimized the use of postoperative radioactive iodine for diagnostic/therapeutic purposes since the 60's for a variety of reasons.

First of all, when a total thyroidectomy is performed, there should be very little, if any, demonstrable remaining thyroid tissue in the great majority of patients. Therefore, the great majority of patients with total thyroidectomy for thyroid carcinoma should *not* require any radioactive iodine postoperatively, especially when the operation is performed by an experienced endocrine surgeon. The problems with radioactive iodine administration for diagnostic and therapeutic purposes, in terms of stunning of thyroid tissue or tumors, which compromises the effectiveness of subsequent therapeutic administration of radioactive iodine (11,12,13), in terms of an increased incidence of gastric carcinoma (14), in terms of long-term cardiovascular problems (15), in terms of remote and almost insignificant incidence of leukemia, not to mention the severe symptoms of a profound hypothyroid state given the preparatory period before the administration of radioactive iodine are well known.

Fortunately, with the advent of recombinant TSH, the preparatory hypothyroid state will be eliminated. The results of the "minimal use" of radioactive iodine for diagnostic and therapeutic purposes over long-term follow-ups have been documented and have proved to be favorable (16).

In recent years, we have relied on Sestamibi scanning for the detection of remnants of thyroid in the thyroid bed or to evaluate cervical adenopathy. However, this entails the use of a radioactive substance and the diagnostic effectiveness of Sestamibi in such a setting has not been fully documented.

Therefore, the importance of echographic examination of the neck in patients following a lobectomy or a total thyroidectomy cannot be overstated.

Ultrasound examination will detect and characterize small remnants in the thyroid bed after a lobectomy; it will characterize the contralateral remnant in terms of texture, the presence or subsequent emergence of small nodules and assist greatly in the determination of the indications for a contralateral thyroid lobectomy (to achieve a total thyroidectomy) in patients who may have only microcarcinomas found in the specimen of the original lobectomy. Furthermore, long-term follow-up of thyroid remnants and the detection of emerging or remaining adenopathy in the ipsilateral or contralateral side is crucial information in the evaluation of such patients. Obviously, the information obtained by ultrasonographic examination has to be correlated with the circulating quantitative thyroglobulin measurements, fine needle aspiration of nodules in the contralateral lobe, and fine needle aspiration of emerging cervical adenopathy.

An illustrative example is that of a patient with cervical adenopathy developing years after total thyroidectomy, who had negative radionuclide scans, equivocal fine needle aspiration biopsies, and almost non-detectable circulating thyroglobulin. The only finding in this patient was significant adenopathy seen on US examination that was not responding to TSH suppression over a number of years.

The decision to recommend a resection and to find metastatic carcinoma in lymphoid tissue in this patient was primarily based on US examination. We have seen several similar cases (Illustration - Case 3).

HYPERPARATHYROIDISM/PARATHYROID GLANDS

Evaluation of hypercalcemia

Some years ago, in a prestigious Midwestern hospital, patients with hypercalcemia were worked up for several weeks on a metabolic ward to characterize the hypercalcemia and determine whether it was caused by hyperparathyroidism. The work up included calcium balance studies in patients equilibrated on a diet which had been assayed for calcium content, bone biopsies, phosphate clearances, and elaborate renal function studies.

In the same hospital, just a few years ago, the work up of a patient with hypercalcemia consisted merely of an ultrasound examination of the neck, "on the way to the operating room for a parathyroidectomy."

The importance of modern US with high resolution was not lost on those same clinicians/investigators. The primary tool to establish the diagnosis of hyperparathyroidism in hypercalcemic patients was an ultrasound examination demonstrating a parathyroid tumor.

For a number of years, we have espoused the same methodology. We establish the diagnosis of hyperparathyroidism in hypercalcemic patients with the demonstration of a parathyroid tumor (s). The importance of US in the diagnosis of hyperparathyroidism cannot be overstated. It is simple, cost effective, and reproducible. Furthermore, US examination is critical in patients with elusive, *intrathyroid* parathyroid tumors (Cases 7 and 8).

In addition, US provides information regarding the thyroid gland, which may be chronically inflamed or contain incidental nodules in a higher percentage of patients with hyperparathyroidism (2,3,6,7,10).

Although the great majority of patients with primary hyperparathyroidism harbor a single adenoma, 20 to 30% may have additional involved parathyroid glands which may cause a persistence or the recurrence of the disease in the foreseeable future. US examination is one of the most effective ways of determining the state of the remaining parathyroid glands preoperatively.

If a parathyroid tumor cannot be visualized by ultrasound examination of the neck, then one must consider this as an important signal in looking for ectopic parathyroid tumors in the anterior superior mediastinum still accessible through a cervical incision, or deeper and lower in the mediastinum, a situation which may lead to the possibility of a mediastinal exploration. The need for a Sestamibi parathyroid scan is highly advisable in such patients where the ultrasound examination does not demonstrate a parathyroid tumor.

In patients with renal (secondary) hyperparathyroidism, the requirement for parathyroidectomy is commensurate with the size of the enlarged parathyroid glands, which should total to an estimated weight of 1 gram, according to some nephrologists. Therefore, the importance of US in patients with renal hyperparathyroidism is primarily based on the confirmation of the diagnosis and indications for parathyroidectomy, according to the estimated weight/size of the four parathyroids. In such patients, the parathyroid glands are seldom ectopic, all four of them have to be addressed and in this day and age, the authors prefer to do a total parathyroidectomy with autotransplantation of the most normal appearing parathyroid tissue that can be found.

Preoperative Evaluation of Parathyroid Tumors
Parameters such as size, location, relationship to the recurrent nerves, fibrosis surrounding atypical (potential carcinoma) tumors are of great importance to the operating endocrine surgeon. The visualization of the other parathyroids, if at all possible, provides a clue as to whether the parathyroidectomy should be unilateral, with a limited incision, or bilateral, to decide whether any of the other parathyroids are enlarged or beginning to develop hyperplasia and therefore should be evaluated and possibly resected to prevent long-term recurrences.

As stated earlier, the ultrasonographers in our office, with long-term experience, had never seen a parathyroid tumor, let alone a normal parathyroid gland, prior to their experience with us. Currently, we are able to visualize at least one, if not more, parathyroid glands, in addition to the parathyroid tumor in the great majority of patients, and thus are guided by US to determine the extent of the operation and "exploration."

An antiquated axiom in parathyroid operations is that if three normal parathyroid glands are found and "the adenoma" is missing, the surgeon should perform a thyroid lobectomy on the side of the missing parathyroid gland, with the hope of discovering an unsuspected intrathyroid parathyroid tumor.

With the preoperative US in patients with hyperparathyroidism, the thyroid gland should be meticulously examined. Therefore, where three normal parathyroid glands are found and the "adenoma" is missing, if the examination of the thyroid by US has not disclosed any abnormality, there would be no point in performing an unnecessary thyroid lobectomy. Conversely, the presence of a well delineated, sonolucent area within the thyroid parenchyma in such a patient would necessitate the resection of that thyroid lobe or a partial lobectomy, if only because the lesion would be a coexisting thyroid lesion, if not an intrathyroid parathyroid tumor (Illustration - Cases 7 and 8).

Finally, the presence of coexisting thyroid pathology and lymph node pathology is important information for preoperative planning and would require further intraoperative evaluation and management.

Postoperative Evaluation
Since the advent of limited or mini-parathyroidectomies, the persistence or recurrence of hyperparathyroidism is not uncommon. Therefore, it is important to examine patients after parathyroidectomy not only chemically but also by US to establish the postoperative state of the remaining parathyroid glands in order to establish baseline imaging for future comparison if and when such patients develop persistent/recurrent hypercalcemia/hyperparathyroidism.

ILLUSTRATIVE CASES

Case 1. Normal Parathyroids

This case illustrates that an experienced ultrasonographer can visualize *normal* parathyroid glands during the course of an ultrasound examination of the thyroid gland.

This patient suffers from Hashimoto's thyroiditis and has a fibrotic thyroid gland. Three normal sized parathyroids are seen: the left superior, left inferior, and right inferior glands, measuring respectively 8 x 3 mm, 6 x 4 mm, and 8 x 4 mm.

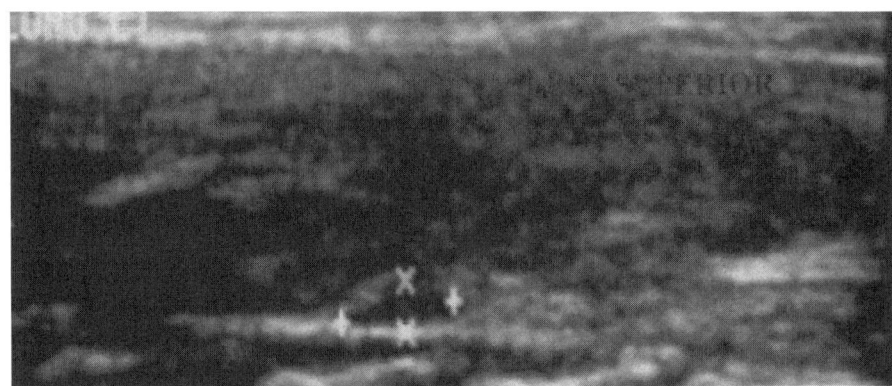

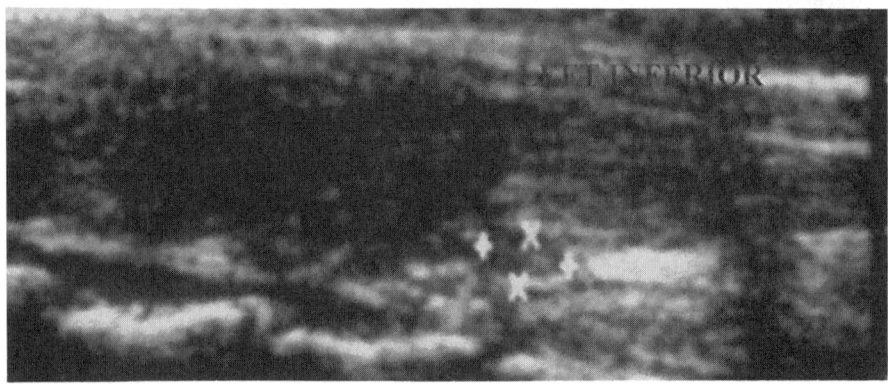

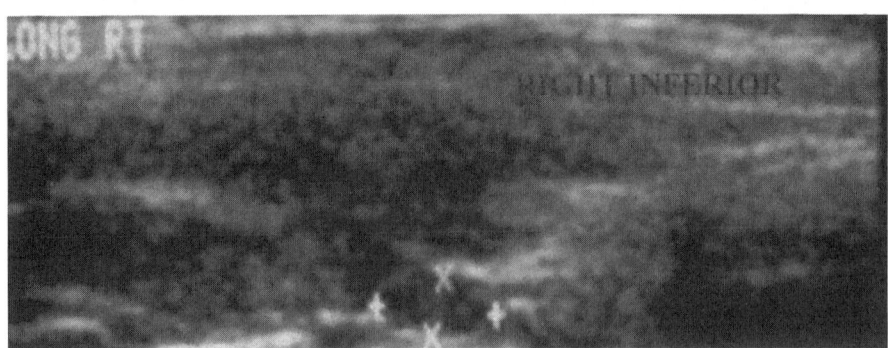

Case 2. Effects of TSH Suppression on a Thyroid Nodule

This case illustrates the importance of US examination in the evaluation of thyroid nodules and their response to TSH suppression therapy. In May of 1997, this 53-year-old lady developed a thyroid nodule in the left lobe. A fine needle aspiration biopsy was read as "aspirate consistent with a Hürthle cell neoplasm." This diagnosis was reviewed by a group of cytologists in another institution. Although there was general agreement between the cytologists in both institutions (cytologists do not like to disagree with each other), there was still sufficient doubt that a medical treatment regimen with increasing doses of T4 was instituted beginning with 0.05 mg daily up to the current 0.137 mg dose.

The ultrasound examinations demonstrate the progressive decrease in size of the tumor from 13 x 11 mm down to 6 x 3 mm over a period of 20 months. The nodule is no longer palpable and we believe that, although this patient was originally referred for a thyroidectomy, with ultrasound confirmation, all the therapy that was required was TSH suppression.

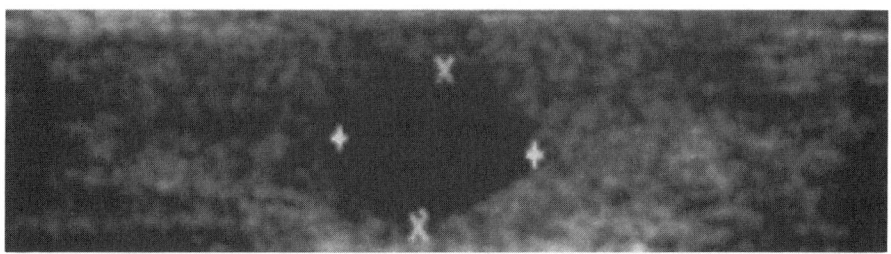

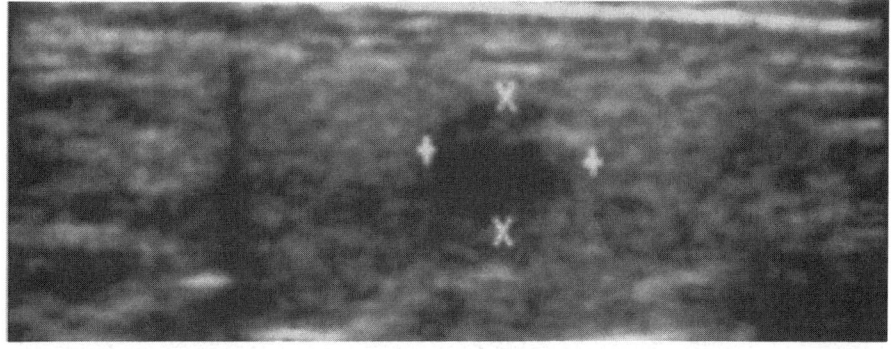

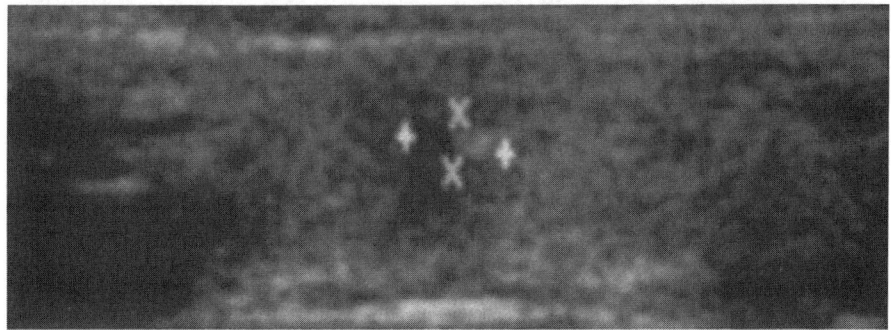

Case 3. Metastatic Thyroid Carcinoma in a Lymph Node Detected Only by Ultrasound

This 30-year-old lady underwent a lateral left neck lymph node excision in 1988. The lesion proved to be thyroid carcinoma in a scalene lymph node. The patient self-referred to another institution for a total thyroidectomy in the same year (1988).

In 1994 her circulating thyroglobulin rose to 5 ng/ml (0-60) from previous non-measurable levels. US examination detected a mass at the base of the left neck, which was barely palpable. A radionuclide scan was negative for any uptake. A fine needle aspiration cytology showed only lymphoid cells.

Since the lesion persisted on ultrasound, a resection was advised and performed in 1996 and the histopathology demonstrated a cystic papillary carcinoma, presumably arising (or persisting) at the site of the original lateral neck node excision in 1988.

The most recent thyroglobulin levels have been between 1 and 2 ng/ml.

The US examinations demonstrate the recurring lesion before and after resection.

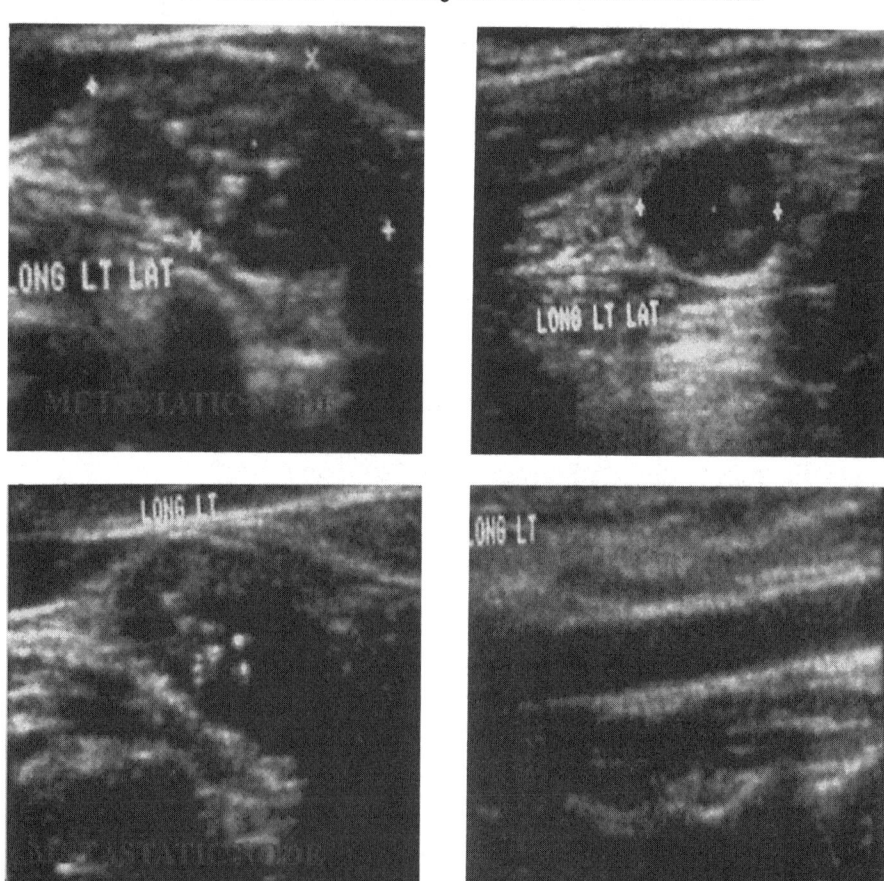

Case 4. Hemorrhage in the Thyroid Gland

A 30-year-old lady on long-term, high dose anticoagulants developed sudden pain and tenderness in the thyroid gland, primarily on the right, but with some extension to the left. This was accompanied by dysphagia and a right vocal cord paresis. She was referred for a fine needle aspiration cytology because of a "cold defect" seen on a thyroid scan.

An ultrasound examination showed large and small cystic lesions primarily on the right. The interpretation was that of a hemorrhage related to the anticoagulation therapy, which could not be discontinued because of a thrombotic diathesis.

On the basis of the US, a fine needle aspiration was declined.

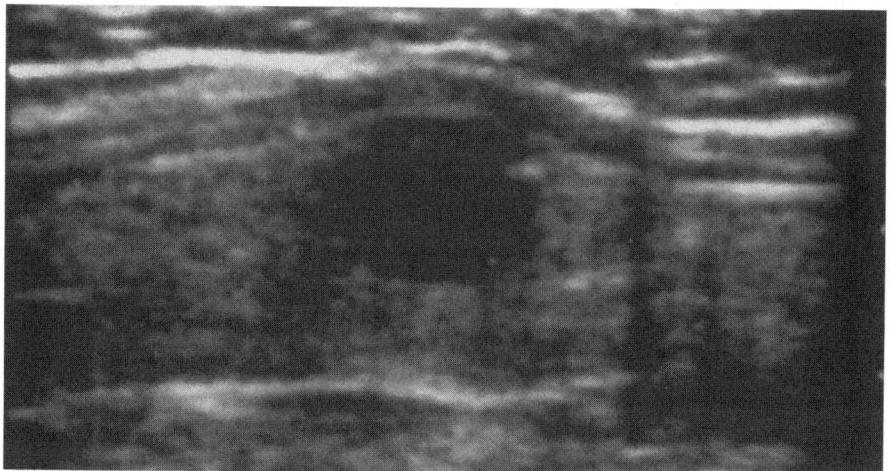

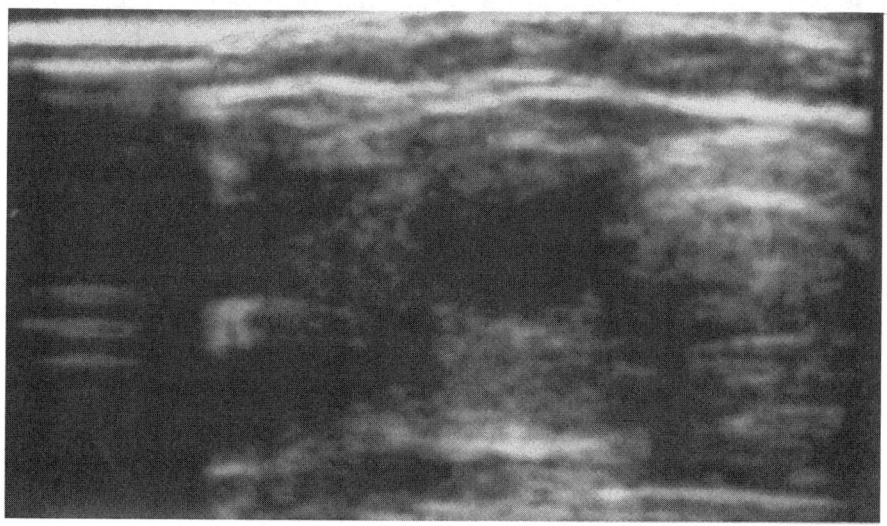

Case 5. Preoperative Recurrent Nerve Paresis

A 35-year-old lady speech pathologist was referred for a thyroidectomy with a tumor of the right lobe and a suspicious cytology. The patient was totally asymptomatic.

An ultrasound examination disclosed bowing and distortion of the posterior surface of the thyroid by the tumor, measuring 27 x 17 mm. This led to an examination of the vocal cords and the discovery of a paresis of the right vocal cord in this totally asymptomatic speech pathologist.

This finding changed the operative approach: a recurrent nerve decompression was planned along with the thyroid lobectomy. Furthermore, any thought of performing a total (*real* total) thyroidectomy simultaneously and thus subject the *left* recurrent nerve to even the slightest possibility of paresis was completely erased. Bilateral cord paresis can be a life threatening complication, especially in this day and age of early postoperative discharge from the hospital.

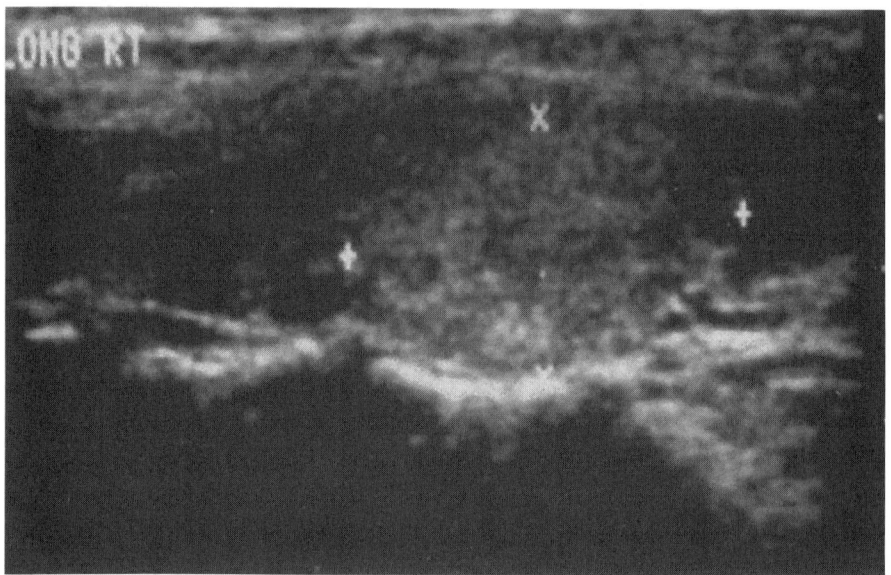

Case 6. Coexisting Parathyroid and Thyroid Tumors

This is a 57-year-old lady with a history of hypercalcemia and documented hyperparathyroidism. The patient was referred for parathyroidectomy. An ultrasound examination disclosed a sizable 19 x 7 mm left superior parathyroid tumor (sonolucent lesion posterior to the thyroid gland). But it also demonstrated that the palpable lesion was a co-existing thyroid tumor measuring 38 x 24 mm, which had been overlooked.

The thyroid tumor is surrounded by a "black" halo a characteristic feature of neoplasia. With the US evidence of a significant thyroid lesion, the patient was prepared for a parathyroidectomy *and* a thyroidectomy. The thyroid tumor proved to be a papillary carcinoma.

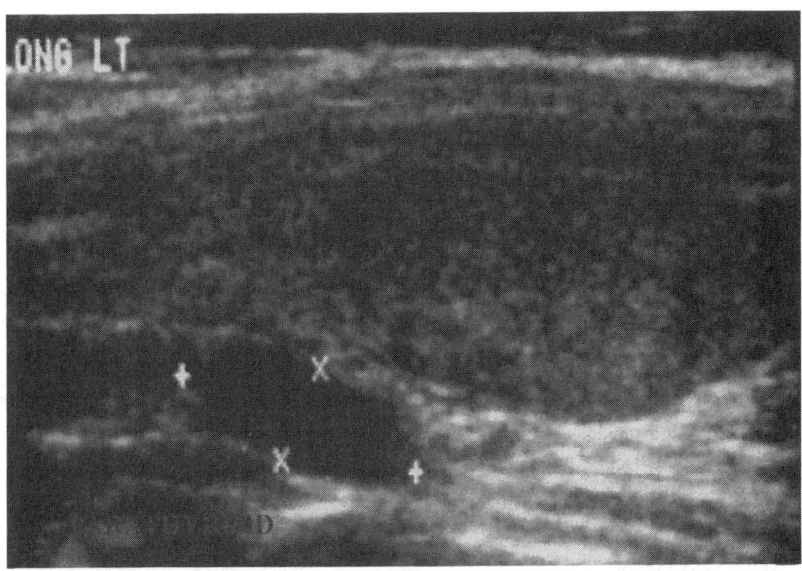

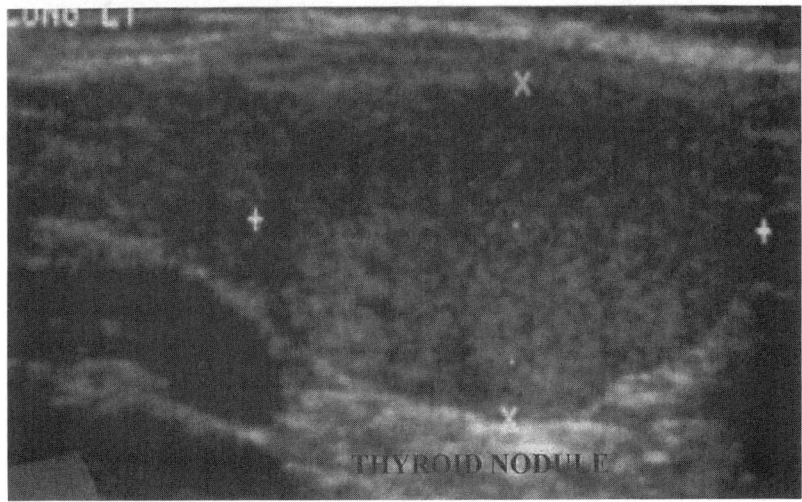

Case 7. Recurrent Hyperparathyroidism/Intrathyroid Parathyroid Tumor

This 61-year-old lady was operated for hyperparathyroidism in *February, 1980*. The right superior gland proved to be a parathyroid tumor and was resected - the left superior and inferior glands were biopsied and proved to be normal.

The right inferior gland could not be located. The patient became eucalcemic after her 1980 parathyroidectomy. However, her circulating parathormone levels remained slightly elevated and her phosphates remained in the lower half of the normal range.

Eighteen years later, in 1998, hypercalcemia was once more documented. The patient was referred back for an evaluation: an ultrasound examination disclosed an *intrathyroid* parathyroid tumor measuring 16 x 9 mm. The patient underwent a partial right thyroid lobectomy with resection of the PTH tumor.

She is now eucalcemic with normal intact PTH and serum phosphates. Over a period of 20 years, this patient proved to have adenomas of the right superior and inferior parathyroids.

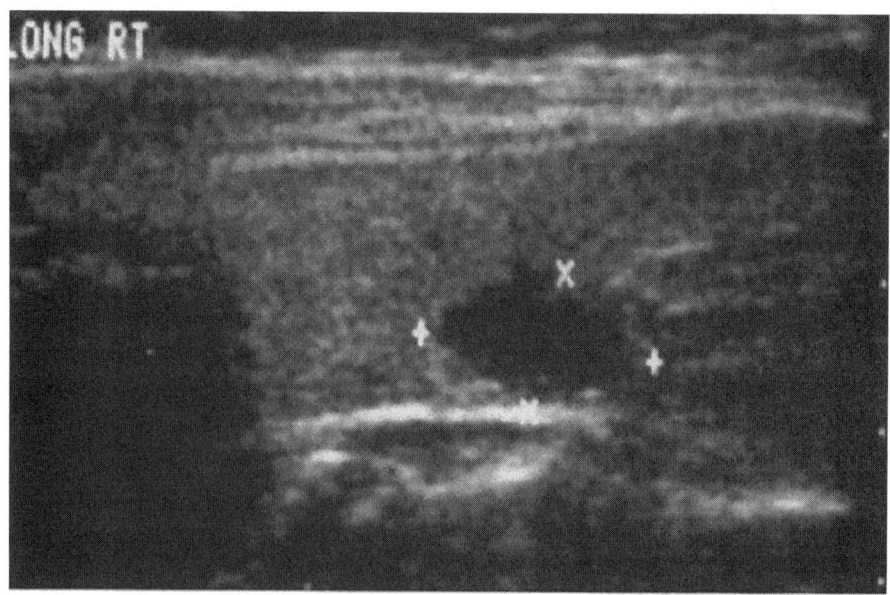

Case 8. Recurrent Hyperparathyroidism/Intrathyroid Parathyroid Tumor

This 64-year-old man, a leading international ecclesiastic whose voice was extremely important, had an extensive bilateral "exploration" for hyperparathyroidism in another institution. Only two parathyroids would be found and they were on the left side. They were normal by inspection and biopsy. The hypercalcemia persisted and the patient was then referred for further management. A Sestamibi scan disclosed uptake on the right consistent with a parathyroid tumor, at a site already extensively dissected by a very competent surgeon. A second exploration with painstakingly tedious dissection to identify and preserve the recurrent nerve was undertaken four months after the first exploration.

A sizable parathyroid tumor of the right inferior parathyroid was resected in July of 1996. The patient became eucalcemic for two years, only to have a recurrence of his hypercalcemia. In December, 1998 an ultrasound examination disclosed an intrathyroid superior PTH tumor measuring 13 x 6 mm. In December, 1998, a third exploration with partial right thyroidectomy disclosed an intrathyroid parathyroid tumor.

The patient is now eucalcemic with a normal circulating intact PTH and, most importantly, a normal voice, confirmed by postoperative laryngoscopy.

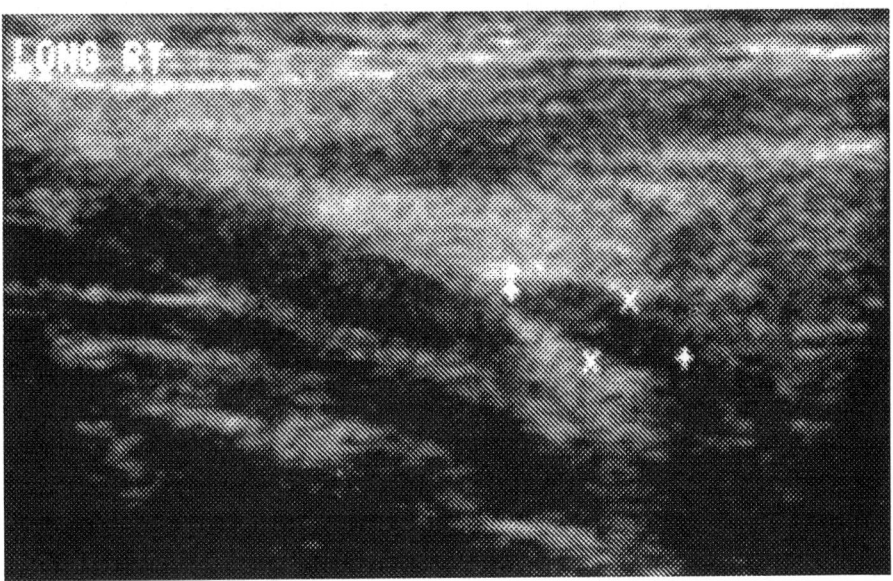

REFERENCES

1. Paloyan, E., American Association of Endocrine Surgeons Presidential Address: The Gatekeepers. *Surgery* 1988; 104:937-9.
2. Walker RP, Paloyan E. The relationship between Hashimoto's thyroiditis, thyroid neoplasia, and primary hyperparathyroidism. *Otolaryngol Clin North Am* 1990; 23; 291-302.
3. Al-Jurf A, Esselstyn CB, Crile G. Thyroid lesions in patients with hyperparathyroidism. *Int Surg* 1979; 64:33-6.
4. Boullon R., DeMoor P. Parathyroid function in patients with hyper-or hypothyroidism. *J Clin Endocrinol Metabol* 1974; 38:999-1004.
5. Calandra DB, Shah K, Lawrence AM, et al. Hyperparathyroidism unmasked by the treatment of hypothyroidism secondary to Hashimoto's thyroiditis. *Surgery* 1984; 96:1015-8.
6. Laing VO, Frame B, Block MA. Associated primary hyperparathyroidism and thyroid lesions. *Arch Surg* 1969; 98:708-12.
7. Lever EG, Refetoff S, Strauss FH, et al. Coexisting thyroid and parathyroid disease: are they related? Surgery 1983; 94:893,900.
8. Lever EG. Primary hyperparathyroidism masked by hypothyroidism. *Am J Med* 1983; 74:144-7.
9. Walker RP, Oslapas R, Ernst K, et al. Hyperparathyroidism induced by hypothyroidism. *Laryngoscope* 1993; 103:263-8.
10. LiVolsi VA, Feind CR. Parathyroid adenoma and nonmedullary thyroid carcinoma cancer. *Cancer* 1976; 38:1391-3.
11. Park H, Perkins OW, Edmondson JW, et al. Influence of diagnostic radioiodines on the uptake of ablative dose of iodine-131. *Thyroid* 1994; 4:49.
12. Park H. Stunned thyroid after high dose 131I scanning. *J Clin Nucl Med* 1992; 17:501.
13. Park H, Park Y, Zhou X, et al. Detection of thyroid remnant/metastasis without stunning: An ongoing dilemma. *Thyroid* 1997; 7:277.
14. Hall P, Holm L. Late consequences of radioiodine for diagnosis and therapy in Sweden. *Thyroid* 1997; 7:205.
15. Franklyn JA Maisonneuve P, et al. Mortality after the treatment of hyperthyroidism with radioactive iodine. *N Eng J of Med* 1998; 338(11): 712-8.
16. McHenry C, Jarosz H, Lawrence AM, Paloyan E. Improving postoperative recurrence rates for carcinoma of the thyroid gland. *Surgery* 1989; 169:429-434.

7

Thyroid Fine Needle Aspiration Biopsy

Hossein Gharib, M.D., F.A.C.P., F.A.C.E.
Consultant
Division of Endocrinology, Metabolism, Nutrition, and Internal Medicine,
Mayo Clinic and Mayo Foundation
Professor of Medicine
Mayo Medical School
Rochester, Minnesota, 55905 USA

Nodular thyroid disease is defined as the presence of single or multiple palpable or nonpalpable nodules within the thyroid gland. Thyroid nodules are common in clinical practice. Solitary palpable thyroid nodules are found in 4% to 7% of the adult population in North America (1-5). The prevalence of nodules increases linearly with age, in women, in iodine-deficient areas, and in populations exposed to ionizing radiation (2,3). Epidemiologic studies suggest that the annual incidence of thyroid nodules is 0.1% per year, which translates into approximately 275,000 new nodules in the United States, with an estimated 10% lifetime expectancy of a nodule developing (1). From a clinical standpoint, fewer than 5% of palpable nodules are malignant.

Fine-needle aspiration (FNA) biopsy of the thyroid has been established as a useful procedure in the primary diagnosis of nodular thyroid disease, and it has had a dramatic impact on the care of patients with thyroid nodules (6-8). FNA biopsy is now regarded as the most useful and accurate method for investigating thyroid nodules and has become an integral part of nodule work-up.

This chapter reviews the biopsy techniques, cytopathologic interpretation, FNA results, diagnostic pitfalls, cystic nodules, complications, and indications for rebiopsy and briefly mentions ultrasonographically guided FNA (UG-FNA) results.

BIOPSY

In contrast to biopsy with large needles and tissue examination, FNA biopsy permits aspiration of material and cytologic examination of the specimen.

Aspiration techniques were developed and used in Sweden in the 1960s; however, the technique has gained wide acceptance in the United States and other countries only during the last 2 decades (9,10).

Biopsy can be performed either in an outpatient setting on an examining table in a physician's office or on a hospital bed. The thyroid gland should be palpated carefully and the nodule or nodules to be aspirated clearly identified. The procedure is explained carefully to the patient to minimize undue anxiety and concern. The patient should be informed that several aspirations will be done. A nurse should always be available to assist with the procedure.

The patient is supine, supported by a pillow under the shoulders, with the neck hyperextended to expose the thyroid. The patient is told to avoid swallowing or talking during the procedure. After the nodule(s) to be aspirated has been identified by palpation, the overlying skin is cleansed with alcohol. Some physicians prefer to use local anesthesia to minimize trauma. After the biopsy has been completed, pressure is applied to all biopsy sites, and after a short period of observation, the patient is dismissed.

Aspiration Technique

There are two methods to examine the thyroid cytologically (2,10). In the aspiration technique, a 27- or 25-gauge 1.5-inch-long needle attached to a 10-mL disposable plastic syringe is used (Figure 7.1*B*). Negative pressure can be applied by using the syringe alone or by using a mechanical syringe holder, such as the Cameco syringe pistol (Precision Dynamics Corporation, Burbank, CA). The use of this pistol-grip syringe holder allows the physician to keep one hand free to identify and to stabilize the area to be aspirated (Figure 7.1*C*). In addition, a newly developed syringe-holding device using a pencil-grip FNA syringe holder has been introduced (TAO and TAO Technology, Inc., Carmel, IN). The advantages of this aspirator appear to be easier manipulation and, possibly, easier needle placement in target tissue. The needle is inserted rapidly into the nodule without suction; after the needle tip is in the nodule, suction is applied while the needle is moved back and forth within the nodule. This maneuver permits cellular material to be dislodged and, thus, sucked into the needle. The procedure is stopped when material appears in the needle hub, and the suction is released by allowing the syringe plunger to return to its normal position. The needle is then withdrawn and removed from the syringe, and the syringe is filled with air by retracting the plunger. The needle is reattached to the syringe, and, this time with the bevel pointing down, one drop of aspirated material is placed on each of several glass slides (Figure 7.1*E*). Smears are prepared by using two glass slides similar to those used to make blood smears (Figure 7.1*F*). Immediately, the slides are placed in bottles of 95% ethyl alcohol or sprayed with Papanicolaou fixative. Usually, 2 to 4 slides per aspiration (total, 8 or 12 slides per biopsy) are prepared (1,2). Specimens should be obtained from both the center and the periphery of (large) nodules.

Although some cytologists require air-dried smears, most U.S.-trained cytologists prefer wet-fixed smears prepared with a modified Papanicolaou stain in the cytology laboratory. For cystic lesions, a larger needle, for example, a 22- or 21-gauge needle, is used; the volume and color of the aspirated fluid are recorded. Cystic fluid is saved in a plastic cup and transferred to the cytology laboratory for concentration by filtration or centrifugation.

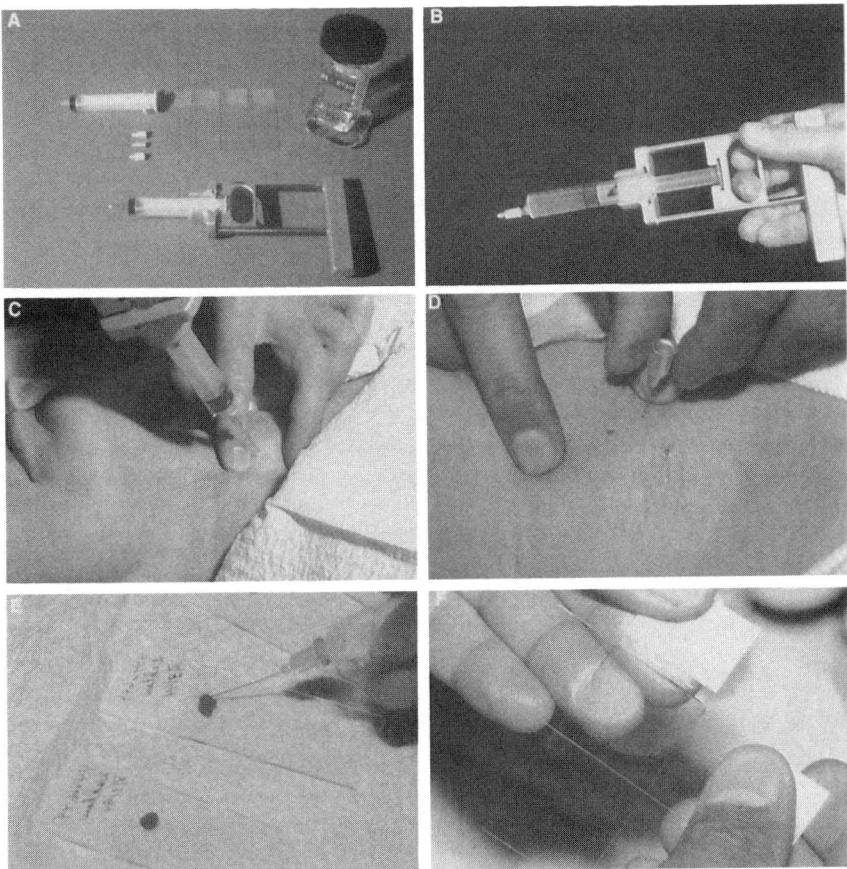

Figure 7.1 Biopsy techniques. A: Equipment includes plastic syringes, 25- or 27-gauge needles, glass slides, alcohol bottles, and a syringe pistol. **B:** Syringe is attached to pistol and held with one hand. **C:** Fine needle aspiration procedure in supine patient with extended neck; one hand of physician is free to locate nodule while needle is inserted. **D:** Nonaspiration technique using 25-gauge needle. The needle is moved back and forth; when aspirate appears in the hub, the needle is withdrawn. **E & F:** With the bevel pointing down, one drop of aspirate is expelled onto each of several glass slides. Smears are prepared by using a second glass slide. Prepared slides should be placed immediately in bottles of alcohol.

Nonaspiration Technique

The purpose of this technique is to minimize trauma to thyroid tissue and to decrease contamination with blood (2,11). Essentially, the procedure is the same as that described above, except that no aspiration or suction is applied in obtaining the specimen. To perform this procedure, a 25-gauge needle is held in a pencil-grip fashion (Figure 7.1D) and inserted directly into the nodule and gently moved back and forth. Through the hub, the operator can see material being obtained. The needle is then removed and attached to a syringe with air inside, and the material is expelled onto glass slides. Slides are prepared as described for the aspiration technique.

Nonaspiration biopsy is particularly useful for vascular thyroid lesions when initial biopsy with FNA yields a bloody specimen.

CYTOPATHOLOGIC DIAGNOSIS

Some indications for FNA biopsy are listed in Table 7. 1. These include the detection of a solitary, palpable nodule; the presence of a dominant nodule within a multinodular gland; an enlarging solitary nodule or dominant nodule in a multinodular gland; the presence of a cyst; a diffuse goiter; and the presence of lymphadenopathy in a patient with known papillary or medullary thyroid carcinoma.

Table 7.1 Indications for Thyroid FNA Biopsy

Single nodule
Dominant nodule in MNG
Enlarging nodule
Cyst
Diffuse goiter
Lymphadenopathy in patient with thyroid cancer (PTC, MTC)

FNA, fine-needle aspiration; MNG, multinodular gland; MTC, medullary thyroid carcinoma; PTC, papillary thyroid carcinoma.

Diagnostic or satisfactory aspirates include those yielding "benign," "indeterminate," or "malignant" diagnoses; the rest are labeled "unsatisfactory" or "nondiagnostic" (7,10,12,13). The criteria for judging sample adequacy are somewhat arbitrary and vary from center to center (3,10). However, most authorities consider a specimen satisfactory if there are at least 6 groups or clusters of well-preserved cells, with each group containing 10 to 15 cells. Because most biopsies are performed by endocrinologists, communication between the clinician and the cytopathologist is important in formulating a useful cytologic interpretation.

Benign Cytology

Approximately 60% to 70% of aspirates are negative or benign (12,13). FNA of a benign thyroid nodule yields fragments of follicular cells that appear as scattered cells, clusters, or sheets of follicular epithelial cells. There is often visible colloid that appears as a dense acellular material. Hürthle cells that appear as large oxyphilic cells with glandular cytoplasm may also be present. Clusters of thyroid epithelium have regularly spaced, small round nuclei with stippled chromatin, and the appearance often resembles a "honeycomb" pattern (Figure 7.2). These changes are referred to as "colloid nodules" or "benign thyroid nodules" (Table 7.2).

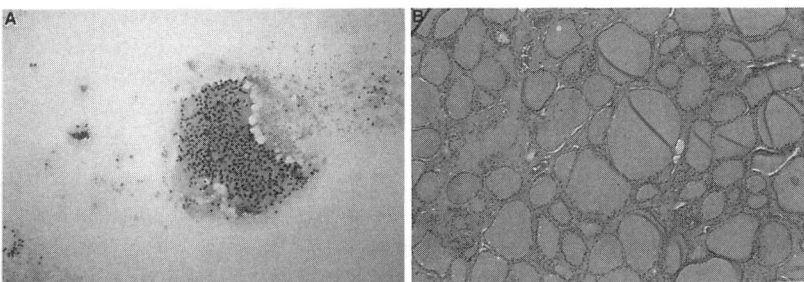

Figure 7.2 Benign colloid nodule A: Cytologic preparation showing diffuse colloid in background and a cohesive group of thyroid cells arranged in honeycomb pattern. (Papanicolaou, x100.) **B:** Histologic section from a patient with colloid goiter showing normal thyroid follicular cells and normal follicles. (H&E, x25.)

Table 7.2 Cytologic Features of Colloid Nodule

Clusters of follicular cells, "honeycomb" pattern
Round to oval nuclei
Abundance of colloid
Foam (degenerating) cells

Chronic lymphocytic thyroiditis (Hashimoto thyroiditis) is characterized by a hypercellular aspirate dominated by a heterogeneous population of lymphocytes. Colloid is usually minimal or absent. The aspirate also usually contains Hürthle cells in large numbers, suggesting a Hürthle cell tumor. However, the presence of Hürthle cells and lymphocytes is characteristic of Hashimoto thyroiditis (Table 7.3 and Figure 7.3). The presence of malignant lymphoma must be considered when reviewing aspirates with lymphocytic cells; the clinical history as well as the details of lymphoid cells are often informative.

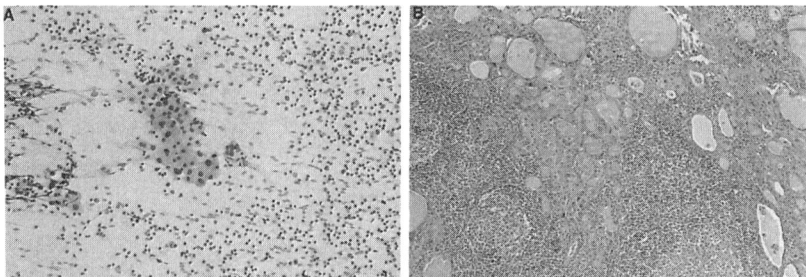

Figure. 7.3 Hashimoto thyroiditis A: Aspirate showing Hürthle cells and an abundance of lymphocytes. (Papanicolaou, x50.) **B:** Histologic section from the same patient as in A illustrating lymphocytic infiltration and lymphoid follicles in normal thyroid parenchyma. (H&E, x20.)

Table 7.3 Cytologic Features of Hashimoto Thyroiditis

Hypercellular aspirate
Abundance of lymphocytes
Hürthle cells
Scant or no colloid

Another benign diagnosis is subacute, or granulomatous, thyroiditis (de Quervain's thyroiditis). This rare form of thyroiditis often presents with a tender gland, symptoms of hyperthyroidism, and an increased erythrocyte sedimentation rate. FNA is usually diagnostic, showing large multinucleated giant cells with a mixture of inflammatory background cells (Figure 7.4). Occasionally, granulomatous reaction suggestive of fibrosis is apparent on the aspirate. Colloid is scant or absent (Table 7. 4).

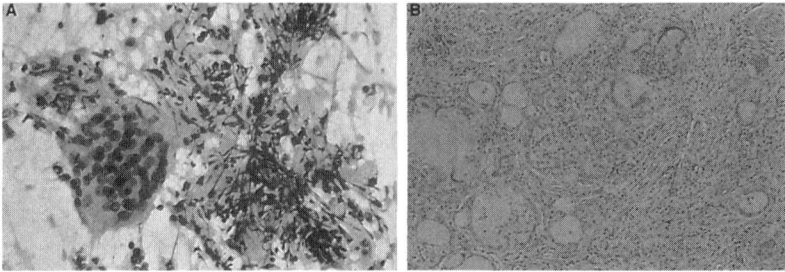

Figure 7.4 Subacute thyroiditis. A: Fine needle aspirate showing a large multinucleated giant cell in a mixed inflammatory background. (Papanicolaou, x250.) **B:** Histologic section from a patient with subacute (granulomatous) thyroiditis showing presence of inflammatory cells and multinucleated giant cells. (H&E, x25.)

Table 7.4 Cytologic Features of Subacute Thyroiditis

Mixed inflammatory background
Large multinucleated giant cells
"Granuloma"
Scant or no colloid

Suspicious Cytology

Ten percent of aspirates are indeterminate, with changes "suspicious for but not diagnostic of malignancy" (4,12,13). Follicular neoplasms are typically hypercellular aspirates with a dispersed microfollicular pattern, nuclear polymorphism, and scant to no colloid (Figure 7.5). Follicular neoplasms cannot be differentiated reliably from well-differentiated follicular carcinomas on cytologic grounds or even with frozen sections (Table 7.5).

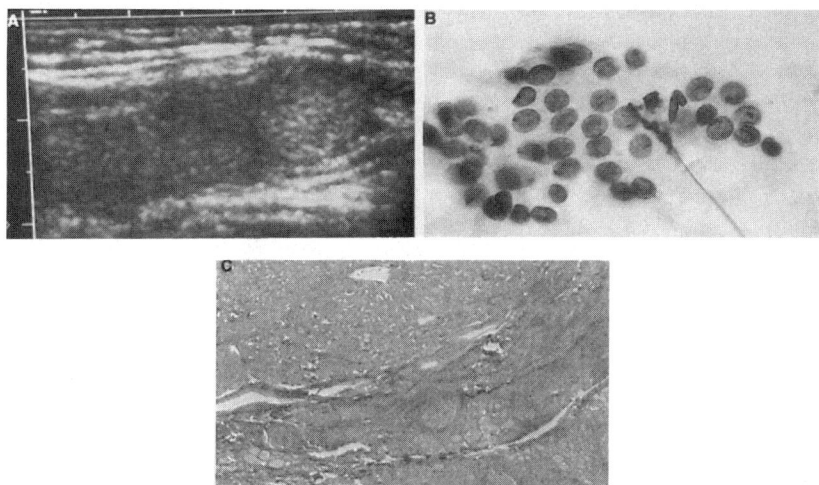

Figure 7.5 Follicular neoplasm in a 41-year-old woman with a recently discovered right thyroid nodule. A: Ultrasonography revealed a 1-cm solid thyroid nodule. **B:** Fine needle aspiration results were suspicious for malignancy, showing hypercellularity, microfollicular pattern, and cellular atypia suggestive of follicular neoplasm. (Papanicolaou, x300.) **C:** Thyroidectomy revealed benign follicular adenoma in Hashimoto thyroiditis without evidence of malignancy. (H&E, x10.)

Table 7.5 Cytologic Features of Follicular Neoplasm

Hypercellular specimen
Microfollicular pattern
Nuclear polymorphism
Scant or no colloid

Hürthle cell neoplasms are characterized by hypercellularity, an abundance of Hürthle cells with granular cytoplasm and enlarged nuclei, and the absence of inflammation and colloid. Hürthle cell tumors may represent either benign or malignant lesions, which can be distinguished only by further histologic examination (Figure 7.6).

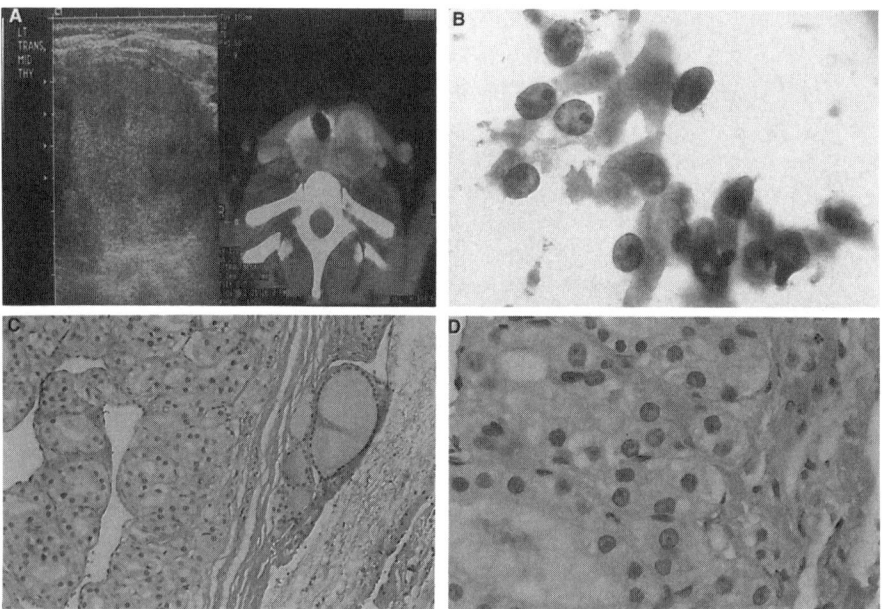

Figure 7.6 Hürthle cell neoplasm in a 74-year-old woman discovered to have a large left thyroid mass with increasing size during the last 6 months. **A:** *Left*, Thyroid ultrasonography showed a solid, 7-cm mass; *right*, neck computed tomography confirmed there was a large solid left thyroid mass, with tracheal deviation to the right. **B:** Fine needle aspirate was suspicious for malignancy, showing "Hürthle cell neoplasm." (Papanicolaou, x300.) **C:** Thyroidectomy revealed a benign Hürthle cell adenoma. (H&E, x50.) **D:** High-power tissue examination showed cellular atypia. (H&E, x150.)

Malignant Cytology

About 5% of satisfactory aspirates are positive or malignant, with papillary thyroid carcinoma being the most common malignancy readily diagnosed cytologically (12,13). The major diagnostic characteristics are large nuclei, nuclear grooves, intranuclear "holes" (or pseudoinclusions), and psammoma bodies (Figure 7.7). Colloid is often absent (but when present, it is viscous) or, with papillary carcinomas, papillary fragments may be seen (Table 7.6).

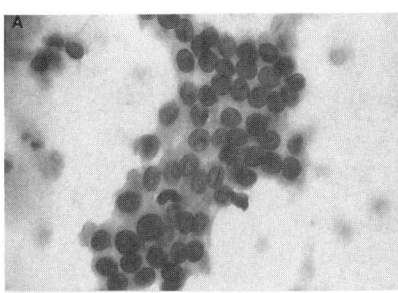 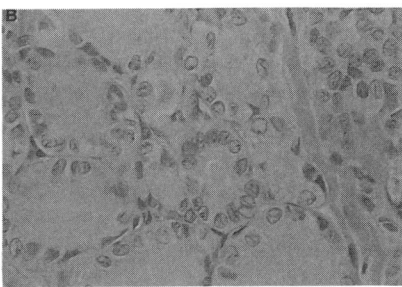

Figure 7.7 Papillary carcinoma. A: Cytologic specimen showing papillary carcinoma with large irregular nuclei, nuclear grooving, pale chromatin, and no colloid. (Papanicolaou, x54.) **B:** Tissue examination showed papillary carcinoma with typical features of "Orphan Annie" nuclei. (H&E, x150.)

Table 7.6 Cytologic Features of Papillary Thyroid Carcinoma

Sheets of cells with papillary configuration
Large, round, irregular nuclei
Pale nuclear chromatin
Intranuclear "holes" (pseudoinclusions)
Psammoma bodies
Viscous colloid

Cytologic features in medullary thyroid carcinoma include hypercellularity, eccentric nuclei in poorly cohesive cells, and the absence of colloid. Multinucleation may be seen (Figure 7.8). Immunoperoxidase staining confirms the diagnosis of medullary carcinoma, but false-positive results may occur. Amyloid, rarely seen in FNA, may resemble colloid, but it stains with Congo red (Table 7.7).

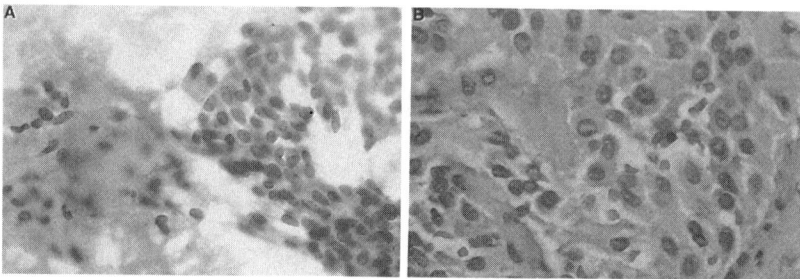

Figure 7.8 Medullary carcinoma. A: Aspirate shows loosely cohesive spindle-shaped nuclei and amorphous material, representing amyloid, intimately associated with the neoplastic cells. (Papanicolaou, x400.) **B:** Thyroidectomy showed round to oval cells with a coarse chromatin pattern and irregular amorphous eosinophilic amyloid. (H&E, x400.)

Table 7.7 Cytologic Features in Medullary Thyroid Carcinoma

Hypercellularity
Poor cell cohesion
Spindle-shaped cells; elongated, eccentric nuclei
Multinucleated cells
Positive staining for calcitonin
Positive staining for amyloid (Congo red)

Anaplastic tumors are rare, often lethal, carcinomas that present with a rapidly enlarging thyroid mass. They are undifferentiated or high-grade adenocarcinomas that typically show marked pleomorphic, bizarre cells (Figure 7.9). They are highly cellular, with large nuclei, prominent nucleoli, and frequent mitotic figures, consistent with an aggressive malignant process (Table 7.8).

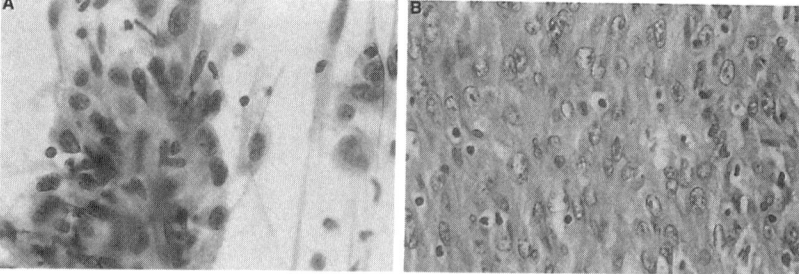

Figure 7.9 Anaplastic carcinoma. A: Large pleomorphic and bizarre cells. There is abundant cytoplasm and nuclei characteristic of malignant cells. (Papanicolaou, x150.) **B:** Tissue examination revealed epithelioid cells and mitotic figures consistent with anaplastic cancer. (H&E, x200.)

Table 7.8 Cytologic Features in Anaplastic Carcinoma

Marked pleomorphism
Large, irregular nuclei
Prominent nucleoli
Mitotic figures
Absence of colloid

Overlapping Cytologic Criteria

Powers and Frable (8) have discussed cytologic diagnostic pitfalls in thyroid FNA interpretation, summarized in Table 7. 9. These include cystic changes that may be seen in degenerating benign colloid goiters, papillary carcinomas that have undergone cystic degeneration, or thyroglossal duct cysts. Papillary formations or configurations are common in papillary carcinomas but may also be present in benign nodular goiters, Hürthle cell tumors, or even follicular cell tumors. Hürthle cells may be seen in Hürthle cell neoplasms, Hashimoto thyroiditis, nodular goiters, or even papillary thyroid carcinomas. Intranuclear inclusions are not specific and are seen in different thyroid neoplasms (Table 7. 9).

Table 7.9 Overlapping Cytologic Criteria in Thyroid FNA

Cystic change
Degeneration in nodular goiter, PTC, FTC, TGDC
Papillary formations
PTC, nodular goiter, HCT, FTC
Hürthle cells
HCT, Hashimoto thyroiditis, nodular goiter, PTC
Intranuclear inclusions
PTC, FTC, MTC

FNA, fine-needle aspiration; FTC, follicular thyroid carcinoma; HCT, Hürthle cell tumor; MTC, medullary thyroid carcinoma; PTC, papillary thyroid carcinoma; TGDC, thyroglossal duct cyst.
Modified from Powers and Frable (8). By permission of Butterworth-Heinemann.

FNA RESULTS

Many studies have analyzed FNA data and have established that thyroid aspiration cytology is a reliable diagnostic procedure (7,12,14-16). In 1991, Caruso and Mazzaferri (15) reported on 9 series, including more than 9,000 patients, with the following diagnoses: 17% benign, 22% suspicious, and 4% malignant. In 1993, Gharib and Goellner (14) reported on more than 18,000 FNA biopsies in 7 large series from several countries: 69% were benign, 27% were suspicious or nondiagnostic, and only 4% were malignant. Analysis of these data revealed that the sensitivity of FNA ranged from 65% to 95% and the specificity, from 72% to 100%. The predictive value of a positive or suspicious cytologic result was 50%, the false-negative rate was 1% to 11%, and false-positive rates ranged from 0% to 10%. The overall accuracy for cytologic diagnosis approaches 95% (Table 7. 10).

Table 7.10 FNA Results[*]

Result	
Satisfactory	85%
Unsatisfactory	15%
False-negative	< 2%
False-positive	< 5%
Sensitivity	80%-90%
Specificity	90%-95%
Accuracy	95%

FNA, fine-needle aspiration.
[*]See references 3,7,14,15.

More recently, Baloch et al. (16) performed FNAs on 616 patients in a 3.5-year period and reported the following diagnoses: 69% benign, 16% neoplasm/malignant, 11% nondiagnostic, and 4% indeterminate. On comparing discrepant diagnoses between cytologic and histologic specimens, overlapping cytologic features in follicular lesions and inadequate/suboptimal specimens accounted for diagnostic misinterpretations. Overall, Baloch et al. concluded that FNA is an effective management tool in thyroid nodules.

These results and those of many similar FNA reports/reviews confirm the diagnostic accuracy and reliability of FNA. In centers with accumulated experience with FNA, the technique has become reliable, reproducible, and effective in the management of thyroid nodules (3-5,17). FNA diagnoses also can assign probabilities of malignancy for thyroid nodules. For example, the probability of malignancy is < 1% for benign aspirates, 29% for "suspicious" specimens, and almost 100% for specimens with malignant cytologic findings (6).

DIAGNOSTIC PITFALLS

The diagnostic pitfalls were reviewed recently by Singer (5) and include indeterminate cytologic results, false-negative results, nondiagnostic specimens, and inexperienced cytologists (Table 7. 11). The indeterminate group, described above, includes specimens with cellular neoplasms, cellular atypia, and features that are not clearly diagnostic but variably suggestive of malignancy (1,7,9,13).

Table 7.11 Diagnostic Pitfalls in Thyroid FNA

Indeterminate cytology
False-negative results
Nondiagnostic material
Inexperienced cytologist

FNA, fine-needle biopsy.
Data from Singer (5).

False-negative results mean "missed cancer," whereas false-positive results lead to thyroidectomy for benign lesions. False-negative results can be due to sampling or interpretive errors (or both). Regardless of the cause, false-negative results should be kept as low as possible.

Investigators who frequently use FNA have suggested some steps to minimize false-negative rates (5,10,18-20). The adequacy of sampling improves by aiming the needle at the peripheral portion rather than the central (degenerating) area of the nodule. A minimum of 2 and a maximum of 6 punctures per nodule is suggested, with 2 to 4 being the number used by most. It is essential that samples be obtained from different areas. Musgrave et al. (21) reported that regular 4-quadrant sampling (12, 3, 6, and 9 o'clock) improves the diagnostic accuracy of FNA. Some have suggested the use of larger (21- or 18-gauge) needles, even in combination with FNA, to obtain tissue fragments in order to reduce nondiagnostic rates and to evaluate follicular lesions. These techniques cause more pain and complications. McHenry et al. (22) reviewed the causes of nondiagnostic aspirates and offered some suggestions for improving results. The diagnostic criteria require that an adequate number of thyroid cells and groups must be present. Whereas a few benign cells do not exclude cancer, a few malignant cells are considered diagnostic of a malignant lesion. Sampling errors are more likely to occur with nodules < 1 cm or > 4 cm in diameter. The true frequency of false-negative results is not known, because in most recent FNA series not all patients screened by FNA subsequently had surgery.

Aspirates with too few cells are considered inadequate for diagnosis and are referred to as either "nondiagnostic" or "unsatisfactory" (14). This category accounts for 5% to 20% of all aspirates. Although such aspirates may be called "negative for malignancy" because no malignant cells are seen, they, in fact, are unsatisfactory (nondiagnostic) because they contain few or no cells for diagnosis. Reaspiration is often useful and results in satisfactory specimens in at least half the cases. However, despite good techniques and acquired experience, 5% to 10% of nodules still remain nondiagnostic. UG-FNA, scan, and risk-factor analysis are often helpful in these cases (1,23).

Cystic Nodules

Thyroid cysts pose a special problem. On palpation, cysts are discrete, smooth, and resilient lesions, and on aspiration, they yield fluid, macrophages, some colloid, and inflammatory cells. Usually, there are no thyroid follicular cells, and the aspirates are nondiagnostic; these account for the majority of unsatisfactory specimens. The diagnosis and management of cystic lesions remain difficult and a matter of controversy.

Cysts are believed to represent degenerative changes within colloid nodules. The incidence of surgically removed nodules reported as cysts varies from 5% to 25% (13,24). Cystic lesions are usually defined as nodules that yield ≥ 1 ml of fluid on aspiration. Although most cysts are benign, cystic changes may occur in both benign and malignant lesions (Table 7.9).

The volume, viscosity, and color of the fluid may be suggestive of the type of lesion present, but none of these excludes malignancy. A crystal-clear fluid suggests parathyroid origin; parathyroid hormone levels are often markedly elevated. Commonly, cystic fluid is clear and amber; hemorrhagic fluid is less frequent but has a higher risk for malignancy (13,24). MacDonald and Yazdi (25) reported 2% malignancy in nondiagnostic aspirates; these aspirates were acellular. They recommended rebiopsy for acellular aspirates and excision if they were still nondiagnostic.

Cysts that disappear after aspiration are almost always benign. A single aspiration seldom cures cysts; recurrences are reported in 40% to 60% of patients (24). Thyroxine therapy is ineffective in shrinking cysts or in preventing recurrence. Surgical excision is commonly recommended for persistent or recurrent cysts, cysts > 4 cm in diameter, and cysts with nondiagnostic or abnormal cytologic findings (13,24).

Sclerosing agents have been used to shrink cysts. Injection of tetracycline into cysts never gained wide acceptance. Currently, alcohol ablation, known as "PEI" (percutaneous ethanol injection), is recommended by some (26). PEI requires ultrasonographic guidance and repeated administration of ethanol, and it may be associated with significant, albeit transient, side effects. The cure rate is reportedly as high as 90%. PEI can be reserved for patients refusing surgery or for those who are poor surgical candidates. It is discussed in detail in Chapter 12.

When reaspiration under direct palpation is still unsuccessful, UG-FNA can be successful, as indicated in Figure 7.10.

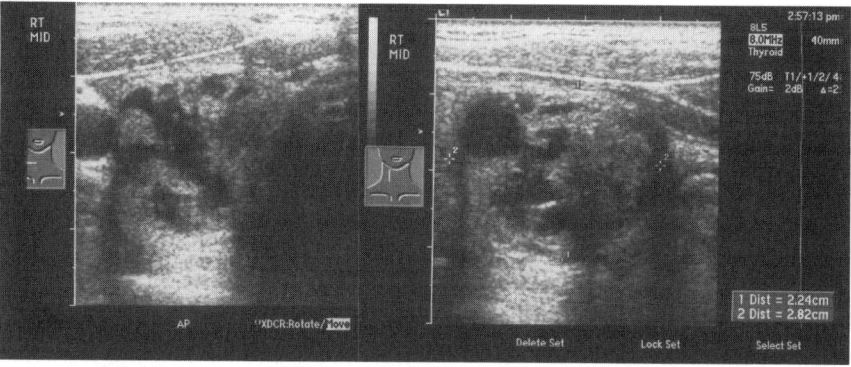

Figure 7.10 Nondiagnostic cytologic results in a 66-year-old man with a right thyroid nodule and normal serum level of thyroid-stimulating hormone. Twice, palpation-guided fine needle aspiration biopsy was nondiagnostic, yielding cystic fluid and foam cells. Transverse (*left*) and longitudinal (*right*) ultrasonograms of the right thyroid lobe showed a 2.2- x 2.8- x 2.1-cm complex nodule containing solid and cystic components in the right thyroid. Results of ultrasonographically guided fine needle aspiration with a 25-gauge needle were consistent with a benign colloid nodule. Medical management was recommended.

COMPLICATIONS OF FNA

Most centers report that FNA is an extremely safe procedure and not associated with any major complications (7,8,10,13). Minor pain or hematoma is frequent but never major. The fear of needle tract implantation has not proved to be a problem, but occasionally, a report reminds us of this very unusual complication (27). Patients who take anticoagulants or salicylates can undergo biopsy without bleeding. The use of a 27- or 25-gauge needle is encouraged because pain, hematoma, and complications are less likely to occur with small-sized needles.

REBIOPSY

Indications for rebiopsy are listed in Table 7.12 and include enlarging nodule, recurrent cyst, nondiagnostic initial aspirate, nodule unresponsive to thyroxine suppressive therapy, and a clinically suspicious but cytologically benign nodule. It generally is recommended that FNA of thyroid nodules be repeated 1 year after the initial report of benign cytology (28). This is particularly useful for practices in which this procedure is introduced, allowing for acquisition of experience and expertise.

Table 7.12 Indications for Rebiopsy

Enlarging nodule
Recurrent cyst
Nondiagnostic initial aspirate
Nodule unresponsive to T_4 therapy
Clinically suspicious, cytologically benign nodule

T_4, thyroxine

However, a recent report by Lucas et al. (29) and *Thyroid* Feb. '99 suggested that reaspiration is of limited usefulness in patients with benign nodular thyroid disease. In their experience, reaspiration results were identical to those of the first biopsy in 90.5% of cases; in the other 9.5%, the cytologic diagnosis remained "benign" but changed from colloid nodule to cystic nodule. There were no false-negative results. In the opinion of the author, routine reaspiration after 1 year is good practice and reduces the false-negative rate. Subsequent FNA biopsies are not recommended unless the nodule(s) grows.

UG-FNA

Recent experience indicates that UG-FNA biopsy may be preferred to direct-palpation biopsy in some circumstances (30-33). For example, UG-FNA is more accurate for nodules < 1 cm in diameter. UG-FNA must be performed for thyroid incidentalomas, because they are nonpalpable, and for nodules that are difficult to palpate. UG-FNA is also useful when rebiopsy of thyroid cysts still yields inadequate specimens. Ultrasonographic guidance can help direct the needle into the solid portions of a complex nodule, thereby increasing the likelihood of obtaining a satisfactory aspirate. Some of the more common clinical indications for UG-FNA are listed in Table 7. 13.

Table 7.13 Indications for Ultrasonographically Guided FNA

Nondiagnostic aspirate on rebiopsy
Difficult-to-palpate nodule
Incidentaloma
Palpable nodules ≤ 1 cm
Nonpalpable adenopathy
Alcohol ablation

FNA, fine needle biopsy.

Nondiagnostic results continue to be a problem in thyroid FNA biopsy. Despite experience and careful biopsy techniques, it is not unusual to have a 5% to 10% incidence of unsatisfactory or nondiagnostic results. UG-FNA will help secure a diagnosis in most cases. When UG-FNA fails to make a cytologic diagnosis, management becomes case-specific, depending on nodule size, patient's age, nodule function on scan, and so forth. Because the frequency of malignancy in nondiagnostic nodules may be 2% to 10%, it is prudent to excise nondiagnostic nodules. If nonoperative management is selected, follow-up with rebiopsy is suggested.

The combined use of ultrasonography and FNA seems to be gaining popularity in most clinics, and this technique is discussed in detail in another chapter.

CONCLUSIONS AND RECOMMENDATIONS

Most reported FNA series have suggested that 10% to 20% of aspirates have suspicious cytologic results, and among these, 20% or more prove to be malignant (2,5,12,13,16). Therefore, most authorities agree that suspicious follicular neoplasms should be removed surgically. We and others have shown that the use of a pertechnetate scan in this setting can be misleading and is not recommended (9,17). To help resolve the dilemma of suspicious cytologic results, factors that predict malignancy, nuclear DNA analysis, thyroperoxidase MoAb 47, and other techniques have been studied (34-36). Final results are still pending. Some investigators have attempted to separate benign from malignant follicular neoplasms on the basis of results other than cytologic findings. More data are required to evaluate these initial reports.

Thyroid FNA biopsy has proved to be a safe, reliable, and cost-effective means of evaluating thyroid nodules (1,3,4,9,14). This procedure has become an integral part of thyroid nodule evaluation and management. In experienced hands and with cytopathologic expertise, false-negative and false-positive results are minimal. Other limitations of FNA biopsy, including nondiagnostic or suspicious cytologic results, continue to pose problems. However, with continued use of UG-FNA and with the development of techniques to separate benign from malignant follicular neoplasms, it is hoped that in the near future we will have fewer problems in this regard. It is recommended that FNA biopsy be used routinely as the initial test for diagnosing and treating nodular thyroid disease (Figure 7.11).

Figure 7.11 Recommended approach to a patient with a clinically solitary thyroid nodule.

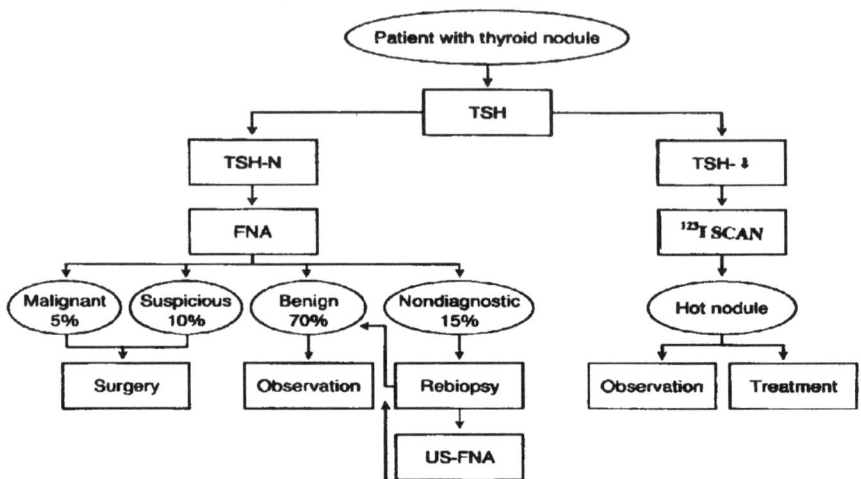

After taking the history and performing a physical examination, the serum level of thyroid-stimulating hormone (TSH) is measured. If this level is normal, fine needle aspiration (FNA) biopsy is performed. Approximately 70% of nodules are benign and managed medically. The remaining 15%, comprising malignant and suspicious cytologic categories, are treated surgically. Nondiagnostic FNAs (15%) are repeated; ultrasonographic (US)-FNA is often diagnostic. A small group of patients with nondiagnostic aspirates even after US-FNA receive treatment based on clinical features related to the probability of cancer.

In most series, the diagnostic accuracy of thyroid FNA has approached 95% (1,9). The positive predictive value of FNA is better than that of pertechnetate scanning and ultrasonographic imaging (37). FNA is inexpensive and improves patient selection for thyroid surgery. Although the total exclusion of false-negative results is nearly impossible, efforts should be made to minimize this problem. Some steps for doing this are listed in Table 7. 14.

Table 7.14 Some Steps That Improve Accuracy of FNA and Lead to Better Nodule Management

Step	Explanation
Endocrinologist performs biopsy	Offers better thyroid examination, accumulates experience with FNA
Experienced cytologist reviews slides	Improves cytologic interpretation
Careful with small (< 1 cm) or large (> 4 cm) nodules	Increased chance of misdiagnosis, UG-FNA improves accuracy
2-4 aspirates from different nodule sites	Improves cytologic sampling
Rebiopsy if cytologic results are nondiagnostic	Half are diagnostic on reaspiration
Nondiagnostic cytologic results are not negative	5%-10% of nondiagnostic nodules harbor malignancy
Aspirates with no follicular cells are nondiagnostic	These should not be considered "negative for malignancy"
Excise large (> 4 cm) or recurrent cysts	Higher likelihood of malignancy
Excise nodules yielding "suspicious" cytologic findings	10%-30% chance of malignancy
Excise clinically suspicious, cytologically benign nodules	Consider cytologic results false-negative until proved otherwise

FNA, fine-needle aspiration; UG-FNA, ultrasonographically guided FNA. Modified from Gharib (9). By permission of Mayo Foundation for Medical Education and Research.

Thyroid FNA biopsy has significantly influenced the care of patients with thyroid nodules. If FNA is used as the initial diagnostic test, fewer patients are referred for surgery than if clinical examination, radioisotope scan, or ultrasonography, or combinations of these are used. In most large series, FNA has resulted in 25% fewer operations for benign goiters, and the frequency of thyroid carcinomas found among surgical specimens has increased from < 15% to 40% to 50% (38,39). Garcia-Mayor et al. (39) recently stated that "the most important impact for the use of FNAB [biopsy] is the simplification of our clinical practice." Furthermore, routine application of FNA decreases the cost of patient care by at least 25% (1,9).

Surgical treatment is usually recommended for nodules with a diagnosis of Hürthle cell or follicular cell neoplasm on FNA biopsy. The extent of surgical resection is a matter of controversy. If at operation the lesion is benign, complete lobectomy with or without isthmectomy is considered sufficient treatment. If the nodule is benign but the gland is multinodular, subtotal thyroidectomy would be a reasonable approach. However, if malignancy is detected on histologic examination, near-total thyroidectomy is the current practice for papillary or follicular carcinomas and total thyroidectomy for medullary thyroid carcinoma. In the latter case, central compartment node dissection should be carried out simultaneously with thyroidectomy.

Thyroid FNA biopsy has 2 objectives. One is to reliably identify benign nodules (the majority), thereby avoiding unnecessary thyroid surgery. The other is to identify malignant lesions and provide guidance for surgical planning. Both objectives can be achieved by acquiring good biopsy technique and experience in combination with expertise in cytopathology. FNA biopsy is now an integral part of nodule work-up. Despite certain limitations, cytologic diagnosis has improved and simplified management of nodular thyroid glands.

REFERENCES

1. Gharib H (1997) Changing concepts in the diagnosis and management of thyroid nodules. *Endocrinol Metab Clin North Am* 26:777-800.
2. Gharib H (1997) Management of thyroid nodules: another look. *Thyroid Today* 20:1-11.
3. Burch HB (1995) Evaluation and management of the solid thyroid nodule. *Endocrinol Metab Clin North Am* 24:663-710.
4. Mazzaferri EL (1993) Management of a solitary thyroid nodule. *N Engl J Med* 328:553-559.
5. Singer PA (1996) Evaluation and management of the solitary thyroid nodule. *Otolaryngol Clin North Am* 29:577-591.
6. Gharib H (1996) Diagnosis of thyroid nodules by fine-needle aspiration biopsy. *Curr Opin Endocrinol Diabetes* 3:433-438.
7. Atkinson BF (1993) Fine needle aspiration of the thyroid. *Monogr Pathol* 35:166-199.
8. Powers CN, Frable WJ (1996) Fine Needle Aspiration Biopsy of the Head and Neck. Boston, Butterworth-Heinemann,
9. Gharib H (1994) Fine-needle aspiration biopsy of thyroid nodules: advantages, limitations, and effect. *Mayo Clin Proc* 69:44-49.
10. Solomon D (1993) Fine needle aspiration of the thyroid: an update. *Thyroid Today* 16:1-9.
11. Santos JE, Leiman G (1988) Nonaspiration fine needle cytology. Application of a new technique to nodular thyroid disease. *Acta Cytol* 32:353-356.
12. Gharib H, Goellner JR, Johnson DA (1993) Fine-needle aspiration cytology of the thyroid. A 12-year experience with 11,000 biopsies. *Clin Lab Med* 13:699-709.
13. Gharib H, Goellner JR (1995) Fine-needle aspiration biopsy of thyroid nodules. *Endocr Pract* 1:410-417.
14. Gharib H, Goellner JR (1993) Fine-needle aspiration biopsy of the thyroid: an appraisal. *Ann Intern Med* 118:282-289.
15. Caruso D, Mazzaferri EL (1991) Fine needle aspiration biopsy in the management of thyroid nodules. *Endocrinologist* 1:194-202.
16. Baloch ZW, Sack MJ, Yu GH, Livolsi VA, Gupta PK (1998) Fine-needle aspiration of thyroid: an institutional experience. *Thyroid* 8:565-569.
17. Daniels GH (1996) Thyroid nodules and nodular thyroids: a clinical overview. *Compr Ther* 22:239-250.
18. Hall TL, Layfield LJ, Philippe A, Rosenthal DL (1989) Sources of diagnostic error in fine needle aspiration of the thyroid. *Cancer* 63:718-725.
19. Bisi H, de Camargo RY, Longatto Filho A (1992) Role of fine-needle aspiration cytology in the management of thyroid nodules: review of experience with 1,925 cases. *Diagn Cytopathol* 8:504-510.
20. Caraway NP, Sneige N, Samaan NA (1993) Diagnostic pitfalls in thyroid fine-needle aspiration: a review of 394 cases. *Diagn Cytopathol* 9:345-350.
21. Musgrave YM, Davey DD, Weeks JA, Banks ER, Rayens MK, Ain KB: (1998) Assessment of fine-needle aspiration sampling technique in thyroid nodules. *Diagn Cytopathol* 18:76-80.

22. McHenry CR, Walfish PG, Rosen IB (1993) Non-diagnostic fine needle aspiration biopsy: a dilemma in management of nodular thyroid disease. *Am Surg* 59:415-419.
23. Schmidt T, Riggs MW, Speights VO Jr (1997) Significance of nondiagnostic fine-needle aspiration of the thyroid. *South Med J* 90:1183-1186.
24. Sarda AK, Bal S, Dutta Gupta S, Kapur MM (1988) Diagnosis and treatment of cystic disease of the thyroid by aspiration. *Surgery* 103:593-596.
25. MacDonald L, Yazdi HM (1996) Nondiagnostic fine needle aspiration biopsy of the thyroid gland: a diagnostic dilemma. *Acta Cytol* 40:423-428.
26. Papini E, Pacella CM, Verde G (1995) Percutaneous ethanol injection (PEI): what is its role in the treatment of benign thyroid nodules? *Thyroid* 5:147-150.
27. Hales MS, Hsu FS (1990) Needle tract implantation of papillary carcinoma of the thyroid following aspiration biopsy. *Acta Cytol* 34:801-804.
28. Wiersinga WM (1995) Is repeated fine-needle aspiration cytology indicated in (benign) thyroid nodules? *Eur J Endocrinol* 132:661-662.
29. Lucas A, Llatjos M, Salinas I, Reverter J, Pizarro E, Sanmarti A (1995) Fine-needle aspiration cytology of benign nodular thyroid disease. Value of re-aspiration. *Eur J Endocrinol* 132:677-680.
30. Cochand-Priollet B, Guillausseau PJ, Chagnon S, Hoang C, Guillausseau-Scholer C, Chanson P, Dahan H, Warnet A, Tran Ba Huy PT, Valleur P (1994) The diagnostic value of fine-needle aspiration biopsy under ultrasonography in nonfunctional thyroid nodules: a prospective study comparing cytologic and histologic findings. *Am J Med* 97:152-157.
31. Danese D, Sciacchitano S, Farsetti A, Andreoli M, Pontecorvi A (1998) Diagnostic accuracy of conventional versus sonography-guided fine-needle aspiration biopsy of thyroid nodules. *Thyroid* 8:15-21.
32. Sabel MS, Haque D, Velasco JM, Staren ED (1998) Use of ultrasound-guided fine needle aspiration biopsy in the management of thyroid disease. *Am Surg* 64:738-741.
33. Carmeci C, Jeffrey RB, McDougall IR, Nowels KW, Weigel RJ (1998) Ultrasound-guided fine-needle aspiration biopsy of thyroid masses. *Thyroid* 8:283-289.
34. Schlinkert RT, van Heerden JA, Goellner JR, Gharib H, Smith SL, Rosales RF, Weaver AL (1997) Factors that predict malignant thyroid lesions when fine-needle aspiration is "suspicious for follicular neoplasm." *Mayo Clin Proc* 72:913-916.
35. Backdahl M, Wallin G, Lowhagen T, Auer G, Granberg PO (1987) Fine-needle biopsy cytology and DNA analysis. Their place in the evaluation and treatment of patients with thyroid neoplasms. *Surg Clin North Am* 67:197-211.
36. Faroux MJ, Theobald S, Pluot M, Patey M, Menzies D (1997) Evaluation of the monoclonal antibody antithyroperoxidase MoAb47 in the diagnostic decision of cold thyroid nodules by fine-needle aspiration. *Pathol Res Pract* 193:705-712.
37. Jones AJ, Aitman TJ, Edmonds CJ, Burke M, Hudson E, Tellez M (1990) Comparison of fine needle aspiration cytology, radioisotopic and ultrasound scanning in the management of thyroid nodules. *Postgrad Med J* 66:914-917.
38. Hadi M, Gharib H, Goellner JR, van Heerden JA (1997) Has fine-needle aspiration biopsy changed thyroid practice? *Endocr Pract* 3:9-13.
39. Garcia-Mayor RV, Perez Mendez LF, Paramo C, Luna Cano R, Rego Iraeta A, Regal M, Sierra JM, Fluiters E (1997) Fine-needle aspiration biopsy of thyroid nodules: impact on clinical practice. *J Endocrinol Invest* 20:482-487.

8

Ultrasound-Guided Fine Needle Aspiration Biopsy of Thyroid Nodules

Richard S. Haber, MD
Mount Sinai School of Medicine,
New York, NY 10029 USA

INTRODUCTION

Cytologic examination of fine needle aspiration (FNA) specimens from thyroid nodules is the key test for the evaluation of thyroid nodules, and the results are critical in the selection of patients with nodules for thyroid surgery. Although needle placement for FNA is traditionally and most commonly guided by nodule palpation alone, the widespread availability of thyroid ultrasonography has made possible a technical refinement of this technique, needle placement under ultrasonographic guidance. Ultrasound-guided FNA is often valuable, and sometimes essential, in obtaining accurate diagnostic material. This chapter reviews the role of ultrasound-guided fine needle aspiration (UG FNA) in the diagnosis of thyroid nodules.

ADVANTAGES OF ULTRASOUND-GUIDED FINE NEEDLE ASPIRATION BIOPSY

Ultrasonographic guidance for FNA biopsy of thyroid nodules provides several advantages over the traditional palpation-guided method.

Accurate Needle Placement in Palpable Nodules

UG FNA provides confirmation that the needle tip is in fact located within a palpable nodule, rather than in adjacent tissue. When guided by palpation only, it may be difficult to determine the correct depth of penetration, especially with relatively small nodules <1.5 cm in diameter, and even with larger nodules. Erroneous needle placement into the tracheal lumen may be obvious when the patient begins to cough, and the aspiration yields only air. But at other times, erroneous palpation-guided needle placement is likely to be unrecognized, and yields either nondiagnostic specimens lacking thyroid cells, or potentially false-negative cytology resulting from biopsy of normal adjacent thyroid tissue.

FNA Biopsy of Nonpalpable Nodules

Ultrasonographic guidance is necessary for FNA biopsy of nonpalpable nodules, which are typically discovered during thyroid ultrasonography, carotid artery ultrasonography, or other neck imaging procedures such as computerized tomography or magnetic resonance imaging. Small nonpalpable nodules less than 1 cm in diameter are generally not palpable. Since they are exceedingly common (1), FNA biopsy is not generally recommended for such nodules, but ultrasonographic guidance must be applied in those cases in which FNA is indicated. The results of UG FNA in such nodules have been reported in two large series (2,3). In addition, experienced thyroid ultrasonographers have found that even relatively large thyroid nodules as large as 5 cm may be nonpalpable due to an obese or muscular body habitus, posterior location, or location in the upper mediastinum deep to the clavicle and manubrium. The latter situation is common in the elderly, in whom kyphosis may cause much of the thyroid to lie in the upper mediastinum, where it is difficult to palpate, but easily imaged with an ultrasonographic probe placed at the appropriate angle in the lower neck (Figure 8. 1).

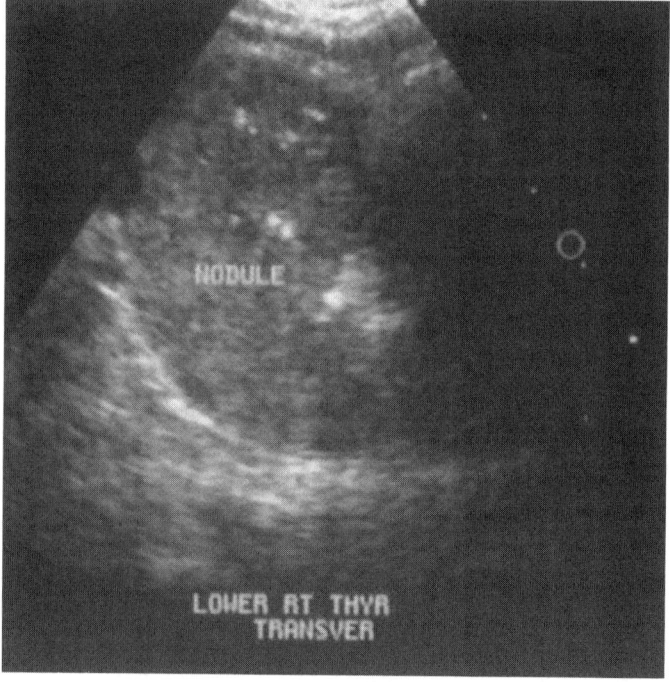

Figure 8. 1 A large (4-cm) nonpalpable lower right thyroid nodule in an 85-year-old man, transverse view. This hypoechoic nodule with several punctate calcifications (bright echoes) lay deep to the right clavicle and could not be appreciated on physical examination, even with swallowing. However, it could be biopsied by FNA using ultrasound guidance. The anechoic area adjacent to the nodule is the acoustic shadow of the tracheal cartilage.

Needle Placement in Partly Cystic Nodules

Many thyroid nodules are predominantly or partly cystic ("complex"), and FNA biopsy of the cystic portion of such nodules almost invariably yields nondiagnostic cytologically inadequate specimens lacking thyroid follicular cells. The accurate cytologic diagnosis of such nodules, which may be malignant, requires sampling of the solid portion to obtain an adequate number of follicular cells. The chances of obtaining a cytologically adequate specimen are greatly enhanced with ultrasonographic guidance, which permits the needle tip to be directed to the solid portions of a complex nodule for FNA biopsy, or to the cystic portions for drainage of fluid (Figure 8.2). For purposes of treating cystic nodules, complete drainage of cyst fluid is facilitated by ultrasound guidance of needle placement. Even in the case of predominantly solid nodules, ultrasonographic guidance for FNA allows placement of the needle tip away from areas of cystic degeneration, and may increase the chance of obtaining adequate specimens (see below).

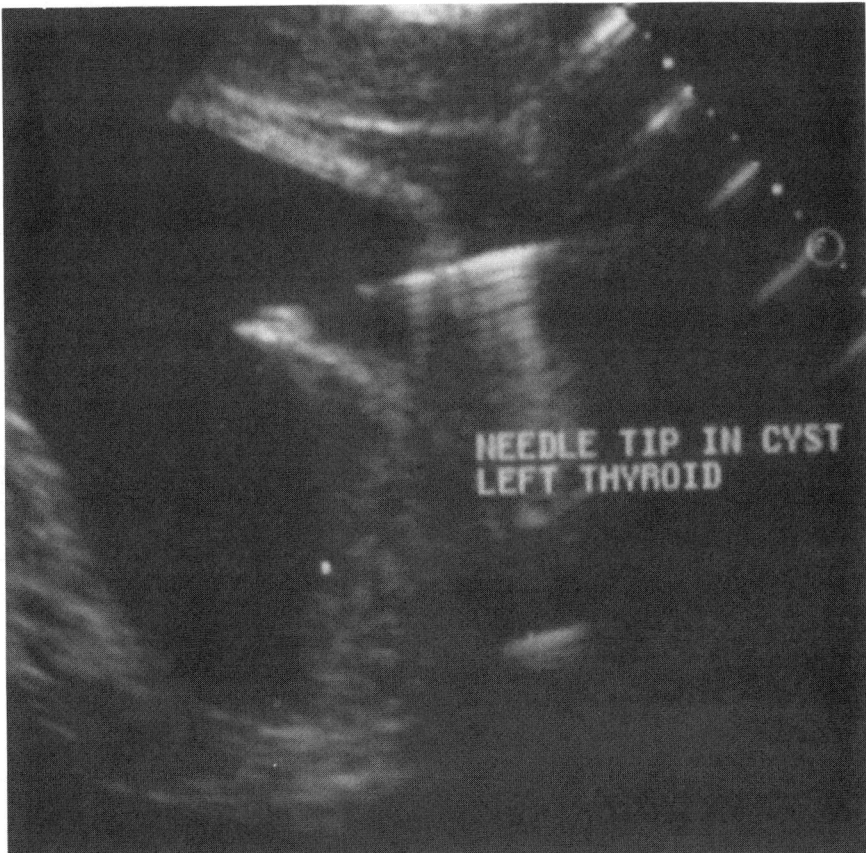

Figure 8.2 Ultrasound guidance for FNA of a partly cystic nodule, transverse view. This 3-cm nodule in a 35-year-old man had a large anechoic cystic component and a solid hyperechoic component seen at the lower right of the nodule image. In this image the needle tip is directed at the cystic component, and is seen as a bright echo. The shaft is seen as well, and artefactual echo signals are visible below the image of the needle shaft.

Safety

FNA biopsy of the thyroid is a remarkably safe procedure, but in some cases concern about proximity of a nodule to surrounding great vessels (common carotid artery, jugular vein, or subclavian vessels) may inhibit application of the procedure. Ultrasonographic guidance provides re-assurance that these vessels are avoided, and makes possible safe FNA biopsy of nodules immediately adjacent to them.

A not uncommon complication of FNA biopsy is local bleeding from small blood vessels in the path of the needle. The author has found that this event may not be recognized by external inspection, but may be quite obvious during ultrasonographic monitoring of an FNA procedure (Figure 8. 3). Because such bleeding in the neck may lead to pain and swelling, it is best to apply pressure and abort further passes with the needle when such a hematoma is recognized by ultrasonography.

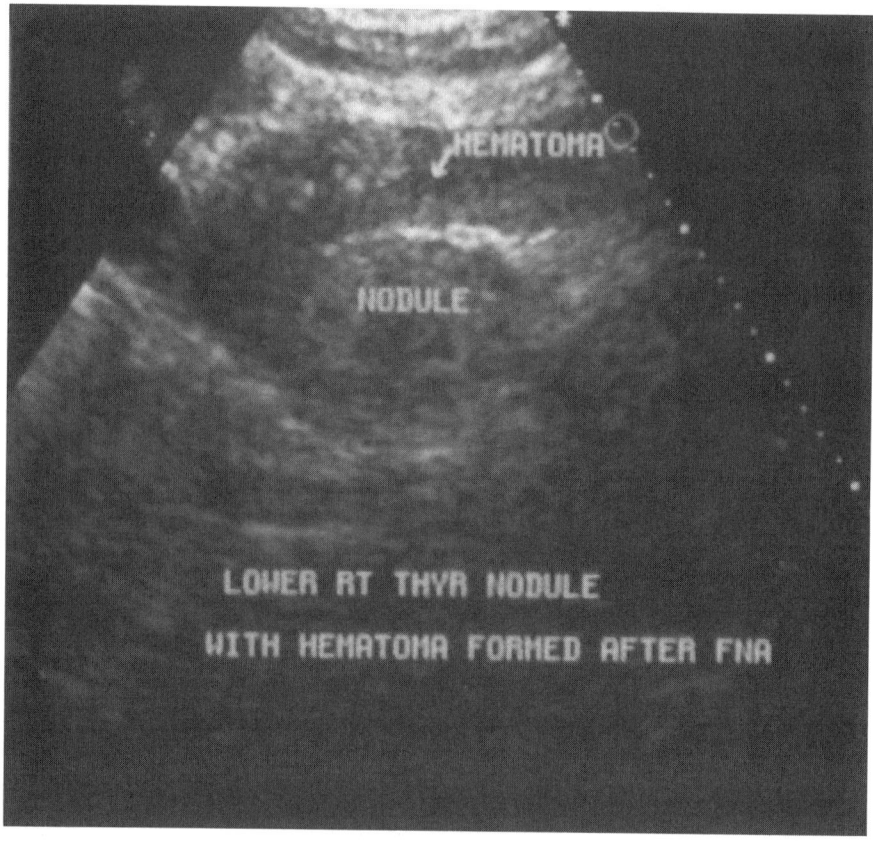

Figure 8.3 Hematoma detected sonographically during FNA of a right thyroid nodule, transverse view. A hypoechoic band anterior to the thyroid gland appeared rapidly during the ultrasound-guided FNA procedure. No hematoma was visible externally.

TECHNICAL ASPECTS

Equipment
Thyroid ultrasonography is performed with high-resolution 7.5-10 MHz transducers appropriate for superficial structures. These transducers (probes) are of two types: linear phased-array, and angular (sector) phased-array. The contact surface for linear-type probes is a bar extending several centimeters, producing a two-dimensional image of tissue directly beneath the length of the probe. This type of probe is often recommended for routine thyroid imaging because its geometry permits imaging of the entire length of a thyroid lobe. The sector-type probe has a dome-shaped contact surface that makes contact with the skin at one point, and generates a wedge-shaped image radiating from this contact point. Because of this narrower contact surface, the sector-type probe is easier to move along the contours of the neck and can be more easily directed at nodules lying deep to the clavicle. It is also convenient for real-time ultrasound guidance, because the needle may be placed relatively close to the center of the image. For these reasons the author prefers the sector-type probe for UG FNA. However, a small linear-type probe would provide the same advantages (4).

As in traditional palpation-guided FNA, 22- to 25-gauge needles are used. The larger 22-gauge needles generate stronger echoes, and are more easily visualized during real-time imaging. Many manufacturers of ultrasound equipment offer biopsy needle guides for attachment to the probe, which assist the operator in aligning the needle with the plane of the two-dimensional image. The author prefers the greater flexibility obtained with freehand placement of the needle.

Method
There is no single standard technique for ultrasound-guided FNA. Ultrasound guidance is optimally performed in real time with direct visualization of the needle tip within the nodule, as described below. Alternatively, ultrasound may be used to localize a target nodule beforehand, with a mark placed on the skin to guide the needle.

The author uses the following real-time guidance method, with a sector-type probe, and a 22- or 25-gauge needle attached to a 10-cc syringe. The probe is protected from contamination with body fluids by a latex cover available from ultrasound equipment suppliers.

The patient is asked to lie supine with the neck extended, and the skin over the nodule is cleansed with iodine solution. Sterile ultrasound transmission gel is applied, the thyroid gland is scanned, and the target nodule is localized. An optimal route of approach for the needle is determined, avoiding the sternocleidomastoid muscle laterally. At this point an assistant is asked to hold the ultrasound probe directly over the nodule, and the biopsy operator aligns the needle shaft with the plane of the ultrasound image (indicated by a marker on the side of the probe). The needle is passed through the skin immediately adjacent to the probe and in alignment with the image plane, at an appropriate oblique angle to the skin according to the depth of the target area. When properly aligned with the plane of the image, the needle tip appears as a bright echo (Figure 8.4 and Figure 8.5).

Since the needle tip will not be visualized if it lies outside the plane of the ultrasound image, it may be necessary to manipulate the probe and/or needle to obtain alignment. The forward movement of the needle tip is monitored on the screen until the tip reaches the target area, at which time material is aspirated, and the needle is withdrawn.

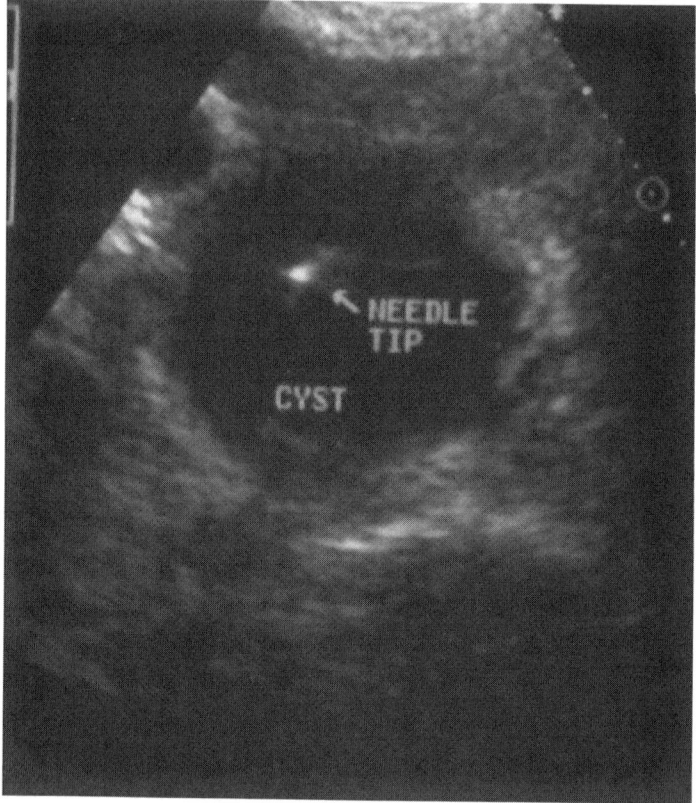

Figure 8.4 Ultrasound-guided FNA of a cystic thyroid nodule, transverse view. The needle tip appears as a bright echo within the anechoic cyst cavity.

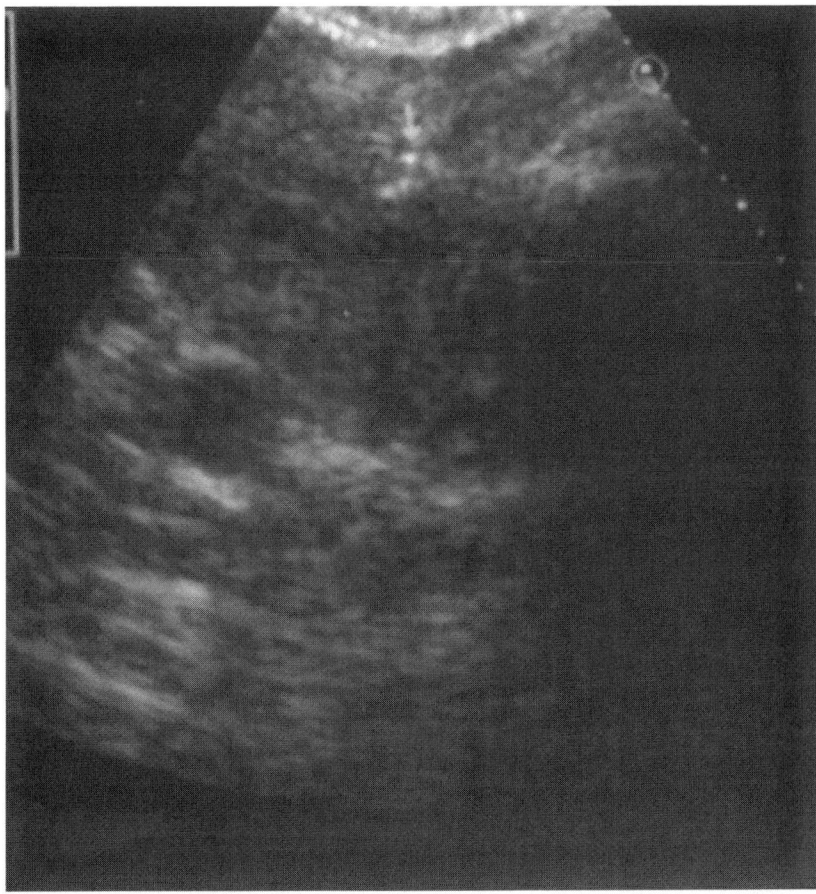

Figure 8.5 Ultrasound-guided FNA of a solid thyroid nodule, transverse view. The arrow indicates the needle tip, seen as a bright echo within the hypoechoic nodule. Several adjacent less bright echoes represent calcifications within the nodule.

Achieving alignment of the needle with the image plane is the most difficult technical aspect, and requires experience. If the operator has difficulty in aligning the needle tip with the image plane, excessive manipulation of the needle within the thyroid gland may cause local bleeding, leading to a bloody aspirate without sufficient follicular cells. As mentioned above, needle guides are available to facilitate this alignment, but since the angle of approach is fixed by the guide, there is loss of flexibility in adjusting the depth of the target area.

ULTRASOUND-GUIDED VS. PALPATION-GUIDED FNA

There are several theoretical reasons why ultrasound-guided FNA might yield superior results to traditional palpation-guided FNA (PGFNA), including fewer false-negative results due to inaccurate placement of the needle tip (improved sensitivity), and fewer nondiagnostic specimens with inadequate cellularity due to inadvertent aspiration of cystic areas. A number of published studies have attempted to compare results using the two methods.

Takashima et al. (5) reported the results of UG FNA in 268 nodules from 210 patients, and compared them with PG FNA results obtained by a head-and-neck surgeon for 62 of the same nodules. The rate of insufficient cellularity (diagnostically inadequate specimens) was only 10/268 (3%) for UG FNA, and 12/62 (19%) for PG FNA ($P<0.001$). They also determined correlation of cytologic diagnoses with final histologic diagnoses for the two methods in 99 nodules which were surgically excised, of which 34 had PG FNA in addition to UG FNA. Sixty-seven (67%) of these nodules were malignant. Excluding inadequate specimens, sensitivity (true positives/[true positives + false negatives]), specificity (true negatives/[true negatives + false positives]), and overall diagnostic accuracy were not significantly different for UG FNA vs. PG FNA (96, 91, and 96% vs. 88, 90, and 88%).

Cochand-Priollet et al. (6) reviewed the results of UG FNA performed by a single radiologist in 132 patients with palpable nodules which were "cold" on radioiodine scanning, all of whom had surgery, and of whom 14% had thyroid cancer. Only 5/132 (4%) cytologic specimens were inadequate, similar to the results reported by Takashima et al. After excluding these insufficient specimens, occult carcinomas, and Hürthle cell tumors, the sensitivity, specificity, and accuracy for cytologic diagnoses in adequate specimens were 95, 88, and 89% respectively. Although no comparison with PG FNA was available in this series, the authors noted that their rate of inadequate specimens was much lower than in previous reports of PG FNA results (6%-32%).

Yokozawa et al. (4) analyzed the results of UG FNA in 1000 patients, obtaining a somewhat higher rate of inadequate specimens (12%). Among the 186 cases which came to surgery, the sensitivity, specificity and accuracy of cytologic diagnoses were 94, 90, and 94% respectively.

Lin et al. (7) reported UG FNA results in 3657 patients with palpable nodules, of whom 378 had surgery. The malignancy rate in the surgical cases was 29%. For the surgical cases the sensitivity, specificity and accuracy of the cytologic diagnoses were 80, 99, and 93% respectively. No data on the rate of inadequate specimens were reported for this series.

Danese et al. (8) studied a series of 9683 consecutive patients with thyroid nodules undergoing either PG FNA (4986) or UG FNA (4697). All aspirates were reviewed by the same cytologist. The rate of inadequate specimens was 8.7% for PG FNA, but only 3.5% for UG FNA, despite the fact that the UG FNA cases included a higher proportion of cystic and partly cystic nodules. For patients who had surgery (18% of whom had cancer), sensitivity, specificity and accuracy of the cytologic diagnoses excluding inadequate specimens were 97, 71, and 76% for UG FNA compared with 92, 69, and 73% for PG FNA.

Carmeci *et al.* (9) compared PG FNA in 370 nodules with UG FNA in 127 nodules, and found that UG FNA was associated with fewer inadequate specimens (7% vs. 16%) and improved sensitivity (100% vs. 89%) and specificity (100% vs. 69%). In this series UG FNA was performed for nonpalpable or difficult-to-palpate nodules (75% of cases), for previously unsuccessful PG FNA, or for nodules discovered incidentally during head-and-neck imaging. Among patients who underwent surgery, patients evaluated by UG FNA had a cancer rate of 59%, compared with 40% for PG FNA, indicating that fewer patients with benign disease were referred for surgery.

Hatada *et al.* (10) evaluated results of UG FNA in 72 palpable nodules and PG FNA in 94 palpable nodules, and found that UG FNA was associated with fewer inadequate specimens (17% vs. 30%), improved sensitivity (62% vs. 45%), and improved specificity (74% vs. 51%). They also noted that the improved diagnostic sensitivity for the detection of malignancy was most evident in smaller nodules (<2 cm), suggesting that without ultrasound guidance erroneous needle placement may have resulted in false-negative results for smaller malignant nodules.

Ideally, a meaningful comparison of UG FNA vs. PG FNA cytology results would require that both techniques be applied to the same series of nodules, with the same operator performing the aspiration, and the same cytologist performing the interpretation. None of the above studies meet these ideal criteria, but among studies comparing the two methods, it appears that UG FNA is superior to PG FNA in terms of rates of inadequate specimens, sensitivity, and specificity (summarized in Table 8. 1).

Table 8.1. Summary of Studies Comparing Cytologic Results of Palpation-guided (PG FNA) vs. Ultrasound-guided (UG FNA) Fine Needle Aspiration Biopsy of Thyroid Nodules

	Reference	PG FNA	UG FNA
Inadequate specimens (%)	(5)	19	3
	(8)	8.7	3.5
	(9)	16	7
	(10)	30	17
Sensitivity (%)	(5)	88	96
	(8)	92	97
	(9)	89	100
	(10)	45	62
Specificity (%)	(5)	90	91
	(8)	69	71
	(9)	69	100
	(10)	51	74

INDICATIONS FOR ULTRASOUND- VS. PALPATION-GUIDED FNA

Indications for utilizing ultrasound guidance for FNA of thyroid nodules can be categorized as absolute indications, when ultrasound guidance is critical, and relative indications, when ultrasound guidance is optional (Table 8.2).

Table 8.2 Indications for Ultrasound Guidance for FNA

Absolute Indications	Relative Indications
Nonpalpable nodules	Palpable nodules <1.5 cm
Difficult-to-palpate nodules	Previous inadequate sample
Partly cystic (complex) nodules	Proximity to major vessels

A decision of whether to utilize ultrasound guidance for FNA of a thyroid nodule is obviously dependent on the availability of a skilled operator who can reliably perform the procedure. In the setting of an office practice, the availability of an ultrasound apparatus would appropriately lower the threshold for using ultrasound guidance compared with offices lacking ultrasound capability. Since the available data strongly suggest that ultrasound guidance has the ability to decrease the rate of inadequate specimens and improve diagnostic accuracy, it is not unreasonable, and potentially cost-effective, to routinely utilize the method in offices where it is available.

REFERENCES

1. Mazzaferri, E.L. (1993) Management of a solitary thyroid nodule. *N. Engl. J. Med.* 328:553-559.
2. Hagag, P., Strauss, S., Weiss, M. (1998) Role of ultrasound-guided fine-needle aspiration biopsy in evaluation of nonpalpable thyroid nodules. *Thyroid* 8:989-995.
3. Leenhardt, L., Hejblum, G., Franc, Fediaevsky, L.D., Delbot, T., Le Guillozic, D., Ménégaux, F., Guillausseau, C., Hoang, C., Turpin, G., Aurengo, A. (1999) Indications and limits of ultrasound-guided cytology in the management of nonpalpable thyroid nodules. *J. Clin. Endo. Metab.* 84:24-28.
4. Yokozawa, T., Miyauchi, A., Kuma, K., Sugawara, M. (1995) Accurate and simple method of diagnosing thyroid nodules by the modified technique of ultrasound-guided fine needle aspiration biopsy. *Thyroid* 5:141-145.
5. Takashima, S., Fukuda, H., Kobayashi, T. (1994) Thyroid nodules: Clinical effect of ultrasound-guided fine needle aspiration biopsy. *J. Clin. Ultrasound* 22:535-542.
6. Cochand-Priollet, B., Guillausseau, P.-J., Chagnon, S., Hoang, C., Guillausseau-Scholer, C., Chanson, P., Dahan, H., Warnet, A., Tran Ba Huy, P., Valleur, P. (1994) The diagnostic value of fine-needle aspiration biopsy under ultrasonography in nonfunctional thyroid nodules: a prospective study comparing cytologic and histologic findings. *Am. J. Med.* 97:152-157.
7. Lin, J.-D., Huang, B.-Y., Weng, H.-F., Jeng, L.-B., Hsueh, C. (1997) Thyroid ultrasonography with fine-needle aspiration cytology for the diagnosis of thyroid cancer. *J. Clin. Ultrasound* 25:111-118.
8. Danese, D., Sciacchitano, S., Farsetti, A., Andreoli, M., Pontecorvi, A. (1998) Diagnostic accuracy of conventional versus sonography-guided fine-needle aspiration biopsy of thyroid nodules. *Thyroid* 8:15-21.
9. Carmeci, C., Jeffrey, R.B., McDougall, I.R., Nowels, K.W., Weigel, R.J. (1998) Ultrasound-guided fine-needle aspiration biopsy of thyroid masses. *Thyroid* 8:283-289.
10. Hatada, T., Okada, K., Ishii, H., Ichii, S., Utsunomiya, J. (1998) Evaluation of ultrasound guided fine-needle aspiration biopsy for thyroid nodules. *Am. J. Surg.* 175:133-136.

9

TECHNIQUES OF ULTRASOUND-GUIDED FNA BIOPSY

Tamotsu Yokozawa, M.D.
Kanji Kuma, M.D.
Kuma Hospital
Kobe, 650-0011, Japan.
Masahiro Sugawara, M.D.
VA Medical Center & UCLA School of Medicine
West Los Angeles, CA 90073, USA

INTRODUCTION

The use of ultrasound guided fine needle aspiration (UG FNA) biopsy has increased because its accuracy in diagnosing thyroid nodules far exceeds that of conventional blind biopsy. We use a drill-spin technique for UG FNA (1,2,3,4), and have applied this technique to more than 14,000 patients with a wide variety of thyroid nodules. Because of the accuracy of diagnosing thyroid nodules using this technique, the number of unnecessary operations has decreased and the number of microcancers has increased in our hospital. In this chapter, we describe our drill-spin technique of performing UG FNA biopsy and a practical approach to different types of thyroid nodules.

PREPARATION FOR UG FNA BIOPSY

Before performing UG FNA biopsy, the procedure needs to be fully explained to the patient. The presence of an ultrasound machine and knowledge of a needle stick to the neck are always frightening to the patient. The following is our approach to patients before UG FNA. First, we show patients an ultrasound picture of the thyroid gland and explain the biopsy sites. The actual conversation is: "This is a safe procedure because the biopsy is performed with direct visualization of the thyroid gland. You may feel a tiny needle stick almost the same as drawing blood. Do not swallow saliva during the needle stick." Supportive measures, such as holding a patient's hand by the nursing staff, can be of great help for nervous patients. UG FNA biopsy is often difficult in small children; it is essential for parents to hold small children during the procedure.

Positioning of monitor and patient

Note that the physician, monitor, and patient make a convenient triangle for the procedure (Fig.4.1). We recommend a semi-reclining position in a reclining chair, since this position is comfortable for patients. More importantly, it allows the biopsy to be done easily by watching the needle track on the monitor. If a patient is supine, it requires that the physician frequently switch back and forth from the monitor to the neck in order to watch the needle progress. (Figure 9.1)

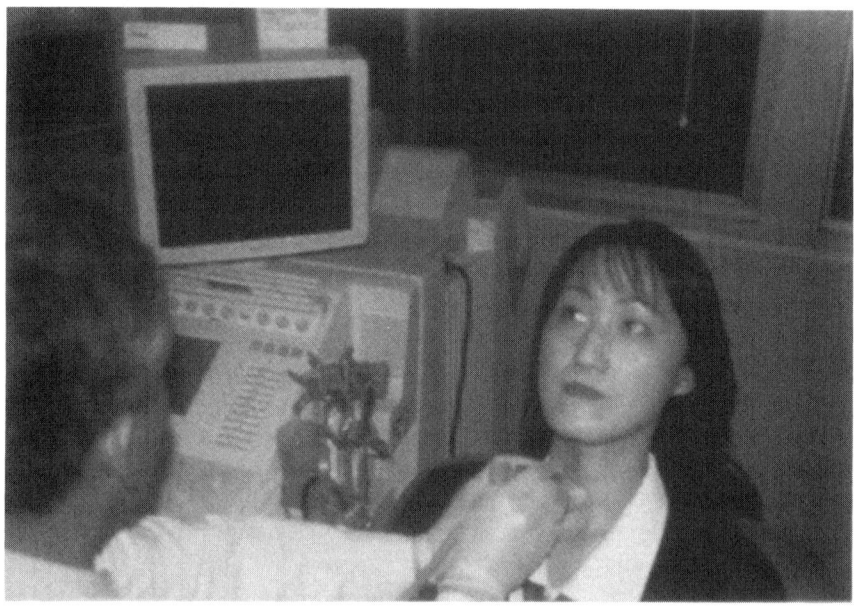

Figure 9.1 Semi-reclining position for UG FNA biopsy. Note the triangle formed by the physician, patient and ultrasound monitor.

Ultrasound scanner and transducers

The ultrasound scanner we are currently using is the Toshiba Power Vision 7000 (Fully Digital Ultrasound System) equipped with a 7.5 MHz transducer (PLK-703AT) (Figure 9.2). It is important that the scanner gives a clear visualization of the thyroid gland and needle tip on the monitor. A digital system is superior to an analog system; however, the digital type is more expensive than the conventional type. In our previous experience, we used a small-sized transducer because of the convenience for biopsy (1,2,3). Our present transducer has a 4.5 x 1.0 cm contact surface, and this size is also convenient (4). (Figure 9.2)

139

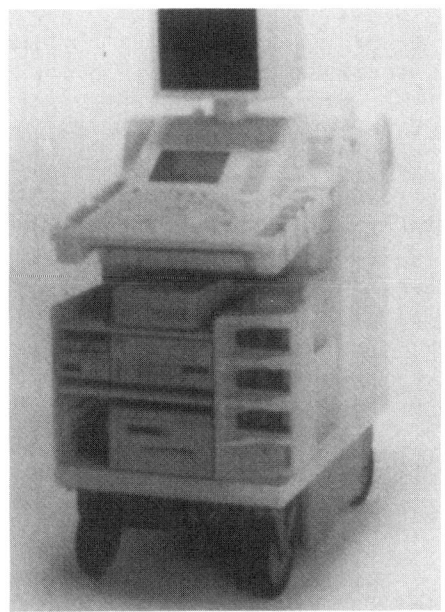

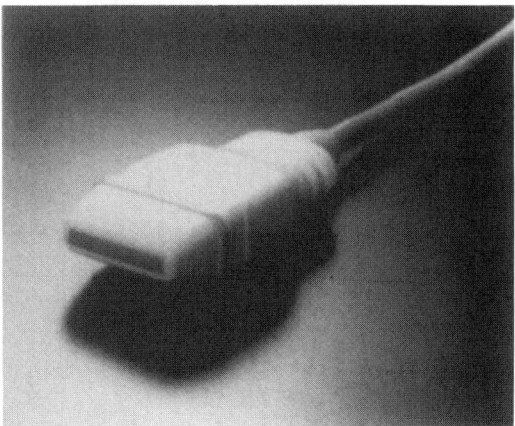

Figure 9.2 Toshiba Power Vision 7000 (Fully Digital Ultrasound System) equipped with a 7.5 MHz transducer (PLK-703AT).

Skin preparation for biopsy

Cleaning of the skin can be done using alcohol or Betadine followed by an alcohol swab. There is a debate about whether an anesthetic should be used. In our experience, we do not use a local anesthetic, and most patients tolerate it well.

TECHNIQUE OF UG FNA

After determining the biopsy sites, a 22 to 25 gauge needle attached to a 10 cc syringe should be placed just above the transducer. It is important to place the needle in the center of the transducer rather than the corner of the transducer. This allows the needle to be inserted almost perpendicular to the neck, and the tip of the needle is observed on the monitor until it reaches the biopsy site. The needle tip is clearly visible as a bright spot on the monitor screen. When it has reached the biopsy site (Figure 9.3A), the transducer is removed, and the syringe-needle unit is fixed with the physician's left hand. Then, suction is applied by pulling the piston portion of the syringe up to the 1 or 2 cc level using the right hand. While maintaining the suction by pulling the piston portion of the syringe with the right hand, the outer part of the syringe that is connected to the needle is spun 2 to 3 times using the left thumb and index finger (Figure 9.3B). This drill-spin technique cuts thyroid tissue by a spinning needle, and abundant cell material can be obtained. It is essential that the syringe-needle unit be kept in the same position and angle while the outer part of the syringe is spun. After samples are obtained, specimens are put on a glass slide. The drill technique was initially described by Miller as a rotation technique (5). Since biopsy sites are frequently small and well-focused areas, this drill-spin technique is more useful than the multiple poking technique. For a demonstration of the technique, a videotape (VHS) is available on request (see footnote).

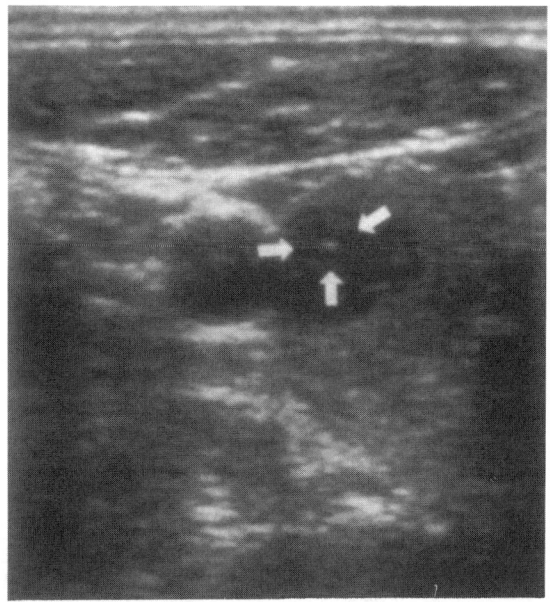

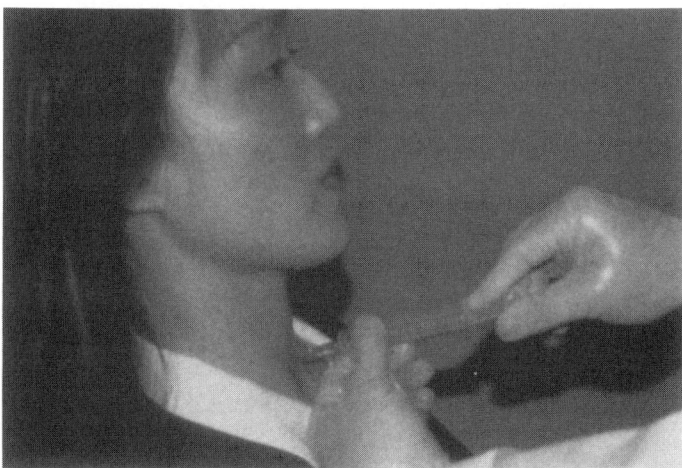

Figure 9.3 A: Localization of needle tip at the biopsy site. The arrows indicate location of needle tip. **B:** Drill-spin technique. After the needle tip is confirmed to be in the biopsy site, the syringe-needle unit should stay in this position all the time. Then, apply suction by pulling the piston portion up to the 1 to 2cc mark: Note that suction is applied by right hand fingers. Maintaining suction, the syringe-connected needle should be spun 2 to 3 turns using left hand fingers. This procedure cuts tissue and samples can be obtained.

PREPARATION OF SLIDES FOR CYTOLOGICAL EXAMINATION

Although there is no harm in making many slide preparations, one of the features of UG FNA biopsy is not having to make as many smear samples as with conventional FNA because the samples are obtained from the most suspected areas. Several techniques are available for making slides for cytological examination (5). Our technique is shown in figure 9.4. The biopsy sample should be placed in the center of the glass slide. The blood component on the glass slide is removed quickly by wiping it with soft tissue paper. Then, the cell component is spread with another glass slide, which is gently placed on top of the sample. After separating the two glass slides, cells can be processed for cytological examination. The advantage of this technique over the sliding technique is the central localization of the sample, allowing clusters of cells to be seen. This permits the cytologist to focus on a relatively small area rather than the entire slide. Another advantage is the minimum destruction of cell components when compared with the sliding smear method.

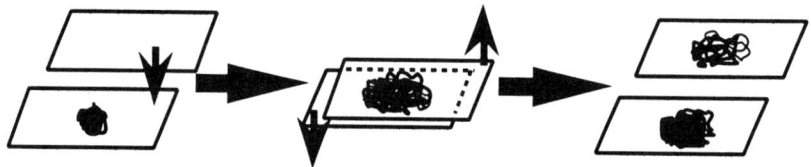

Figure 9.4 Our method of making glass slide preparations for cytological examination.

OTHER METHODS OF PERFORMING UG FNA BIOPSY

Table 9.1 summarizes other methods of performing UG FNA biopsy that have been published. As noted, UG FNA biopsy has been done exclusively in the supine position using an analog type of ultrasound equipment. The approach for aspiration was either perpendicular or oblique, and needle size varied from 22 to 25 gauge. We currently use a 22gauge needle for this biopsy; its advantage is that it obtains abundant cells. However, a disadvantage is that the specimens are sometimes bloody. Several institutions use a needle steering device, although we have not used it because of its limited flexibility. Complications such as minor bleeding and pain are infrequent. Because there is direct visualization of the thyroid gland, accidental damage to the trachea, carotid artery, and recurrent nerve damage can be avoided. (Table 9.1)

Table 9.1 Techniques for Performing UG FNA Biopsy.

No.	Year	Reference and Country	Total cases	Position			Equipment		Approach for aspiration		Size of needle (gauge)	With a needle-steering	No. of passes
				Reclining	Sitting	Supine	Digital	Analog	Perpendicular	Oblique			
1	1993	Boland, et al. (6), U.S.A.	96	-	-	O	-	O	-	O	22-25	O	≥ 2
2	1993	Rosen, et al. (7), Canada	59	-	-	O	-	O	-	-	22-25	-	-
3	1994	Cochand-Priollet, et al. (8), France	132	-	-	O	-	O	-	-	23	-	3
4	1994	Quinn, et al. (9), U.S.A.	102	-	-	O	-	O	-	O	21	O	3
5	1994	Kuma, et al. (1), Japan	134	-	-	O	-	O	O	-	22, 23	-	1or 2
6	1994	Sanchez, et al. (10), U.S.A.	25	-	-	O	-	O	-	O	25	O	4
7	1995	Ito, et al. (11), Japan	197	-	-	O	-	O	-	O	22	O	1 (?)
8	1995	Yokozawa, et al. (2), Japan	1000	-	O	-	-	O	O	-	22	-	1 or 2
9	1995	Hanbidge, et al. (12), U.S.A.	123	-	-	-	-	O	-	-	23, 27	-	4
10	1996	Yokozawa, et al. (3), Japan	678	-	O	-	-	O	O	-	22	-	1 or 2
11	1997	Lu, et al. (13), Republic of China	9	-	-	O	-	O	-	O	-	O	1-3
12	1997	Sabel, et al. (14), U.S.A.	79	-	-	O	-	O	-	O	20	O	-
13	1997	Rodriguez, et al. (15), Spain	89	-	-	O	-	O	-	-	-	-	-
14	1998	Danese, et al. (16), Italy	4697	-	-	O	-	O	-	-	21-23	-	mean 4.8
15	1998	Hatada, et al. (17), Japan	70	-	-	O	-	O	-	O	22	O	-
16	1998	Carmeci, et al. (18), U.S.A.	127	-	-	O	-	O	-	-	22 or 25	-	4
17	1998	Khurana, et al. (19), U.S.A.	119	-	-	O	-	O	-	-	22	-	mean 3
18	1998	Yokozawa. (4), Japan	≥13423	O	-	-	O	-	O	-	22	-	1 or 2
19	1999	Leenhardt, et al. (20), France	450	-	-	-	-	O	-	-	25	-	-

RECOMMENDED TECHNIQUES FOR DIFFERENT TYPES OF THYROID NODULES

One of the advantages of UG FNA biopsy is the ability to choose the biopsy site after ultrasound analysis. Table 9.2 shows common ultrasound findings of thyroid nodules with corresponding possible diagnoses and the recommended or preferred biopsy site. Because ultrasound is not definitive in diagnosing cancer, a FNA biopsy is necessary to confirm the diagnosis. Figures 9.5 to 9.11 demonstrate ultrasound findings of representative thyroid nodules and recommended biopsy sites, which were determined after actual visualization of the nodular lesions in surgical specimens and comparison with corresponding preoperative ultrasound findings.

Table 9.2 Ultrasound Findings of Thyroid Nodules and Biopsy Sites*

Ultrasound findings	Possibility	Biopsy sites
Round and anechoic area	Cyst or Adenomatous nodule	Any place
Mixed solid and cystic nodule	Cystic benign nodule or Cystic carcinoma	Put needle in the root of polyp-like lesion
Round and hypoechoic solid nodule	Follicular adenoma or Adenomatous nodule or Carcinoma	Any place (Avoid too much suction)
Solid nodule with irregular border or presence of psammoma calcification	Carcinoma	Aim at peripheral hypoechoic lesion

* This classification was based on the comparison between ultrasound findings and histological diagnoses of more than 1000 cases.

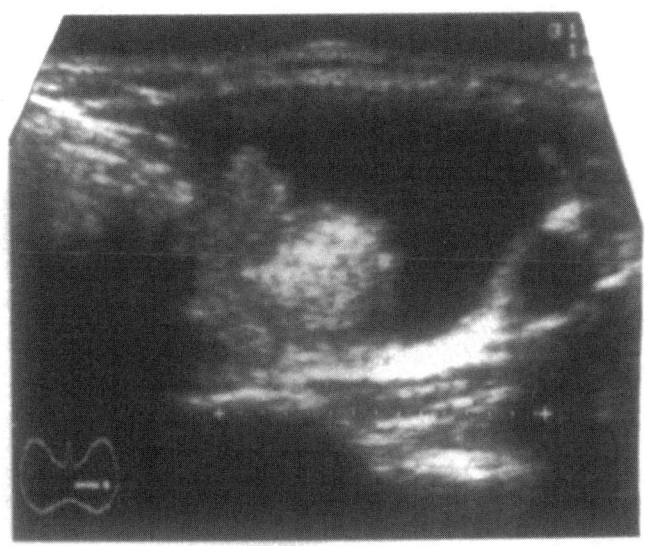

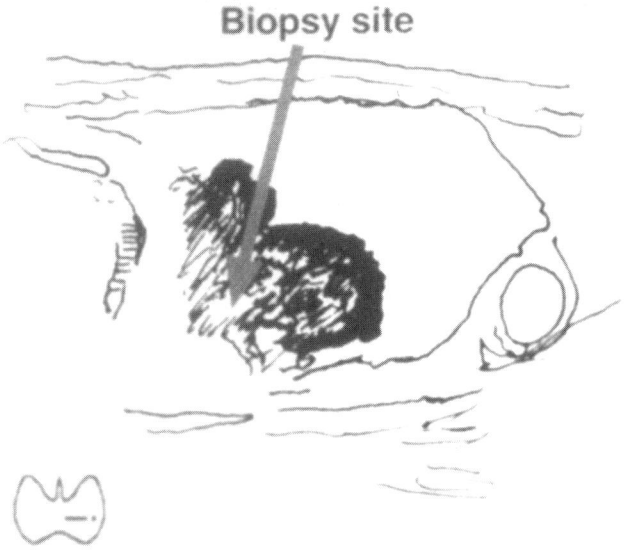

Figure 9.5 Cystic Nodule. The concern is whether or not a cystic nodule contains a papillary carcinoma; the incidence of papillary cancer in a cystic nodule has been reported to be 1 to 3% (2,24-26). UG FNA is the most powerful tool for diagnosing cystic carcinoma. As the ultrasound demonstrates, the nodule grew into the cystic lumen. The needle should be directed to the root of the pedicle, where cancer cells are frequently found (2). The portion of the pedicle facing the cystic lumen tends to contain degenerative cells.

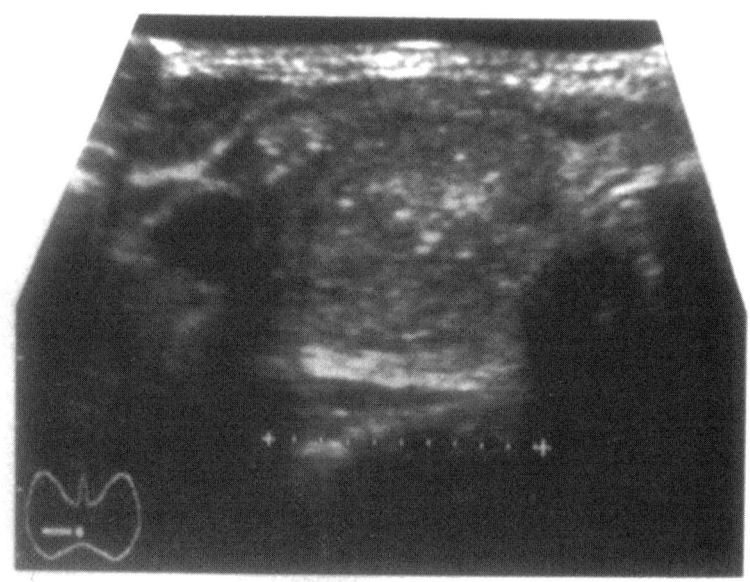

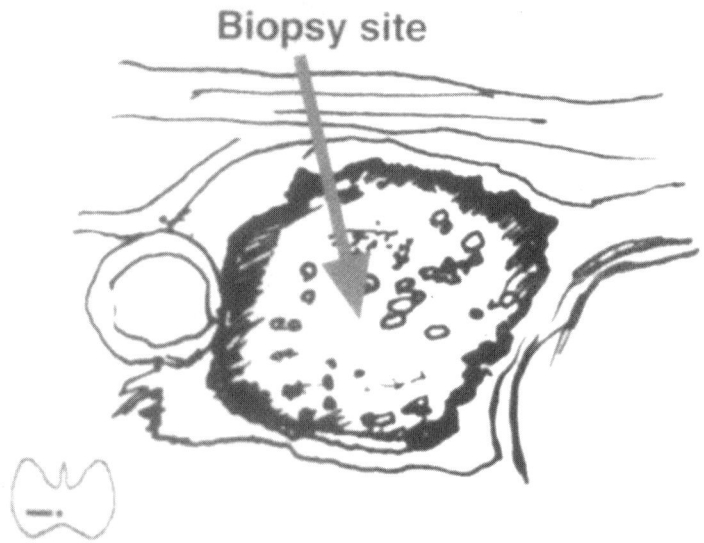

Figure 9.6 Papillary Carcinoma. Ultrasound shows a relatively hypoechoic mass, suggesting a tumor. The biopsy site should be in the peripheral portion of the mass, since cancer cells tend to proliferate peripherally and not centrally. Based on our experience, areas where psammoma bodies are present are also good places to biopsy. This biopsy showed papillary carcinoma.

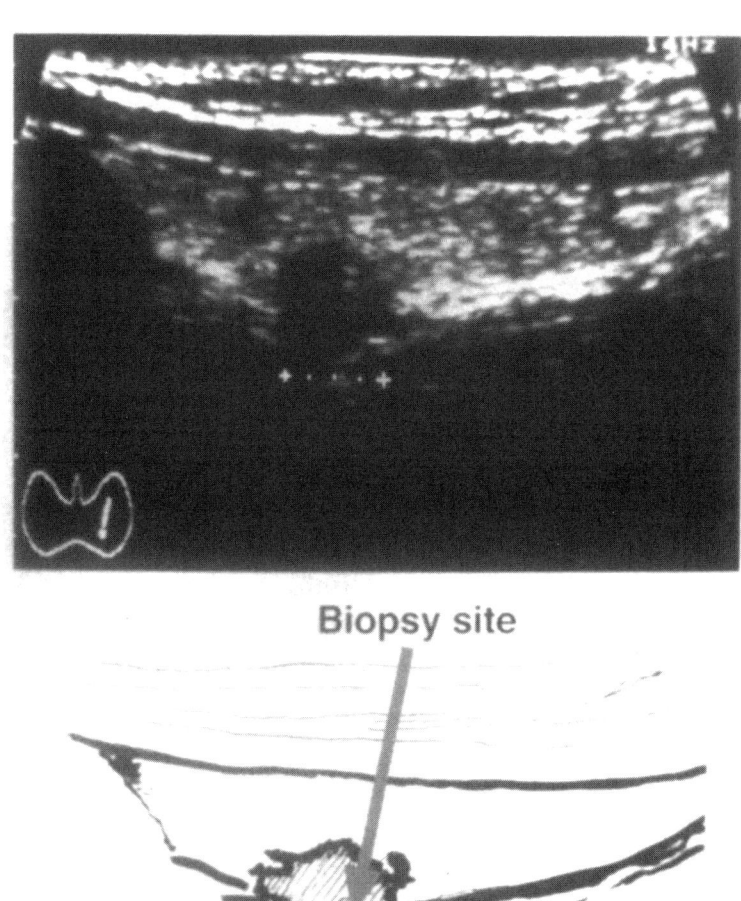

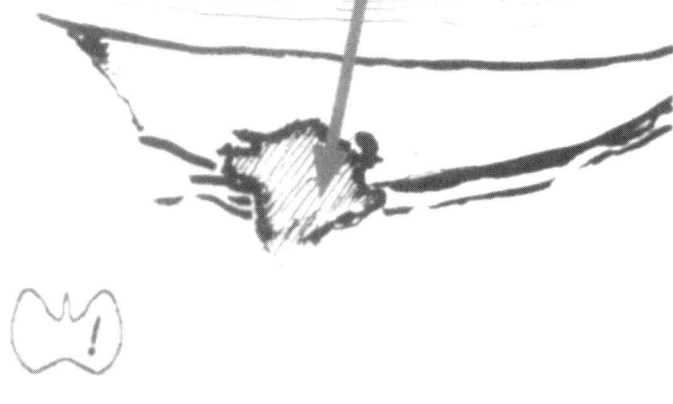

Figure 9.7 Papillary Carcinoma with Recurrent Nerve Invasion. The recurrent nerve is not visualized by ultrasound, but its location can be suspected by careful observation of the sonography. A small hypoechoic mass that is suspected to be extrathyroidal invasion of the recurrent nerve is seen. Although a biopsy can be obtained from any portion, peripheral portions of the mass are preferred.

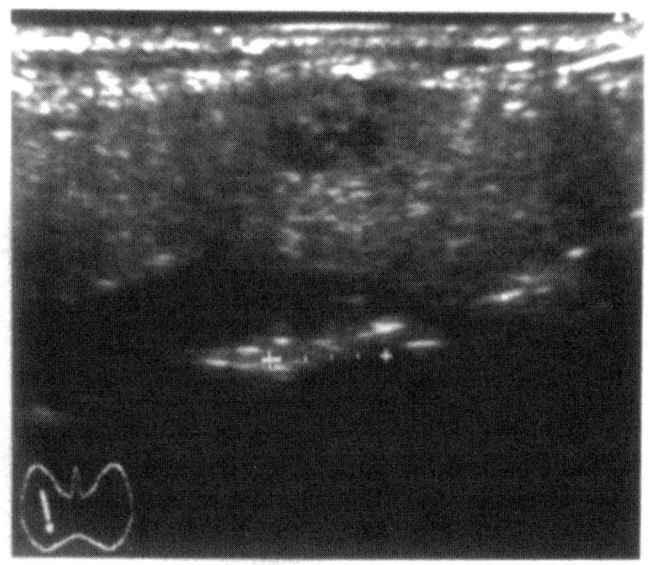

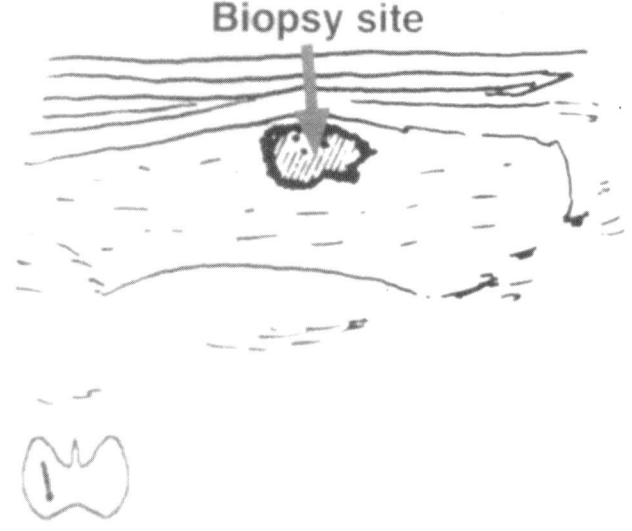

Figure 9.8 Microcancer. This case was a micro medullary carcinoma. This patient had no palpable mass, and the ultrasound was performed because of a family history of medullary carcinoma. When the size of the lesion is less than one centimeter in diameter, a drill-spin technique is a must.

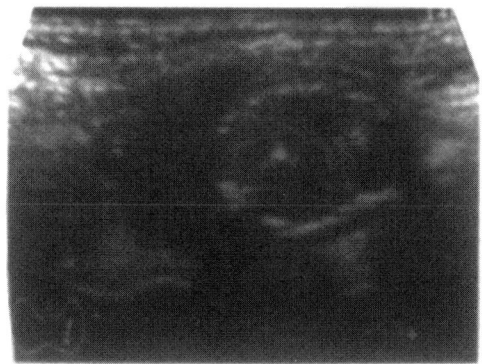
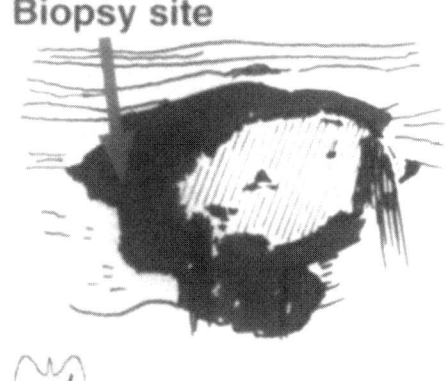
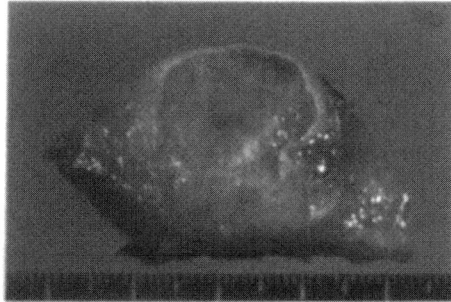

Figure 9.9 Tumor with a calcified capsular membrane. Calcification is seen in the capsular membrane of the mass both on ultrasound and the gross specimen. The biopsy site should be outside the membrane since the needle may not penetrate through the calcification. This case was a follicular carcinoma.

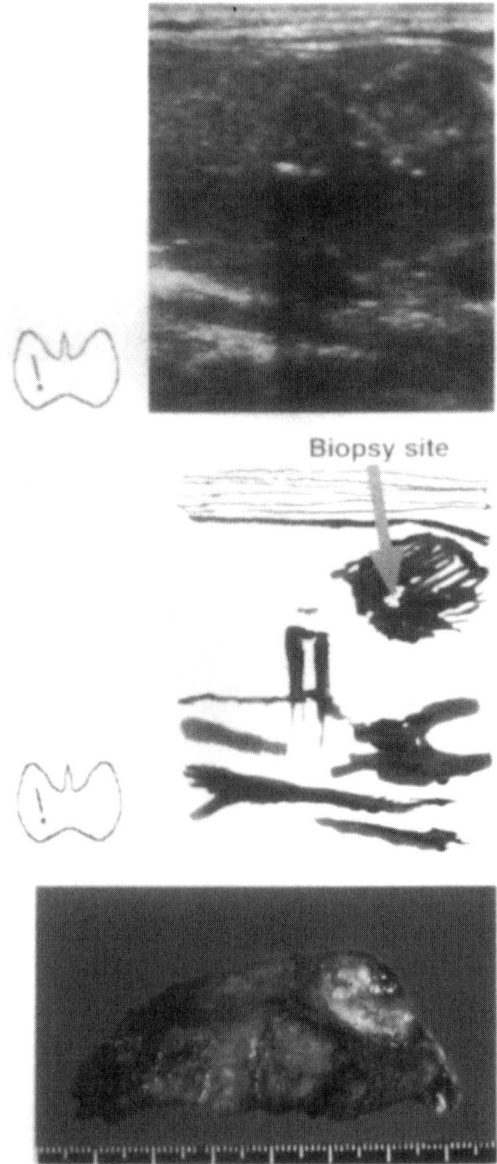

Figure 9.10 Cancer Associated with Hashimoto Thyroiditis. Thyroid cancer associated Hashimoto thyroiditis is difficult to detect by ultrasound because Hashimoto thyroiditis presents a diffuse hypoechoic picture. In this case the biopsy was taken from the irregularly shaped and more pronounced hypoechoic area associated with Hashimoto thyroiditis.

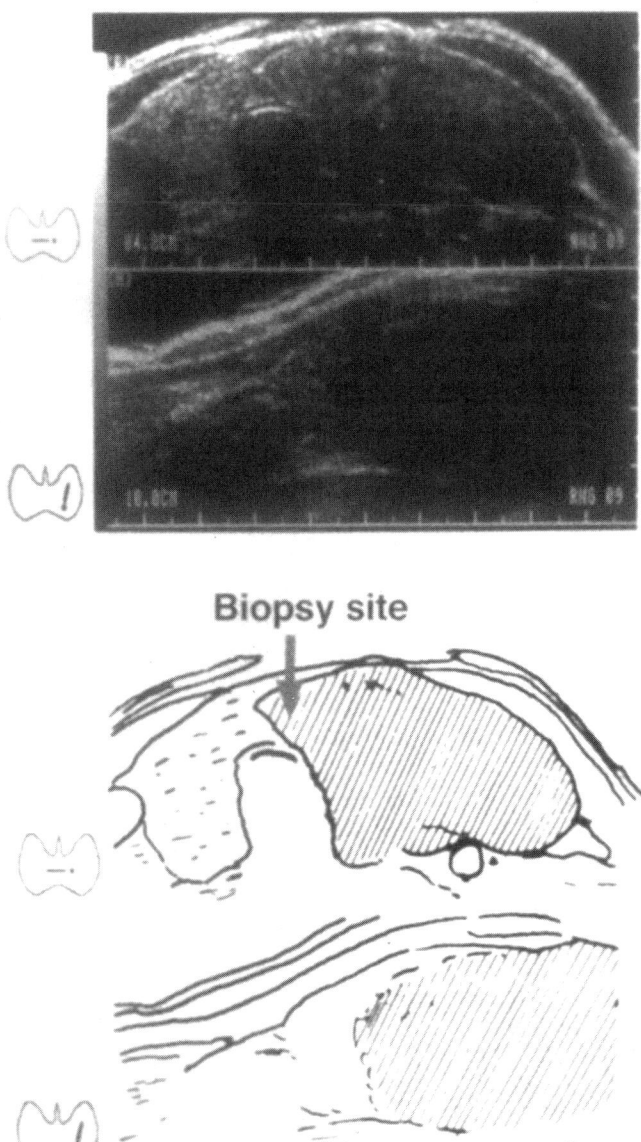

Figure 9.11 Thyroid Lymphoma. Thyroid lymphoma occurs exclusively in the thyroid gland of Hashimoto thyroiditis. The packed lymphoma cells produce a pseudocystic picture on ultrasound. The biopsy site is in the peripheral portion of the hypoechoic area.

PITFALLS OF UG FNA BIOPSY

Because superficial tumors are difficult to visualize using less than a 20MHz transducer, a tumor located just under the skin (i.e., lymph node metastasis), should be biopsied without using ultrasound guidance. Bloody samples always interfere with cytological interpretation; therefore, one should try to avoid blood vessels, which can be identified using Doppler equipment. An alternative approach is to biopsy without using suction, which will minimize bleeding as described originally by Santos (22). An annoying problem of FNA is a non-diagnostic sample or insufficient material; however, the number of non-diagnostic samples is decreased by using UG FNA (2,3). If the needle is in the correct location, diagnostic samples can be obtained more than 95% of the time. In nodules that are malignant, the likelihood of obtaining sufficient cells is even greater. In fact, cancer cells are relatively easily obtained by FNA. Based upon our experience, the presence of calcification and small nodules are the most common causes of insufficient material on FNA (2-4).

Footnote. Address for VHS request: Dr. T. Yokozawa, Kuma Hospital, 8-2-35 Shimoyamate Dori, Chuo-ku, Kobe, 650-0011, Japan

REFERENCES

1. Kuma, K., Matsuzuka, F., Yokozawa, T., Miyauchi, A., Sugawara, M. (1994) Fate of untreated benign thyroid nodules: results of long-term follow-up. *World J. Surg.* 18:495-499.
2. Yokozawa, T., Miyauchi, A., Kuma, K., Sugawara, M., (1995) Accurate and simple method of diagnosing thyroid nodules by the modified technique of ultrasound-guided aspiration biopsy. *Thyroid* 5:141-145.
3. Yokozawa, T., Fukata, S., Kuma, K., Matsuzuka, F., Kobayashi, A., Hirai, K., Miyauchi, A., Sugawara, M. (1996) Thyroid cancer detected by ultrasound-guided fine needle aspiration biopsy. *World J. Surg.* 20:848-853.
4. Yokozawa, T., Kuma, K. (1998) Use of fine needle aspiration and ultrasound-guided aspiration biopsy. *Thyroidol. Clin. Exp.* 10:103-108.
5. Miller, J.M. (1996) Techniques of fine-needle aspiration biopsy. In: Kini, S.R. ed., *Thyroid*. 2nd ed. New York: Igakushoin, 5-12.
6. Boland, G.W., Lee, M.J., Mueller, P.R., Mayo-Smith, W., Dawson, S.L., Simeone, J.F. (1993) Efficacy of sonographically guided biopsy of thyroid masses and cervical lymph nodes. *Am. J. Roent.* 161:1053-1056.
7. Rosen, I.B., Azadian, A., Walfish, P.G., Salem, S., Lansdown, E., Bedard, Y.C. (1993) Ultrasound-guided fine needle aspiration biopsy in the management of thyroid disease. *Am. J. Surg.* 166:346-349.
8. Cochand-Priollet, B., Guillausseau, P.J., Chagnon, S., Hoang, C., Guillausseau-Scholer, C., Chanson, P., Dahan, H., Warnet, A., Tran Ba Huy, P.T., Valleur, P. (1994) The diagnostic value of fine-needle aspiration biopsy under ultrasonography in nonfunctional thyroid nodules: a prospective study comparing cytologic and histologic findings. *Am. J. Med.* 97:152-157.
9. Quinn, S.F., Nelson, H.A., Demlow, T.A. (1994) Thyroid biopsies: fine needle aspiration biopsy versus spring-activated core biopsy needle in 102 patients. *J. Vasc. Interv. Radiol.* 5:619-623.

10. Sanchez, R.B., vanSonnenberg, E., D'Agostino, H.B., Shank, T., Oglevie, S., Laoide, R., Fundell, L., Robbins, T. (1994) Ultrasound guided biopsy of nonpalpable and difficult to palpate thyroid masses. *J. Am. Coll. Surg.* 178:33-37.
12. Ito, M., Yamashita, S., Ashizawa, K., Namba, H., Hoshi, M., Shibata, Y., Sekine, I., Nagataki, S., Shigematsu, I. (1995) Childhood thyroid diseases around Chernobyl evaluated by ultrasound examination and fine needle aspiration cytology. *Thyroid* 5:365-368.
13. Hanbidge, A.E., Arenson, A.M., Shaw, P.A., Szalai, J.P., Hamilton, P.A., Leonhardt, C. (1995) Needle size and sample adequacy in ultrasound-guided biopsy of thyroid nodules. *Can. Assoc. Radiol. J.* 46:199-201.
14. Lu, C.P., Chang, T.C., Wang, C.Y., Hsiao, Y.L. (1997) Serial changes in ultrasound-guided fine needle aspiration cytology in subacute thyroiditis. *Acta Cytol.* 41:238-243.
15. Sabel, M.S., Haque, D., Velasco, J.M., Staren, E.D. (1998) Use of ultrasound-guided fine needle aspiration biopsy in the management of thyroid disease. *Am. J. Surg.* 64:738-741
16. Rodriguez, J.M., Reus, M., Moreno, A., Martinez, M., Soria, T., Carrasco, L., Parrilla, P. (1997) High-resolution ultrasound associated with aspiration biopsy in the follow-up of patients with differentiated thyroid cancer. *Otolaryngol. Head Neck Surg.* 117:694-697.
17. Danese, D., Sciacchitano, S., Farsetti, A., Andreoli, M., Pontecorvi, A. (1998) Diagnostic Accuracy of conventional versus sonography-guided fine-needle aspiration biopsy of thyroid nodules. *Thyroid* 8:15-21.
18. Hatada, T., Okada, K., Ishii, H., Utsunomiya, J. (1998) Evaluation of ultrasound-guided fine needle aspiration biopsy for thyroid disease. *Am.J. Surg.* 175:133-136.
19. Carmeci, C., Jeffrey, R.B., McDougall, I.R., Nowells, K.W., Weigel, R.J. (1998) Ultrasound-guided fine-needle aspiration biopsy of thyroid masses. *Thyroid* 8:283-289.
20. Khurana, K.K., Richards, V.I., Chopra, P.S., Izquierdo, R., Rubens, D., Mesonero, C. (1998) The role of ultrasonography-guided fine needle aspiration biopsy in the management of nonpalpable and palpable thyroid nodules. *Thyroid* 8:511-515.
21. Leenhardt, L., Hejblum, G., Franc, B., Fediaevsky, L.P., Delbot, T., Guillouzic, D., Ménégaux, F., Guillausseau, C., Hoang, C., Turpin, G., Aurengo, A. (1999) Indications and Limits of ultrasound-guided cytology in the management of nonpalpable thyroid nodules. *J. Clin. Endocrinol. Metab.* 84:24-28.
22. Santos, J.E.C., Leiman, and G. (1988) Nonaspiration fine needle cytology: application of a new technique to nodular thyroid disease. *Acta Cytol.* 32:353-356.
23. Crile, C. (1966) Treatment of thyroid cysts by aspiration. *Surgery* 59:210-212.
24. Miller, J., Zafar, S., Karo, J. (1974) The cystic thyroid nodule. *Radiology* 110:257-261.
25. Rojeski, M.T., Gharib, H. (1985) Nodular thyroid disease. Evaluation and management. *N. Engl. J. Med.* 313:426-436.

10

THE ROLE OF ULTRASOUND IN MANAGING THYROID CANCER

H. Jack Baskin, M.D., F.A.C.E.
Florida Thyroid and Endocrine Clinic
Orlando, FL 32804, USA

INTRODUCTION

Well-differentiated thyroid cancer is the nineteenth most common cancer with 16,000 new cases each year. It is unique in its behavior in that it frequently occurs in young people and is the second or third most common cancer in the fifteen to thirty year old age group. Although the majority of patients are cured by their initial surgery, the cancer has a propensity to recur or metastasize many years after apparently successful surgery. Therefore, patients require lifelong periodic follow-up, often exceeding fifty years. This presents a challenge to the endocrinologist in charge of their care, not only to observe for recurrence of their cancer, but also to manage their hypothyroidism. A cost-effective approach to the management of these patients using ultrasound is the topic of this chapter.

Most authorities agree that follow-up must be individualized as to the risk of recurrence since this risk varies greatly among patients. Several methods have been developed of classifying which cancers are the most likely to recur. These classifications use the size of the primary tumor, the cell type, the age of the patient, and the extent of invasion or metastasis to categorize patients into various stages. This is of great benefit to the clinician in establishing the intensity with which each patient must be followed.

The management and follow-up of thyroid cancer patients was hampered in the past because of the lack of sufficiently sensitive methods to detect early recurrence. The only diagnostic tool available was the whole body scan (WBS) using ^{131}I after withdrawal from thyroid hormone suppression. This changed in the 1990's when several new probes were developed that aid in the early detection of recurrent thyroid cancer. These include sensitive thyroglobulin (Tg) assays that allow measurement of suppressed Tg levels, recombinant TSH ($_{rh}$TSH) that allows scanning without thyroid hormone withdrawal, neck ultrasound to detect early lymph node recurrence, and ultrasound-guided FNA (UG FNA) biopsy of suspicious lymph nodes.

WHOLE BODY SCANS

For several decades, the only practical test that was available to follow patients who had thyroid cancer was the WBS; but for many reasons, scanning is a poor test for the long term monitoring of these patients. It can only be used in patients who have undergone a total or near-total thyroidectomy and received ^{131}I ablation. It requires referring the patient to a nuclear medicine physician or radiologist and coordinating the withdrawal of the patient's thyroid hormone suppression therapy. This intentional induction of hypothyroidism is uncomfortable to the patient, and theoretically, a possibility exists for thyroid cancer to grow or metastasize when exposed to the increase in endogenous thyroid stimulating hormone while thyroxin suppression is interrupted for scanning. The considerable expense and time loss from work are also considerations that contribute to the loss of follow-up in many patients. Park et al have shown that the ^{131}I used in scanning patients stuns the thyroid tissue making it difficult to treat patients with ^{131}I when the scan is positive (1). Perhaps the greatest drawback of the WBS is its poor sensitivity in detecting recurrent or metastatic thyroid cancer. When pre-treatment scans are compared with post-treatment scans obtained using the treatment dose of ^{131}I, there is a third more cancer seen on the post-treatment scan. Many patients with proven thyroid cancer do not have a positive scan. A WBS became the way to follow thyroid cancer patients by default – there was simply no other method available.

The introduction of $_{rh}$TSH in 1999 has eliminated the need for patients to be taken off their thyroid hormone suppression in order to be scanned; however, it has increased the expense of the WBS without improving its sensitivity. The use of $_{rh}$TSH does not eliminate the need for the patient to have a total or near-total thyroidectomy and ^{131}I ablation, nor does it solve the problem of stunning if the scan is positive and the patient requires treatment with ^{131}I. Certainly, an easier and more cost-effective test for following patients who have had thyroid cancer is desirable.

THYROGLOBULIN

Thyroglobulin is a 19S glycoprotein with more than 3000 amino acids and a molecular weight of 660,000 Dalton, making it the largest protein in the human body. It is formed in the endoplasmic reticulum of the thyroid follicular cell and migrates to the Golgi apparatus to be stored until secreted into the thyroid follicular lumen, where it constitutes most of the colloid (2). Its only known function is to serve as a template for combining iodine and tyrosine into thyroid hormones. The thyroid hormones are synthesized extracellularly in the follicular lumen, rather than in the cell as is the case with all other endocrine glands. For many years, Tg was thought to exist only in the thyroid gland, but in 1961 its presence was demonstrated in the peripheral circulation, where it is released as a by-product of thyroid hormone synthesis. The value of measuring this *prohormone* has become apparent in recent years.

In 1968, Torrigiani, et al developed a radioimmunoassay for measuring Tg and found that patients with Graves' disease, thyroiditis, and all types of goiter, including thyroid cancer, had increased levels of Tg (3). It also increases following a FNA biopsy, and because of its extremely long half-life, remains elevated for several weeks. Measurement of Tg has been helpful in distinguishing thyrotoxicosis factitia, in which Tg levels are low, from other causes of thyrotoxicosis, in which Tg levels are high (4). Persons with athyrotic cretinism were found to have no circulating Tg, a confirmation that only thyroid tissue produces Tg. Tg was also absent in the circulation of patients who had undergone a total thyroidectomy and ^{131}I ablation for thyroid cancer.

Although serum Tg is of no value in diagnosing thyroid cancer preoperatively, in 1975 Van Herle and Uller proposed the concept of using serum Tg as a tumor marker to detect recurrent thyroid cancer in patients who had undergone a total thyroidectomy for thyroid carcinoma (5). They hypothesized that the presence of Tg in the peripheral blood of such patients was an indication of residual, recurrent, or metastatic thyroid cancer.

The original Tg assays were not sensitive enough to measure very low levels of Tg less than 10 ug/L; therefore patients had to be withdrawn from their thyroid hormone suppression in order to determined if their Tg was elevated. In the 1990's sensitive Tg assays that measure Tg as low as 1ug/L were developed. This allows measurement of Tg in patients while they were still taking thyroid hormone suppression (6). The Tg assays varied widely from one laboratory to another. In part, this was due to various Tg sources used for antibody production – some originated from patients with Graves' disease, some came from patients who had thyroid cancer, while others came from autopsy material. An international reference standard was adopted in 1995 resulting in less variation between laboratories. However, because one is looking for a change in Tg from a previous level, it is advisable to be consistent and use the same laboratory, preferably one that retains the previous Tg sample for comparison. Some thyroid cancers produce more Tg than others, and it is an advantage to know the Tg level preoperatively. Therefore, blood should be drawn for a Tg level prior to surgery, keeping in mind that Tg is increased after a FNA biopsy and may remain high for several weeks afterward because of its long half-life. If a cancer is known to be producing a large amount of Tg, a low Tg after surgery is more reassuring.

Improved sensitivity and standardization of the Tg assay have increased reliance on this test in the follow-up of patients who have undergone surgical treatment of thyroid cancer. Increasing numbers of patients are being seen who have rising levels of Tg but a negative WBS; when post-treatment scans are done, they reveal recurrent or metastatic disease, and Tg levels decline after treatment. Thus a rising Tg level is thought to be a more sensitive test to use in the follow-up of patients than the old "gold Standard" WBS.

The sensitive Tg assay has proven to accurately detect over 90% of patients who have recurrent or metastatic thyroid cancer without having to stop thyroid hormone suppression (7). Unlike a WBS, Tg is accurate even in patients who were not treated with ^{131}I ablation (8-10). Levels of Tg less than 3ug/L in patients taking thyroid hormone suppression have generally been considered normal, and patients are followed-up in one year with repeat Tg. A Tg greater than 5ug/L is often associated with recurrent cancer and needs further evaluation to confirm and locate the recurrence.

A rise in the suppressed Tg greater than 5ug/L in a patient whose previous suppressed Tg was normal is a strong signal for recurrent cancer, but a WBS will not always reveal the recurrence. However, if that patient is treated with ^{131}I, it is likely that the post-treatment WBS will identify recurrent or metastatic thyroid cancer. In addition the post-treatment Tg level usually decreases. Therefore, Tg monitoring seems to be a far more sensitive method of following thyroid cancer patients than routine WBS. Whether this earlier recognition of recurrent cancer will result in less mortality is not yet certain (11).

There are two drawbacks to using the Tg to monitor thyroid cancer patients. The presence of anti-Tg antibodies (not anti-microsomal or antithyroid perioxidase antibodies) in the serum interferes with the Tg assay and causes a false increase or decrease in the Tg level. Therefore, anti-thyroglobulin antibodies must be checked in every patient each time the Tg is measured and the Tg assay not be used in those who have this antibody. Recently, a polymerase chain reaction (PCR) based assay for thyroglobulin messenger RNA in the blood has been developed and may prove to be a more sensitive method to detect recurrent cancer, and this test is not affected by the presence of anti-Tg antibodies (12). Although the Tg assay is sensitive in detecting early recurrence of thyroid cancer, the second drawback of Tg is its inability to localize recurrent lesions. Several investigators have shown that ultrasonography can detect >90% of these recurrent tumors.

NECK ULTRASOUND

Physical examination and palpation of the neck, even by experienced endocrinologists, will seldom detect an early recurrence of thyroid cancer. The overlying scar tissue and the propensity of metastatic lymph nodes to recur under the sternocleidomastoid muscle or in the carotid sheath make physical examination of the postoperative neck difficult. Lymph nodes as large as 2.5 centimeters may not be palpable when imbedded under the muscle.

High-resolution, real-time ultrasound using a linear phased-array transducer has proven to be an extremely sensitive method to recognize recurrent or metastatic thyroid cancer in the neck (13). Lymph nodes as small as 0.5 centimeter in size are easily seen with ultrasound. Several investigators have shown that ultrasound will detect three to four times as many recurrent or metastatic cancers as does palpation alone. Simeone, et al reported on 25 postoperative thyroid cancer patients whose ultrasound and UG FNA biopsy revealed thyroid cancer that was later confirmed by surgery, and only eight (32%) of these patients had a palpable mass (14). Gorman, et al identified nine recurrent medullary thyroid cancers using ultrasound, and only three were palpable (15).

Sutton, et al discovered suspicious lymph nodes on ultrasound in 52 patients who had undergone previous surgery for thyroid cancer; only eight of these patients had a palpable mass (16). UG FNA biopsy was performed and 29 (56%) were found to be malignant. Of those that were found to be malignant and had a WBS, 55% had a negative scan. Others have also shown ultrasound to be more sensitive than scanning in detecting recurrent or metastatic cancer in the neck. Antonelli, et al performed ultrasound in 63 patients who had undergone a total thyroidectomy and ^{131}I ablation and had a negative WBS, twelve patients were discovered to have ultrasound evidence of malignancy that was later confirmed surgically (17). Since 90% of recurrent thyroid cancer is in the neck and it is rare for thyroid cancer to metastasize elsewhere without neck involvement; ultrasound of the neck is not only more cost-effective to follow these patients than a WBS; it is also more sensitive.

ULTRASOUND OF THE POSTOPERATIVE NECK

Those who are not familiar with viewing the postoperative neck using ultrasound will find it worthwhile to first examine the ultrasound appearance of the neck of non-cancer patients who have undergone thyroid surgery. It is recommended that the physician perform ultrasound on several patients who have had a hemithyroidectomy or total thyroidectomy for benign disease. This allows one to view the normal postoperative neck without worrying about malignancy (Figure 10.1).

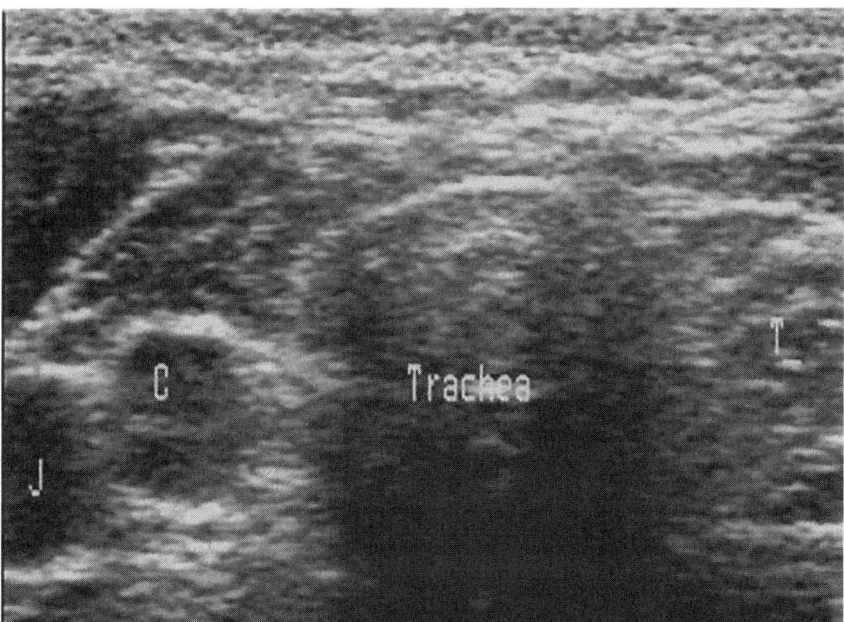

Figure 10.1 Hemithyroidectomy. Patient had right lobe removed for a benign nodule. Left lobe appears normal, but the right lobe and isthmus are absent. Note how the carotid artery (C) and the jugular vein (J) have moved medially in close proximity to the trachea. A small amount of hyperechoic connective tissue is seen in the remaining thyroid bed.

The removal of the thyroid gland allows the common carotid artery and the internal jugular vein to move medially near the trachea. Examination using ultrasound shows some scar tissue in the postoperative thyroid bed that has a uniform echogenic texture and is relatively hyperechoic. A recurrent cancer or metastatic lymph node occurring in this area will appear as a hypoechoic mass and will be well-demarcated from the surrounding hyperechoic structures.

Normal lymph nodes are characteristically oval in their transverse dimension and oblong in their longitudinal dimension. In performing ultrasound in the postoperative thyroid cancer patient, transverse sections of the neck are done. While metastatic lymph nodes may occur anywhere in the neck, they most commonly appear in the thyroid bed or along the jugular chain of nodes. Examination is first made of the thyroid bed where the thyroid gland was resected; then the jugular vein from the head of the clavicle up to the angle of the mandible is examined closely. Particular attention should be paid to the area between the common carotid artery and the internal jugular vein and the area lateral to these vessels. Occasionally, a metastatic lymph node will occur in the posterior triangle of the neck or anterior to the trachea; therefore, these areas need to be examined as well.

As is true with ultrasound of thyroid nodules, the high sensitivity of ultrasound in detecting enlarged lymph nodes is not matched by its specificity in determining if a lymph node is benign or malignant. An UG FNA biopsy of a suspicious lymph node is necessary to confirm the diagnosis. However, several ultrasound characteristics of lymph nodes will often help in determining which lymph nodes need to be biopsied (18).

Size
Several large studies have shown that lymph node size does not correlate with malignancy. Often inflammatory lymph nodes are quite large, while an early metastatic lymph node may be small. Just as is true with thyroid nodules, it is technically difficult to perform FNA biopsy on a lesion less than one centimeter in size and almost impossible if it is less than 0.5 centimeter. One should mark the location of these small suspicious lymph nodes and reexamine them in three to six months; a UG FNA biopsy is indicated if the lymph node enlarges.

Shape
As mentioned earlier, cervical lymph nodes are elongated in the longitudinal plane and are often several centimeters long. They maintain this shape when they enlarge for any reason; therefore, it is not often very helpful to measure their longitudinal dimension. However, when viewed in the transverse plane, cervical lymph nodes are oval with their transverse diameter approximately twice the anterior-posterior diameter (19). When lymph nodes enlarge from inflammation, they generally retain this flattened or oval shape (20).

Malignant lymph nodes are typically more rounded with the anterior-posterior diameter more equal to the transverse diameter (Figures 10.2 and 10.3). This rounded or bulging shape is a strong indication that the lymph node enlargement is due to malignancy. Measure the anterior-posterior diameter of a lymph node and the transverse diameter; and calculate the A-P/T Ratio. Most modern ultrasound equipment has an on-board computer that does this automatically. If the A-P/T Ratio exceeds 0.7, the lymph node should be considered suspicious for malignancy (Figures 10.4 and 10.5) (17). Those that have an anterior-posterior diameter of one centimeter or greater should have an UG FNA biopsy. Suspicious nodes with an anterior-posterior diameter between 0.5 and one centimeter should be marked and re-examined in three to six months.

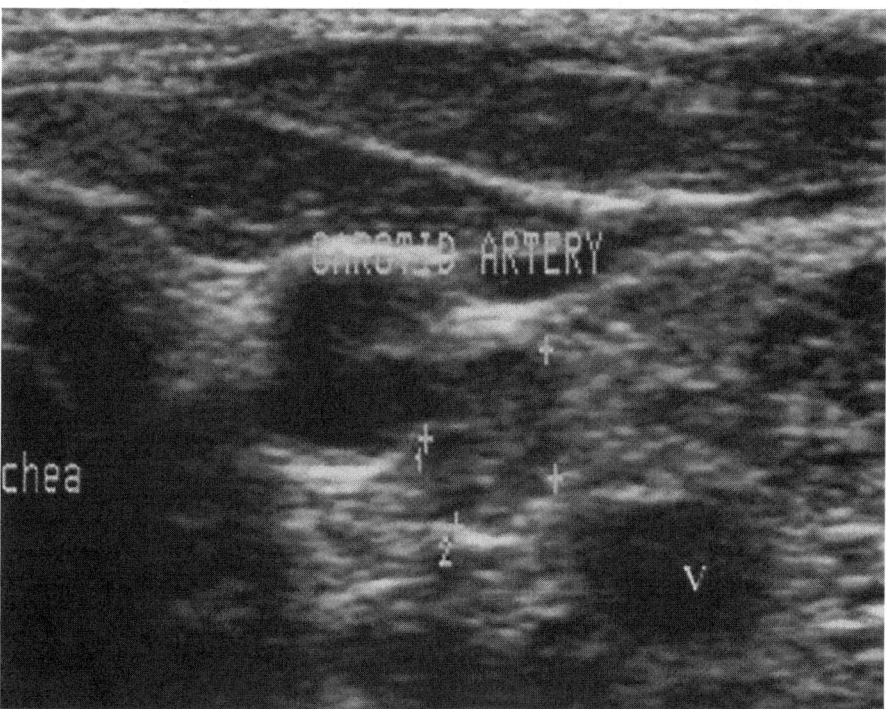

Figure 10.2 Metastatic Lymph Node in Carotid Sheath. Small rounded lymph node marked by calipers in connective tissue between common carotid artery and the internal jugular vein (V). UG FNA biopsy confirmed papillary cancer.

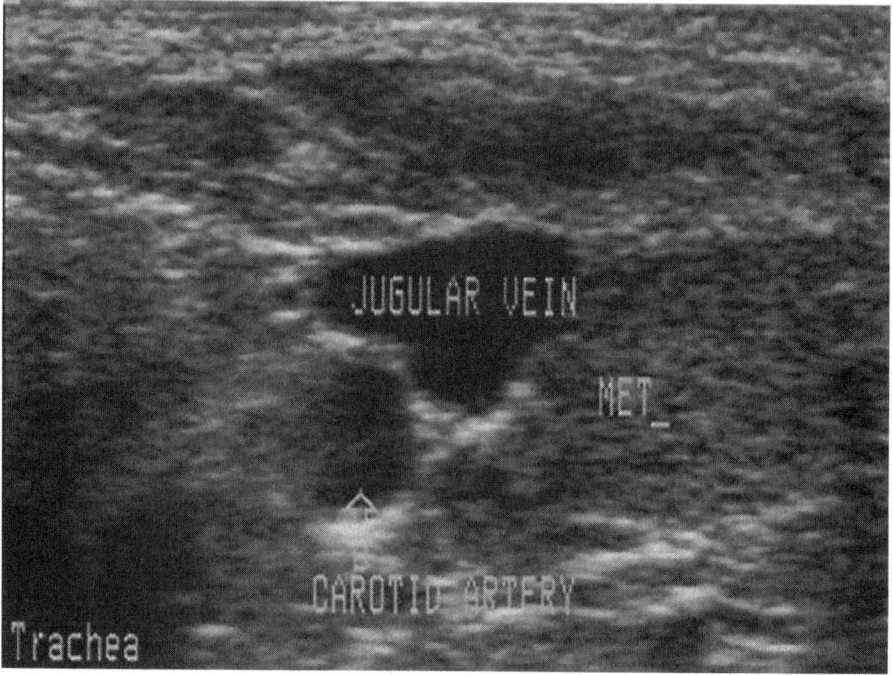

Figure 10.3 Metastatic Lymph Node. Lymph node (MET) lateral to the carotid artery and jugular vein. Note absence of hilar line. Although this node was large, it could not be palpated on physical examination. Malignancy was confirmed by UG FNA biopsy

Calcifications

Analogous to the microcalcifications seen in many malignant thyroid nodules, calcifications are sometimes an indication of malignancy in a metastatic lymph node. They appear as echogenic foci within the lymph node due to punctate flecks of calcium and are frequent in metastasis from medullary cancer. They are occasionally seen in metastasis from papillary cancer, but are not specific for malignancy since calcifications may also be seen in granulomatous lymph nodes.

Hilar Line

Normal and inflammatory lymph nodes frequently have an echogenic line running thorough the middle of the lymph node (Figure 10.6). It is thought to be due to fat within the hilus of the lymph node and is referred to as a hilar line. The presence of a hilar line is a good indication that the lymph node is not malignant. Solbaiti, et al reported a hilar line in only 4% of malignant lymph nodes (21).

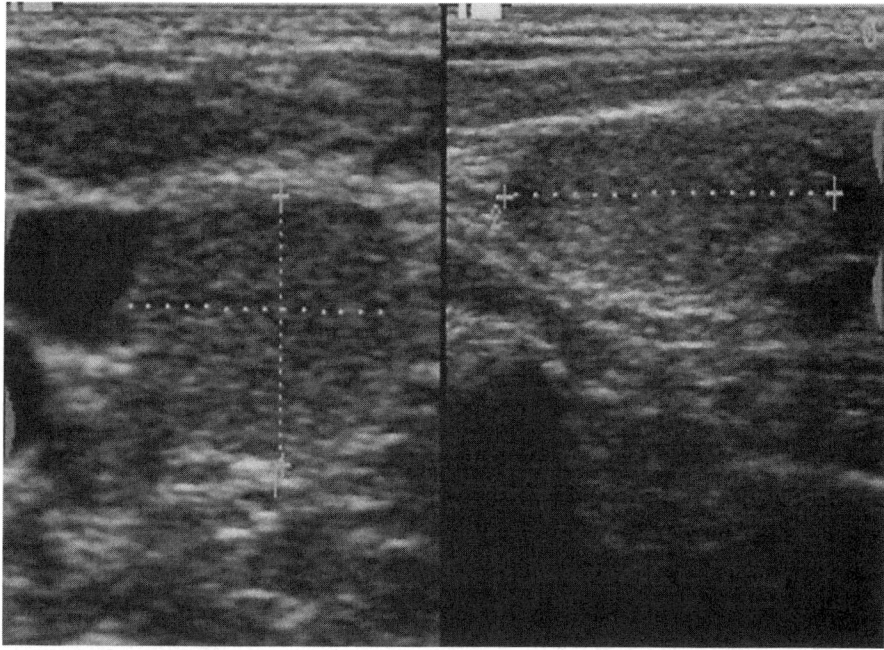

Figure 10.4 Malignant Lymph Node. Transverse and Longitudinal Views. Note the rounded or bulging shape of this node in the transverse view (A-P/T Ratio >0.7), but the flattened shape of the same lymph node in the longitudinal view. Ultrasound of the neck to look for malignant nodes should be done in the transverse view.

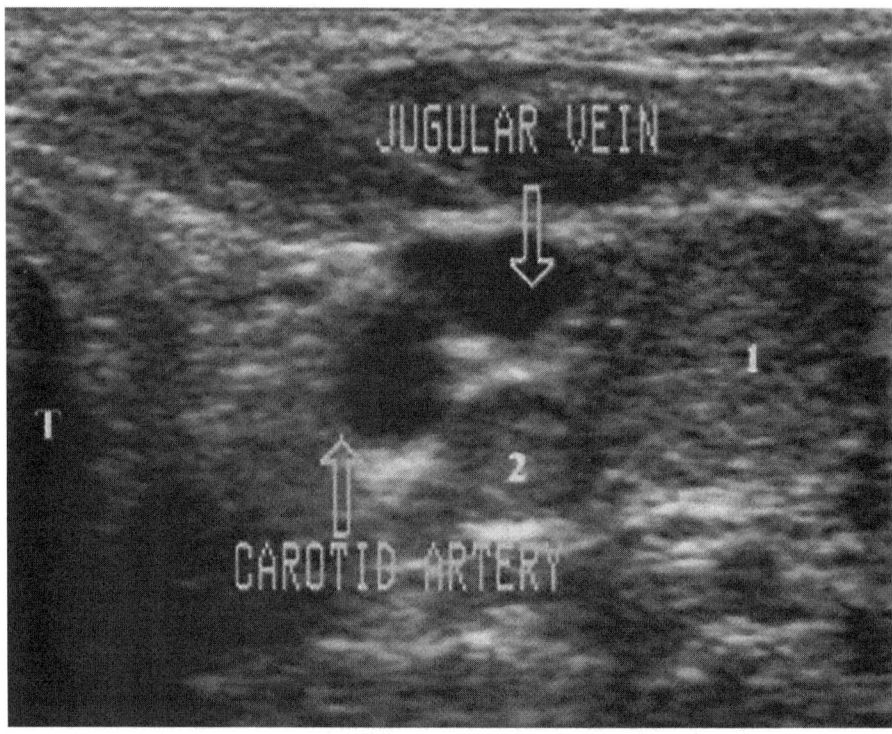

Figure 10.5 Two Malignant Lymph Nodes. Both the large (1) and the small (2) nodes have the typical rounded appearance of metastatic lymph nodes. Papillary cancer was confirmed in both lymph nodes at surgery

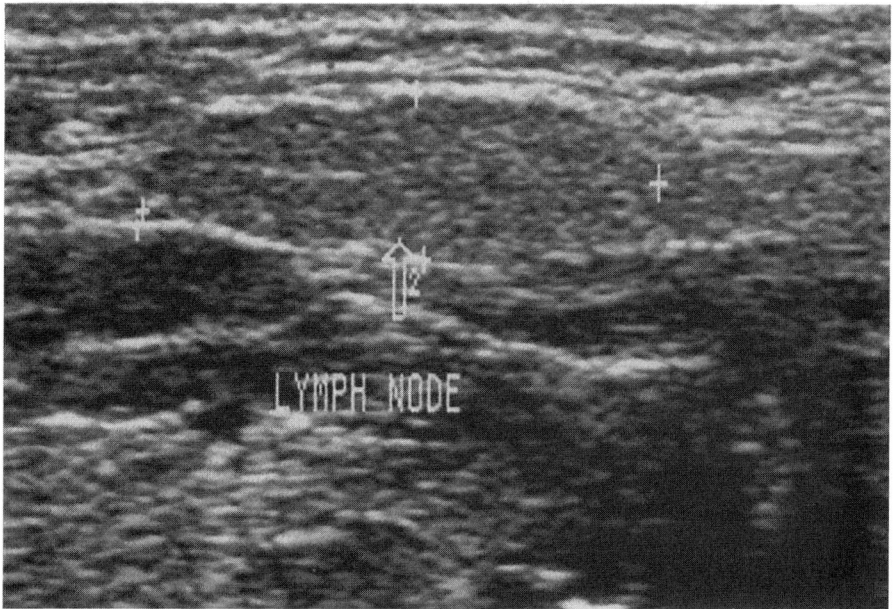

Figure 10.6 Benign Lymph Node. Superficial, benign lymph node in the neck. Note the flattened shape of the node and the partial hilar line.

UG FNA BIOPSY OF CERVICAL LYMPH NODES

Although the shape and the internal structural characteristics of lymph nodes seen with ultrasound are valuable in detecting which lymph nodes are most likely to be malignant, a UG FNA biopsy is necessary to confirm the diagnosis (22). Patients with a suppressed Tg > 3ug/L should undergo ultrasound. If an enlarged rounded lymph node with an oval appearance (A-P/T Ratio >0.7) is discovered, an UG FNA biopsy is indicated. However, some investigators do not feel a biopsy is necessary if a hilar line is present (16).

For those physicians who are accustomed to performing UG FNA biopsies of thyroid nodules, doing an UG FNA biopsy of a cervical lymph node will not present a problem. Just as in performing a biopsy of a thyroid nodule, sterile technique is maintained. Visualization of the biopsy needle in the near field is aided by a jiggling in-and-out motion of the needle (23-24). The bevel of the biopsy needle is observed using ultrasound until it enters the lymph node. A spin and suction technique, rather than a jabbing technique, works best to obtain the specimen. The slides are prepared the same as with thyroid nodule material using Papilliconou fixative.

Frasoldati, et al measured the Tg in the needle wash-out after performing the UG FNA biopsy of the specimen and found markedly increased levels in those that were malignant compared with those that were benign (25). Lee, et al reported a 100%

sensitivity and specificity using this technique along with FNA biopsy and recommend doing it routinely when performing UG FNA biopsy of cervical lymph nodes (26).

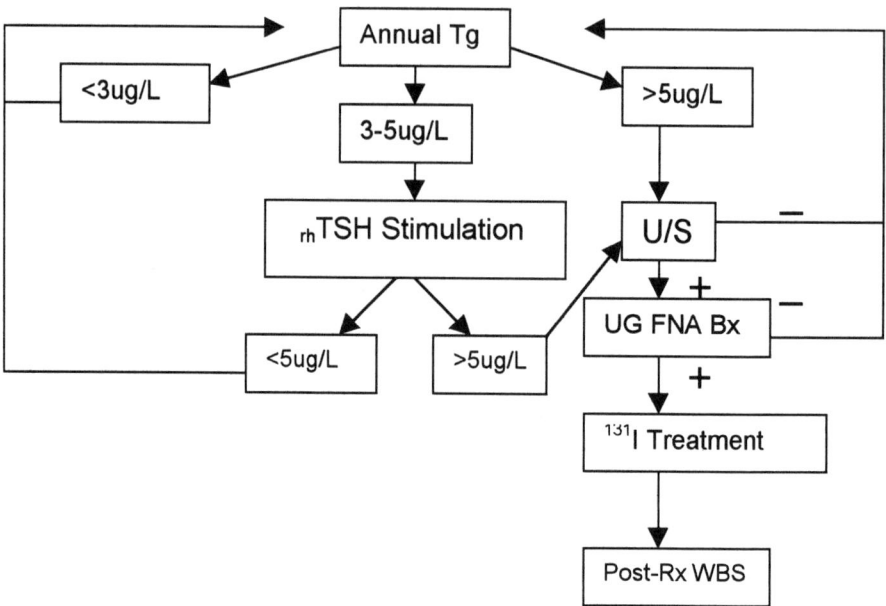

Figure 10.7 Algorithm for Following Thyroid Cancer Patients. This algorithm relies on serial Tg levels to detect recurrent or metastatic cancer after a patient has had one negative WBS. Ultrasound, UG FNA biopsy, and $_{rh}$TSH stimulation of Tg are employed rather than ^{131}I scanning to avoid stunning the thyroid cancer tissue.

Of course, a WBS should always be done after a patient has been treated with ^{131}I.

This algorithm cannot be used if the patient has anti-Tg antibodies, and it is helpful to know that the pre-op Tg was elevated.

SUMMARY

The algorithm in Figure 10.7 is designed to follow patients who do not have anti-Tg antibodies, by relying on serial monitoring of the Tg level while the patient is on l-thyroxin suppression. Once a negative WBS is obtained, no further scanning would be done, unless the patient is again treated with ^{131}I, after which a post-treatment WBS is always ordered. Tg, with $_{rh}$TSH stimulation of Tg when indicated; and ultrasound, with UG FNA biopsy when indicated, replace the routine WBS. This provides a more sensitive and cost-effective method for detecting early recurrence in the postoperative thyroid cancer patient.

REFERENCES

1. Park H., Perkins O., Edmondson J., Schnute R., Manatunga A. (1994) Influence of diagnostic radioiodines on the uptake of ablative dose of iodine-131. *Thyroid* 4; 49-54.
2. Baskin H. (1995) Thyroglobulin: a clinical review. *Endocrine Practice* 1; 365-367.
3. Torrigiani G., Doniach D., Roitt I. (1969) Serum thyroglobulin levels in healthy subjects and in patients with thyroid disease. *J Clin Endocrinol Metab* 29; 305-314.
4. Mariotti S., Martino E., Cupini c., Lari R., Giani C., Baschieri L., Pinchera A. (1982) Low serum thyroglobulin as a clue to the diagnosis of thyrotoxicosis factitia. *NEJM* 307; 410-411.
5. Van Herle A., Uller R. (1975) Elevated serum thyroglobulin. *J Clin Invest* 56; 272-277.
6. Ronga g., Fiorentino A., Paserio E., Signore A., Todino V., Tummarello M., Filesi M., Baschieri I. (1990) Can Iodine-131 whole -body scan be replaced by thyroglobulin measurement in the post-surgical follow-up of differentiated thyroid carcinoma? *J Nucl Med* 31; 1766-1771.
7. Van Sorge-Van Boxtel R., Van Eck-Smit B., Goslings B. (1993) Comparison of serum thyroglobulin, 131I and 201Tl scintigraphy in the postoperative follow-up of differentiated thyroid cancer. *Nucl Med Commun* 14; 365-372.
8. Baskin H. (1994) Effect of postoperative 131I treatment on thyroglobulin measurements in the follow-up of patients with thyroid cancer. *Thyroid* 4; 239-242.
9. Harvey R., Matheson N., Graboeski P., Rodger A. (1990) Measurement of serum thyroglobulin is of value in detecting tumor recurrence following treatment of differentiated thyroid carcinoma by lobectomy. *BR J Surg* 77;324-326
10. Ozata M., Suzuki S., Miyamoto T., Liu R., Fierro-Renoy F., DeGroot I. (1994) Serum thyroglobulin in the follow-up of patients with treated differentiated thyroid carcinoma. *J Clin Endocrinol Metab* 79; 98-105.
11. *Mazzaferri* E. (1995) Editorial: treating high thyroglobulin with radioiodine: a magic bullet or a shot in the dark? *J Clin Endocrinol Metab* 80; 1485-1491.
12. Haber R. (1998) Editorial: the diagnosis of recurrent thyroid cancer- a new approach. *J Clin Endocrinol Metab* 83; 4189-4190.
13. Reading c., Gorman C. (1993) Thyroid imaging techniques Clin *Lab Med* 13; 711-724.
14. Simeone J., Daniels G., Hall D., McCarthy K., Kopans D., Butch R., Mueller P., Stark D., Ferrucci J., Wang C. (1987) Sonography in the follow-up of 100 patients with thyroid carcinoma. *AJR* 148; 45-49.
15. Gorman B., Charboneau J., James E., Reading C., Wold L., Grant C., Gharib H., Hay I. (1987) Medullary thyroid carcinoma: Role of high-resolution US. *Radiology* 162; 147-150.
16. Sutton R., Reading C., Charboneau J., James M., Grant C., Hay I. (1988) US-guided biopsy of neck masses in postoperative management of patients with thyroid cancer. *Radiology* 168; 769-772.
17. Antonelli A., Miccoli P., Ferdeghini M., Di Coscio G., Alberti B., Iacconi P., Baldi V., Fallahi P., Baschieri L. (1995) Role of neck ultrasonography in the follow-up of patients operated on for thyroid cancer. *Thyroid* 5; 25-28.
18. Baskin H. (1996) Thyroid ultrasonography-a review. *Endocrine Practice* 3; 153-157.
19. Vassallo P., Wernecke K., Ross N., Peters P. (1992) Differentiation of benign from malignant superficial lymphadenopathy: the role of high-resolution US. *Radiology* 183; 215-220.
20. McIvor N., Freeman J., Salem S., Elden L., Noyek A., Bedard Y. (1994) Ultrasonography and ultrasound-guided fine-needle aspiration biopsy of head and neck lesions: a surgical perspective. *Laryngoscope* 104; 669-674.
21. Solbiati L., Rizzatto G., Bellotti E. (1988) High-resolution sonography of cervical lymph nodes in head and neck cancer: criteria for differentiation of reactive versus malignant nodes (abstr). *Radiology* 169; 113.
22. Boland G., Lee M., Mueller P., Mayo-Smith W., Dawson S., Simeone J. (1993) Efficacy of sonographically guided biopsy of thyroid masses and cervical lymph nodes. *ARJ* 161; 1053-1056.

23. Matalon T., Silver B. (1990) US guidance of interventional procedures. *Radiology* 174; 43-47.
24. Reading C., Charboneau J., James E., Hurt M. (1988) Sonographically guided biopsy of small (3 cm or less) masses. *ARJ* 151; 189-192.
25. Frasoldati A., Toschi E., Zini M., Flora M., Caroggio A., Dotti C., Valcavi R. (1999) Role of thyroglobulin measurement in fine-needle aspiration biopsies of cervical lymph nodes in patients with differentiated thyroid cancer. *Thyroid* 9; 105-111.
26. Lee m., Ross D., Mueller P., Daniels G., Dawson S., Simeone J. (1993) Fine-needle biopsy of cervical lymph nodes in patients with thyroid cancer: a prospective comparison of cytopathologic and tissue marker analysis. *Radiology* 187; 851-854.

11

PERCUTANEOUS ETHANOL INJECTION OF BENIGN THYROID NODULES AND CYSTS USING ULTRASOUND

Enrico Papini, M.D.
Department of Endocrine, Metabolic and Digestive Diseases
Claudio M. Pacella, M.D.
Department of Diagnostic Imaging,
Ospedale Regina Apostolorum
Albano, Rome, Italy

INTRODUCTION

Ultrasound (US) evaluation of the thyroid gland and US-guided fine needle-aspiration biopsy (FNA) of thyroid lesions have become the natural diagnostic complement of physical examination in endocrinological practice. The safety and ease of FNA have led to the attempt to change this diagnostic technique into an office-based, low-cost, nonsurgical procedure for the treatment of benign thyroid nodules. On the basis of experience in the treatment of hepatocellular carcinomas (1) and of parathyroid tumors (2 - 4), US-guided percutaneous ethanol injection (PEI) was first proposed in 1990 as a possible therapy for autonomously functioning thyroid nodules (AFTN) (5). Since then, several reports have confirmed the feasibility and effectiveness of PEI in the treatment of AFTN (6 - 13), of cystic thyroid nodules (14 - 17) and of benign cold thyroid nodules (18 - 22).

At the present time PEI is performed in clinical practice in Italy and in a few other European (23 - 27) and Japanese centers (28 - 30). The technique is not used in the U.S.A, where no trials on its effects have yet been carried out. This can be attributed to the complications reported during the first years of use of PEI (31), before the technique was perfected. Moreover, a lack of experience in interventional ultrasonography and only partial knowledge of the new procedure prevented many endocrinologists from adopting PEI in their clinical practice.

These reasons explain the American reluctance to abandon in all cases, even the most suitable, surgical and radioiodine treatments for a new therapeutical procedure, still considered experimental and potentially harmful in the USA (32).

This chapter deals in some detail with the actual procedure of PEI, and the hazards involved in its performance. The efficacy, limits and side effects of PEI will be compared with those of radioiodine treatment and surgery in order to identify the specific indications of percutaneous treatment.

Procedure
PEI is performed on outpatients; the patient should not be fasted and can safely go home (or to work) after each PEI session. There is no need of local or general anesthesia, bed rest or observation of the patient after the procedure. In case of mild pain a single dose of an analgesic (aspirin or ketoprofen) is administered by mouth. No preliminary analysis of blood clotting is needed (in our experience hematomas are rare and rapidly self-resolving), but it is advisable to avoid the administration of anticoagulant or antiaggregant drugs the day before treatment and to ask about the presence of clotting disorders.

The time required for the procedure itself is about 15 minutes. As injection is preceded by a careful US and CD examination of the thyroid and followed by examination of the cervical structures, sessions should be scheduled at half-hourly intervals.

Thyrotoxicosis due to conditions for which PEI is not suitable (such as Graves' disease or multiple hyperfunctioning areas) should be excluded beforehand. Coexisting hypofunctioning nodules should be searched for and prior to PEI treatment FNA should be performed on each observed lesion to avoid the risk of later thyroidectomy due to the growth of previously unrecognized suspicious lesions. Indeed, differentiated carcinomas only rarely present as AFTN but malignant nodules are not infrequently associated with hyperfunctioning nodules or with pseudocystic lesions (33).

Fully Informing Patient
Before treatment the patient should be thoroughly informed about the characteristics of the procedure, and the advantages and disadvantages of PEI. In particular, it should be explained that the aim of PEI is to obtain by means of a nonsurgical procedure a rapid and striking decrease of the volume (and, in the case of AFTN, of the function) of thyroid lesions.

The treatment has a very low risk of permanent recurrent nerve damage, with no risk of bleeding, scars or, particularly, late hypothyroidism (34 - 37).

The disadvantages should also be clearly explained: need of repeated treatments, brief pain during alcohol injection, mild cervical tenderness for 24 - 48 hours after the procedure.

In the case of AFTN it should be explained that PEI induces a greater and more rapid volume decrease than 131-I, without the considerable risk of late hypothyroidism associated with the latter therapy (38 - 39). However, it should be pointed out that PEI is more time-consuming, complicated and painful than radioiodine treatment and that it presents a low risk of persistent hyperfunction (particularly low for lesions with a largest diameter of less than 30 mm).

The patient should be informed that recurrent nerve damage, the only dangerous complication of PEI, is quite rare in skilled hands (less than 1 % of patients treated in our last five years' experience). As the severity of damage (almost always temporary (34, 37)) and the time required for resuming nerve function (from a few minutes to three months) are related to the extent of chemical damage induced by alcohol, the patient should be asked to pronounce at regular intervals a word beginning with a vowel ("advance", for example) (35).

It should be explained that the pain induced by ethanol decreases immediately after the injection; the patient should be asked to raise his left hand when pain increases and to lower it when pain subsides (after about 30") after which the treatment can be resumed.

In the case of cystic nodules, it should be stressed that cervical pain is rare (17% of reported cases), short-lasting and mild. Local or general complications are nearly absent (no transient dysphonia and no late hypothyroidism were observed in 123 cases reported from the major trials in this field (15 - 16, 30)). The number of treatments is quite low (one or two sessions in most cases) and the patient should be told that the only therapeutic alternative for recurrent cyst is surgery. Thyroidectomy, however, involves a higher cost, a higher incidence of local complications (permanent recurrent nerve damage, wound bleeding, cosmetic damage from scarring) and the not infrequent occurrence of late hypothyroidism (40). A written informed consent should be signed by the patient before treatment.

Technique of Treatment

1. Autonomously Functioning Thyroid Nodules

PEI can be performed by one operator, who inserts a 22-gauge 75-mm spinal needle (Yale Spinal Needle, Becton Dickinson, Milano, Italy) through a guiding device connected to the probe (US-guided procedure), or by two operators, one handling the probe and the other the needle (US-assisted procedure). Both techniques are effective: the former is less expensive (as only one physician is needed) and, owing to its ease, does not require extensive training. Indeed the needle enters the cervical structures along a pre-determined line and the depth of the needle tip penetration can be calculated in advance. The puncture of the skin by the blunted tip of the spinal needle induces a mild but unpleasant pain that can become intolerable when insertions must be repeated during the same session.

The US-assisted procedure requires two operators trained to work together, but needle insertion can be performed without a fixed entry angle. That offers a wider choice of needle entry points, which is quite important when "difficult" areas of the AFTN are to be treated, and avoids the pain caused by needle penetration through the thick anterior neck muscles. As the probe can be moved freely from the inserted needle, continuous US monitoring of the cervical structures surrounding the nodule is possible. That allows the operator to change the scan axis in order to check more thoroughly for ethanol seepage outside the nodule and to determine when the treatment is completed.

The patient is asked to lie in a supine position, with his neck slightly hyperextended over a small pillow. The sonographer and the real-time ultrasound machine, fitted with a 10 - 13-MHz probe, are to the right of the patient, and the operator is at the patient's head.

After a careful US and CD examination of the thyroid and of the cervical structures, the skin is sterilized with an antiseptic solution, serving also as ultrasonic transmission medium for the probe (which is wrapped in a disposable plastic film). The patient is instructed to swallow only at regular intervals (when indicated by the operator) to avoid unexpected thyroid excursions and sudden needle displacements. A disposable 25-gauge, 50-mm flexible needle (Monoject 200, Sherwood Medical, St Louis, Mo) fitted to a plastic insulin syringe containing 1 ml of 2% Xylocaine is introduced without anesthesia through the skin with a gentle, slow motion. In the US-assisted procedure, the point of insertion on the skin surface and the direction of the needle are determined by means of the acoustic shadow of a thin steel bar placed between the probe and the skin. After a 1 - 2-cm penetration through the skin and the prethyroid muscles, the bar is removed, the position of the needle tip within the thyroid is reevaluated, and its angle is slightly modified to direct the tip precisely into the selected target.

Usually two injections are performed per session: the needle is positioned in the center first of the upper and then of the lower portion of the AFTN. This sequence (well tolerated, as the puncture by the 25-gauge needle is in itself nearly painless) makes possible the destruction of a greater expanse of tissue with small (2 - 4 ml) doses of 95% sterile ethanol (Ethyl-Alcohol, 10 ml vials, SALF, Bergamo, Italy) than the injection of large amounts (five or more ml) of ethanol in a single zone. Moreover, it avoids the risk and the discomfort associated with excessive increase of pressure within the nodule.

To reduce the immediate pain due to ethanol diffusion outside the thyroid (along the needle track), a preliminary bolus of Xylocaine (0.5 ml) is administered. After visualization (usually scanty) of the perfused area, a syringe containing 5 ml of 95% ethanol is then substituted. Under direct sonographic control a limited amount of ethanol (1.0 ml) is slowly (30 - 60") injected into the nodule. Ethyl alcohol distribution is visualized during injection as an inhomogeneous round hyperechoic area. The rapidly vanishing irregular image, 8 - 10 mm in diameter, is replaced by a number of scattered hyperechoic spots, which indicate ethanol deposition within the perfused thyroid tissue. After half a minute, in which the patient has been encouraged to speak and the operators have checked for extra-nodular ethanol diffusion, further slow boluses are administered at regular intervals. Injection ceases after the administration of 2 - 4 ml of ethanol, either when the treated area appears completely perfused, when the hyperechoic spots create an acoustic shadowing, or when the patient is reluctant to continue. In the case of hyperfunctioning thyroid nodules with large cystic areas, complete fluid removal is first effected and a syringe containing ethanol is then substituted for the aspirating syringe without removing the needle.

The needle is left in place for one minute, allowing fluid pressure within the nodule to decrease, and is thereafter withdrawn from the neck while 0.5 - 1.0 ml of Xylocaine is slowly injected.

After two minutes (during which the patient can change his neck position, breathe and swallow freely and is reassured about the progress of the procedure), a second injection is performed on the opposite pole of the AFTN.

Once the session is concluded, the patient is asked to lie in a non-hyperextended position for two to three further minutes, so as to avoid vasovagal reactions, and is thereafter allowed slowly to sit up. A local dressing, to be removed in the evening, is gently applied (pressure must be avoided) and a mild analgesic is administered if pain is still described as intense. After 10 minutes in the waiting room and further reassurance the patient can leave the office.

PEI is given once or twice weekly and treatment is usually completed in 3 - 6 sessions, mainly depending on the size of the hyperfunctioning nodule.

Color-Doppler and Power Doppler evaluation
After the first AFTN treatment, each session should be preceded by a careful CD or PD evaluation of the still vascularized areas. A high vascularity level indicates the presence of areas still unaffected by direct ethanol damage or by infarction due to ethanol-induced thrombosis of the AFTN vessels (41). Hence, during each treatment, needle insertion should be directed to the persistent vascular images within the nodule. In this way CD monitoring reduces the time required for successful treatment, avoiding re-treatment of already necrotized areas and aiming

alcohol diffusion at the still pervious vessels.

CD and PD findings are an early prognostic index of PEI efficacy at the end of treatment (42), when serum TSH levels are still undetectable, thyroid parenchyma is still functionally inhibited on scintiscan and further criteria to assess the completeness of PEI are lacking. The absence or the striking reduction of vascular images, the progressive decrease (30 - 40% versus baseline) of AFTN volume, and changes in tissue echogenicity (nodules more hypoechoic and inhomogeneous than at baseline, with blurred margins and disappearance of fluid collections) suggest that treatments be stopped.

A US and CD examination should be performed after one month, to evaluate the progressive reduction of nodule volume and to complete, if necessary, the treatment with a further injection aimed at the still vascularized areas. Further reduction in nodule volume can be observed by US after six and 12 months.

2. Cystic Thyroid Nodules

Pure intrathyroidal cysts are rare, but complex lesions characterized predominantly by a fluid component are frequent ultrasound findings (43). Most cystic thyroid nodules are benign, representing degenerative changes or bleeding within colloid nodules or adenomas. However, the reported prevalence of malignancy in complex thyroid lesions ranges from 0.9 to 25% of cases (44). Therefore a careful preliminary cytological evaluation is mandatory before performing PEI treatment.

During the first evaluation the cyst fluid should be aspirated completely with a 22-gauge common needle and submitted, after cytocentrifugation, to an experienced cytologist. After careful US and CD examination for possible suspicious areas within the residual solid portion of the nodule, two or more FNA passages are performed with a 27-gauge, 19-mm ultra-thin needle (Microlance 3, Becton Dickinson, Dublin, Ireland) on different zones of the nodule wall until satisfactory smears for cytological evaluation are obtained. Two weeks later, in the event of fluid recurrence and after cytological confirmation of the benign nature of the nodule, PEI treatment is performed.

The PEI procedure for cystic nodules is similar to that adopted for AFTN treatment. After the insertion of a 22-gauge common needle fitted to a 20-ml plastic syringe inserted into a steel syringe holder, a nearly complete fluid removal is slowly performed. When the needle tip is surrounded by a small amount of fluid (less than 1 ml), a syringe containing ethanol is substituted for the aspirating syringe without removing the needle. The utmost attention must be paid to keeping the needle tip in the center of the small residual fluid collection. A quantity of ethanol equivalent to 25% of the volume of aspirated fluid, but not exceeding 10 mL, is then slowly injected (with the precautions described in the paragraph concerning AFTN). When a rapidly refilling area is observed within the lesion, ethyl alcohol should be rapidly and precisely injected into the enlarging zone.

The needle is left in place for one minute, allowing the fluid pressure within the nodule to decrease, and is thereafter withdrawn from the neck while 0.5 - 1.0 ml of Xylocaine is slowly injected.. Care must be taken not to press the treated lesion in any way. The session is concluded as described above.

3. Solid Cold Thyroid Nodules

Due to the relatively high risk of thyroid cancer in cold nodules, prior to PEI FNA should be performed on different areas of the lesion and should be repeated at least twice at different times. PEI should not be carried out until an unequivocally benign cytological diagnosis is obtained. The patient should be informed that ethanol treatment causes cellular damage that could make it difficult to perform a cytological diagnosis in the case of subsequent nodule regrowth (45). In our experience, histological evaluation of resected cold nodules can also be hampered by previous PEI treatments. The patient's willingness to endure a prolonged follow-up should always be assessed.

PEI is performed under ultrasound guidance as described for AFTN. Since most cold thyroid nodules lack a well-defined peripheral capsule, ethanol injection must be carefully monitored and an increase of intranodular volume due to excessive fluid injection must be avoided.

In the case of small nodules a single treatment is usually performed (21). Large locally symptomatic nodules need repeated injections to show a satisfactory clinical improvement (22).

Major Hazards and Possible Mistakes

1. Risk of Vocal cord paresis.

In experienced hands, it is nearly impossible to induce severe adverse reactions, such as tissue fibrosis in the cervical structures surrounding the gland, thromboembolic effects in large neck vessels, or complications requiring hospitalization. However, transient dysphonia (self-resolving in a few hours or months) was first reported in 2 - 5 % of treated AFTN (36). All the affected patients who were examined by an ENT physician had unilateral vocal cord paresis induced either by direct chemical damage of the recurrent laryngeal nerve (caused by ethanol seepage outside the thyroid capsule) or by nerve compression (caused by a sudden increase in intranodular pressure). Although complete recovery from vocal cord paresis was documented by indirect laryngoscopy in almost all the reported cases (34 - 35, 37), special care must be taken to follow these safety rules:

a. Needle tip position should always be carefully checked before ethanol injection. A safe area of injection is obtained when the needle tip is observed at least 3 - 5 mm within the nodule margins both in long and short axis scans. Particular attention should be devoted to posterior and caudal nodules, which are probably close to the ipsilateral recurrent nerve.

b. If, during needle positioning, the tip accidentally goes beyond the posterior margin of the nodule and the thyroid capsule, it is advisable to avoid alcohol injection. Indeed, even if the needle is withdrawn and thereafter correctly positioned within the nodule, ethanol could seep posteriorly through the needle track inducing recurrent nerve damage.

c. When the nodule appears swollen, ethanol injection should be stopped in order to avoid alcohol seepage outside the lesion due to high fluid pressure.

d. After ethanol injection, multiple hyperechoic spots can create acoustic shadowing that hampers clear needle visualization. As swallowing can change the needle tip position, in these cases it is wise to suspend ethanol injection, withdraw the needle and insert it again into a not yet treated part of the lesion.

e. After a few treatments the nodule can become fibrotic and hard to penetrate. A forceful injection of large amounts of ethanol could induce ethanol seepage outside the lesion.

f. It is helpful to ask the patient to speak at regular intervals during the PEI procedure to ensure that the recurrent laryngeal nerve is intact.

2. Neck pain and extraglandular fibrosis.
Retrograde diffusion of ethanol along the needle track causes neck pain (due to chemical irritation of the superficial cervical structures) and mild extraglandular fibrosis. These side effects can be prevented by:
a. avoiding the rapid injection of excessive amounts of ethanol into a single site;
b. waiting a few seconds before retracting the needle at the end of treatment;
c. injecting small amounts (1 ml) of Xylocaine immediately before and during needle withdrawal (35).

3. Worsening of Thyrotoxicosis.
Although PEI is followed by an acute increase in serum thyroglobulin levels (due to ethanol-induced damage of thyroid follicles), only slight increases in serum thyroid hormones are usually observed after the procedure. In very few patients with severe thyrotoxicosis (rare in AFTN) the procedure is followed by transient exacerbation of thyrotoxic symptoms (12). This side effect can be prevented in hyperthyroid patients (especially elderly people with cardiovascular diseases) by means of a short-term pretreatment with beta-blockers and/or methimazole.

4. Driving ability
There is no evidence that serum ethanol level increases after PEI, since a small amount of ethanol is injected into the nodule (35). In our experience, no patient has complained of drowsiness, headache or difficulty with coordination after treatment.

5. Overlooked malignancy

Prior to PEI treatment a careful US evaluation of the thyroid should always be performed. Since thyroid lesions are not surgically removed, FNA should be performed on each observed nodule to avoid later thyroidectomy necessitated by previously unrecognized suspicious lesions, and to prevent the insidious growth and diffusion of overlooked malignancies (46). This hazard, in our opinion, precludes extensive use of PEI in cold solid lesions.

In cystic nodules FNA should be performed (after fluid drainage) on the solid areas of the lesion and should be repeated at least twice at different times.

PEI should not be attempted until an unequivocally benign cytological diagnosis is obtained. Ethanol treatment induces cellular damage that could make it difficult to obtain a cytological diagnosis in the case of subsequent nodule regrowth (45).

6. Hematomas and Thrombosis

These quite rare complications (36) are due to gross mistakes in performing the procedure (accidental puncture of medium- or large-size vessels) or to an attempt to make a sharp change in needle direction without first withdrawing the needle from the neck.

7. Fainting

To avoid vasovagal reactions at the end of the session (11) the patient should be asked to lie in a nonhyperextended position for two to three minutes while breathing and swallowing freely. Then the patient can slowly sit up.

TISSUE CHANGES

The diffusion of absolute ethanol within tissues causes cellular dehydration, protein denaturation and coagulative necrosis. Ethanol drainage into the small vessels is followed by endothelial damage and intraluminal thrombosis. Hence PEI induces a complex pattern of thyroid damage including directly induced coagulative necrosis of thyroid tissue, hemorrhagic infarction (due to vascular thrombosis) and reduction of enzyme activity in the still viable areas surrounding the zones of complete chemical ablation (41). The treated areas are surrounded by a granulomatous reaction with multinucleate giant cells and plump fibroblasts. These findings explain the marked and rapid shrinkage induced by PEI (the final nodule volume is about 30% of the baseline value) and the nonrecurrence of hyperthyoidism in completely cured AFTN (since the treated nodule is gradually substituted by scarring granulation tissue).

In AFTN removed after PEI the necrotic areas were easily distinguished from the surrounding thyroid parenchyma, and the healthy thyroid tissue appeared devoid of regressive or inflammatory features and thrombosis of small vessels. No adhesions or fibrosis were present outside the thyroid capsule in patients correctly treated with PEI. These findings confirm that subsequent surgical treatments are feasible, if needed, after PEI (28, 41).

The absence of lymphocytic infiltration explains the extreme rarity of permanent serum autoantibody surge and consequently of hypothyroidism or Graves' disease even after a prolonged period (4 - 8 years).

ROLE OF PEI IN CLINICAL PRACTICE
Efficacy and limits of PEI
PEI is a low-cost technique because it does not require hospitalization and uses widely available US machines and inexpensive materials. Neither surgical nor nuclear medicine facilities are needed. The endocrinologist and/or the sonographer can themselves perform the treatment as part of their normal routine. However, it is essential that operators be well trained so as to avoid damage to the recurrent laryngeal nerve. Endocrinologists should approach PEI only after acquiring thorough knowledge of sonographic neck anatomy and US-guided biopsy. It is then advisable to start thyroid interventional procedures beginning with the drainage and sclerosis of cystic nodules (the thyroid lesions that are easiest to treat and at the lowest risk of recurrent nerve damage). Thereafter, treatment of small nontoxic AFTN can be undertaken. Beginners should aim only at inducing a decrease in nodule volume. Indeed, complete functional ablation requires several sessions and an almost complete destruction of the AFTN, with greater risk of complications when operators are unskilled.

One of the advantages of PEI is the selective damage to the lesion and the sparing of the surrounding thyroid parenchyma (41), associated with the absence at a prolonged follow-up (8 years, in our experience) of persistent increase in serum autoantibodies and of late hypothyroidism after PEI.

Care in performing the percutaneous procedure avoids damage to the thyroid capsule or the other structures of the anterior cervical region (12). Several patients have undergone surgical excision without any problem after a correctly performed PEI treatment (28, 41). Hence it would seem that an ineffective PEI treatment does not preclude successful subsequent surgical therapy of thyroid lesions, if needed.

Nontoxic AFTN
PEI seems to be especially suited to the treatment of small nontoxic AFTN in young patients.

There are conflicting data on the risk of evolution of toxicity in nontoxic AFTN. The rate of transition from nontoxic to toxic AFTN in follow-up studies (which have generally involved a small number of cases and relatively short periods of time) ranged from 1.2 to 5.7% per year (47 - 48). These data are consistent with a prolonged study that demonstrated the passage of AFTN to overt hyperthyroidism in 16% of cases in 7.5 years (49). In a recent paper (39), however, the use of sensitive TSH and free-T3 determinations demonstrated subclinical hyperthyroidism in 73.5% of AFTN at presentation. During follow-up the progression to thyrotoxicosis was observed in an additional 24.4%. Nodule growth was demonstrated in 33% of cases during 30 months and, interestingly, the occurrence of cystic changes did not normalize hyperfunction in any AFTN.

On the basis of these data, many endocrinologists suggest a conservative management of patients with nontoxic AFTN, since the low rate of toxic evolution does not justify the disadvantages of surgery (50 - 51) and the risk of post-radioiodine hypothyroidism is relatively high when suppression of extranodular tissue function is incomplete (38, 52 - 53).

Young patients with untreated AFTN, however, need long-term (time-consuming and expensive) follow up with repeated clinical, ultrasound and hormonal evaluation because of the risk of progressive increase of nodule size and of progression to hyperthyroidism. Indeed, prolonged subclinical hyperthyroidism may be associated with accelerated bone turnover and progressive reduction of bone mineral content (54). In older patients with subclinical cardiac disease, the erratic hormone secretion of AFTN (often characterized by mild T3-toxicosis) may induce tachyarrhythmia or precipitate cardiac failure (55).

In nontoxic AFTN, usually small in size (maximum diameter <30 mm), PEI is rapid (only 3 – 4 sessions are generally needed) and highly effective against hyperfunction (normalization of serum TSH levels is reported in 68 -100% of the cases) (34 - 37). PEI induces an impressive reduction in nodule volume (after 6 - 12 months the nodule dimensions shrink to 30-40% of the baseline volume) which seems to be greater and to occur sooner than with radioiodine. In our experience, the therapeutic results are long-lasting (unchanged after eight years of follow-up) and are not associated with late thyroid function impairment.

Hence decreasing the volume and function of AFTN by means of a small number of mini-invasive outpatient treatments is more cost-effective and, for the patient, a more attractive option then simply waiting and periodically evaluating clinical and hormonal conditions, with the impending possibility of later ablation and its attendant risk of surgical complications and impaired thyroid function.

Thyroid cysts
PEI is highly effective in the treatment of thyroid cysts and of "complex" thyroid nodules. Although aspiration by itself may cure thyroid cysts (56), recurrences are quite common, and surgery is often the final treatment of large recurring lesions. In a prospective randomized trial PEI proved to be significantly superior to aspiration alone in inducing volume reduction (16). Furthermore, the reported recurrence rate of pure thyroid cysts treated by PEI was 5% in a 6-month survey (15). In a 12-month prospective study only one out of 38 complex (predominantly

cystic) thyroid nodules recurred (16). In these studies no adverse effects were reported and the procedure needed to be performed only once or twice to be completely effective.

Surgery, the only alternative treatment to ethanol injection for recurrent or enlarging thyroid cysts, is more expensive, painful and liable to produce transient or permanent complications (50 - 51) than PEI.

Toxic AFTN

Radioiodine therapy is less complicated and more cost-effective than PEI in the treatment of large toxic AFTN, since repeated PEI sessions are needed to complete the therapy.

The Italian multicenter study (318 patients with a follow-up period of 3 - 12 months) and several long-term studies (34 - 37) confirmed the rapid and persistent efficacy of the procedure. However, the most important factors in predicting the response to PEI were the baseline nodule volume and the skill of the operators. Thyroid nodules less than 10 ml in volume showed complete therapeutic response (i.e. normalization of serum TSH and thyroid hormones, nodule volume decrease, and effacement of the previously hyperfunctioning area at thyroid scintiscan) in most patients. On the contrary, only a minority of nodules with a volume greater than 40 ml was successfully treated. In fact, the volume of thyroid tissue ablated by each procedure is relatively small (41) and large nodules thus require an impracticably high number of injections. The importance of skilled operators was confirmed by the results reported by different centers. Indeed, the reported rate of complete therapeutic response in toxic AFTN ranged from 64 to 85%.

In our opinion, radioiodine is the first-line treatment for large AFTN (maximum diameter >3.0 cm). In these cases, in fact, the necessary number of ethanol injections under US guidance (and, therefore, the cost, discomfort and risk of the procedure) increases, while the probability of complete therapeutic efficacy decreases (it was equal to 50 - 89% of the treated cases in a pool of 11 studies including 394 patients (31)). Thus, PEI treatment of large toxic AFTN should be reserved for selected cases such as patients who are pregnant (57), live in geographical areas devoid of nuclear medicine facilities, are poor risks for surgery, or refuse or present contraindications to irradiation.

Toxic multinodular goiters

PEI is less good than radioiodine in the treatment of patients with toxic multinodular goiter. Toxic multinodular goiters are characterized by multiple discrete foci of autonomy (58), and after successful chemical ablation of the hyperfunctioning area a significant recurrence rate should be expected, due to the other areas of functional autonomy. On the other hand, radioiodine therapy induces a safe and atraumatic control of hyperthyroidism and a slow but progressive decrease of nodular goiter volume (59). Most patients with toxic multinodular goiter are elderly and therefore irradiation and late hypothyroidism are not a problem.

PEI should be reserved for the rare patients who refuse (or do not have access to) 131-I, present an unacceptable surgical risk, and have a toxic multinodular goiter with a dominant hyperfunctioning lesion which causes compressive symptoms.

Cold solid nodules
Palpable cold solid nodules are present in 4 - 7% of the general population (60). FNA has made it possible to select the nodules at low risk of malignancy and has sharply reduced thyroid surgery for solitary nonfunctioning nodules. However, only a subgroup (about 50%) of cytologically benign nodules is responsive to the usual L-T4 suppressive therapy (61). Unresponsive nodules can just be observed over time (many of them however show slow but progressive growth) or can be surgically resected (62). As surgery is not devoid of side effects, including late hypothyroidism, PEI was proposed as a debulking procedure for solitary solid, cytologically benign nodules, which are cold at scintiscan (18). Several trials have confirmed a significant reduction in nodule size after multiple sessions of PEI (20, 22). In a recent study (21) a single dose of ethanol (one third of the nodule volume) was injected into the lesion. Nodule volume decrease was already observable one month after treatment, and after six months the mean nodule volume decrease was 43% versus baseline.

The procedure is effective and could be employed for patients with large nodules who complain of local symptoms and who refuse surgery or are a poor surgical risk and are not responsive to, or whose condition contraindicates levothyroxine suppressive therapy (22).

PEI, however, should be performed only in carefully selected cases of hypofunctioning thyroid nodules because of the relatively high risk of thyroid neoplasia in these cases (63).

Indications for PEI treatment.
In our opinion, PEI should become the first-line treatment of recurrent thyroid cysts (simple or complex), once malignancy has been excluded by careful cytologic evaluation. The lesion is rapidly and definitively treated by PEI, local symptoms subside, the patient is reassured, and the risk of progressive growth leading to surgery is prevented.

Small AFTN (diameter < 3 cm), mainly if not yet completely suppressing the surrounding thyroid parenchyma, are best treated by PEI. Indeed, the avoidance of scarring, the lack of exposure to radiation, the absence of hypothyroidism following the procedure, and the achievement of an effective reduction in the size of the nodule without surgical intervention make this procedure very appealing to young patients.

Radioiodine and surgery remain the treatments of choice for large (> 3 cm) toxic thyroid nodules and toxic multinodular goiters. PEI should be used only in selected cases as a substitute either for surgery (i.e. when patient has had previous neck operation, is a poor surgical risk or refuses surgery), or for ^{131}I therapy (i.e. when patient is pregnant or young, if no nuclear medicine facilities are available or if irradiation is contraindicated).

In our opinion PEI should not be generally used in current clinical practice to ablate cold thyroid nodules. The technique should be reserved to the highly selected (and rare) cases not amenable to the established treatments. Indeed, the relatively high risk of malignancy makes a prolonged and careful follow-up of all treated lesions essential. Moreover cellular changes induced by alcohol make cytological diagnosis less reliable in the case of nodule growth.

Acknowledgments

This chapter was made possible by the essential contributions of all the members of our Departments. In particular, we wish to thank:

Vincenzo Anelli, M.D.; Antonio Bianchini, M.D.; Giancarlo Bizzarri, M.D.; Anna Crescenzi, M.D.; Rinaldo Gugliemi, M.D.; Sara Pacella; Claudio Panunzi, M.D.; Lucilla Petrucci, M.D.; Guido Pisicchio; Roberta Rinaldi, M.D.; Silvia Taccogna, M.D. and Prof. Francesco Nardi, M.D..

An Illustrated Guide to Percutaneous Injection Procedure

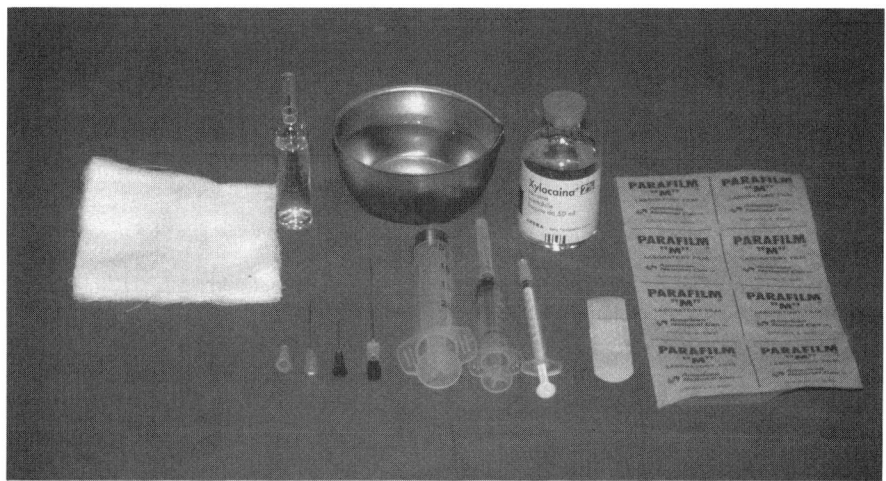

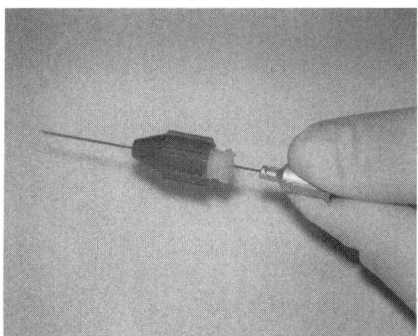
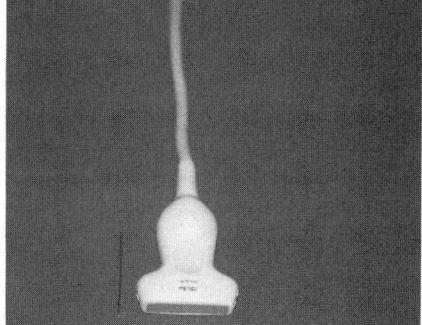

I. MATERIALS

Figure 11. 1: Materials needed for US-assisted PEI treatment. A: 10-ml sterile vial of 95% ethanol, 2% Xylocaine bottle, insulin syringe, disposable 5-ml and 20-ml plastic syringes, 22-gauge 20-mm needle, Monoject 200 (25-gauge 50-mm) needle, Yale spinal (22-gauge 75-mm) needle, 27-gauge 19-mm needle, steel bar, antiseptic solution, plastic film, sterile dressings, disposable gloves, sterile towels. **B:** Monoject 200 is the disposable needle currently most frequently used in our clinical practice. The sharp tip of this ultra-thin flexible needle punctures almost painlessly, thus allowing us to perform multiple treatments during the same PEI session. **C:** The 10 – 13-MHz probe and the steel bar used for the US-assisted procedure.

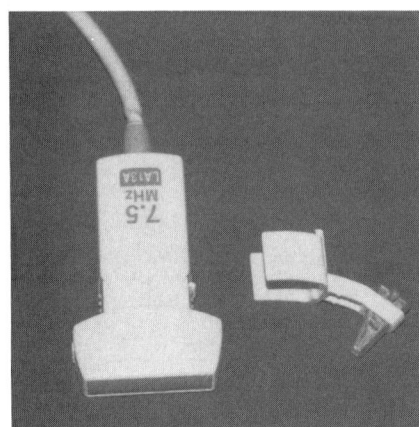
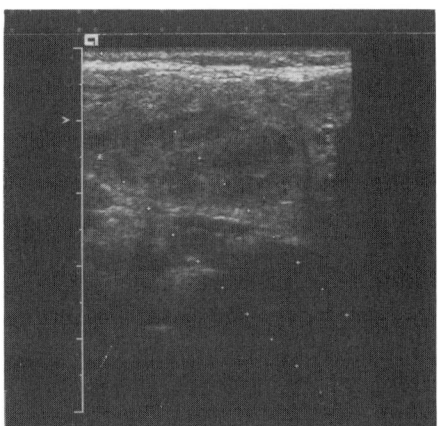
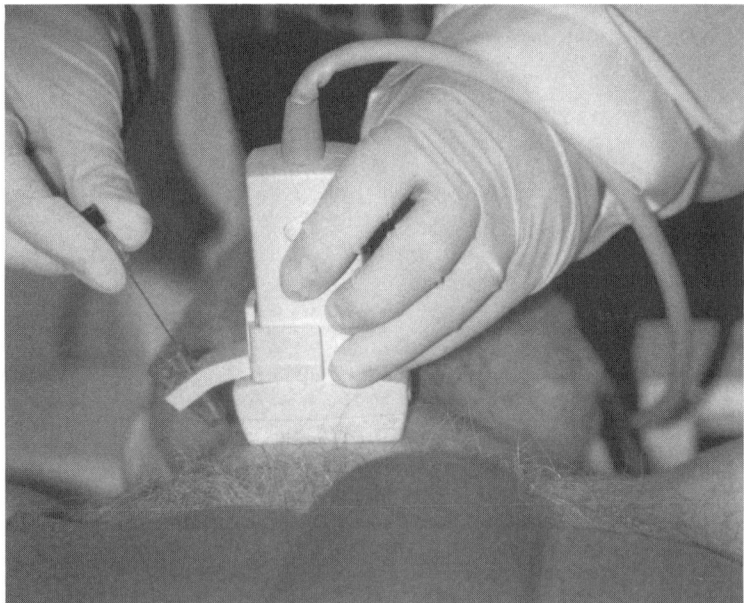

Figure 11. 2: US-guided PEI technique. A: 7.5 - 10-MHz US probe with guiding device for the US-guided PEI treatment. **B**: US image showing the electronic track which guides needle insertion into the target nodule. **C**: Spinal needle insertion through the guiding device. The whole procedure can be performed by a single operator with the aid of a nurse.

185

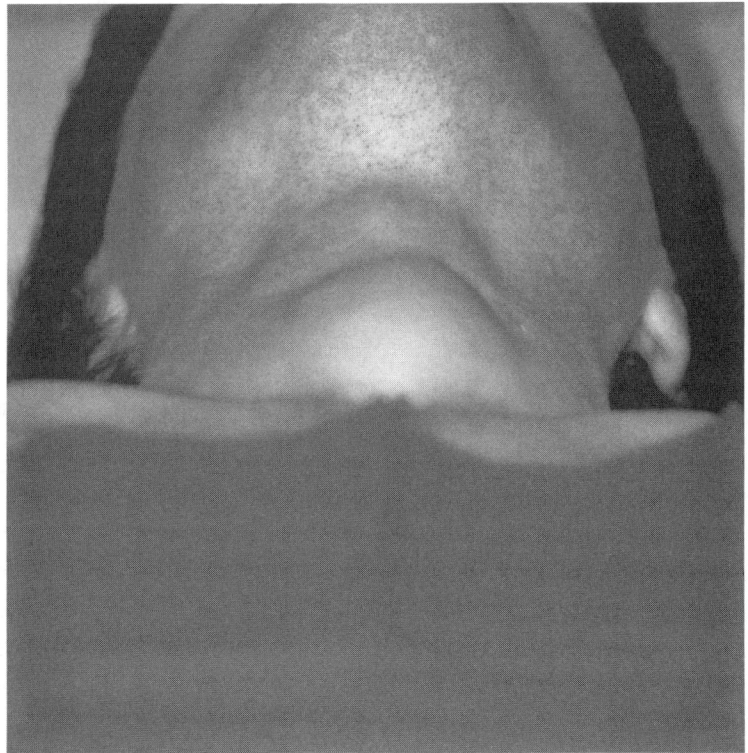

II. PEI TREATMENT OF CYSTIC NODULES
Figure 11. 3: PEI treatment of a large (40 ml) cystic lesion in a 38-year-old man. A: Before treatment a huge cervical lump is observable. The patient had undergone two complete percutaneous drainages of the fluid collection four and two weeks before PEI. Both drainages were rapidly followed by recurrence of bleeding within the pseudocyst.

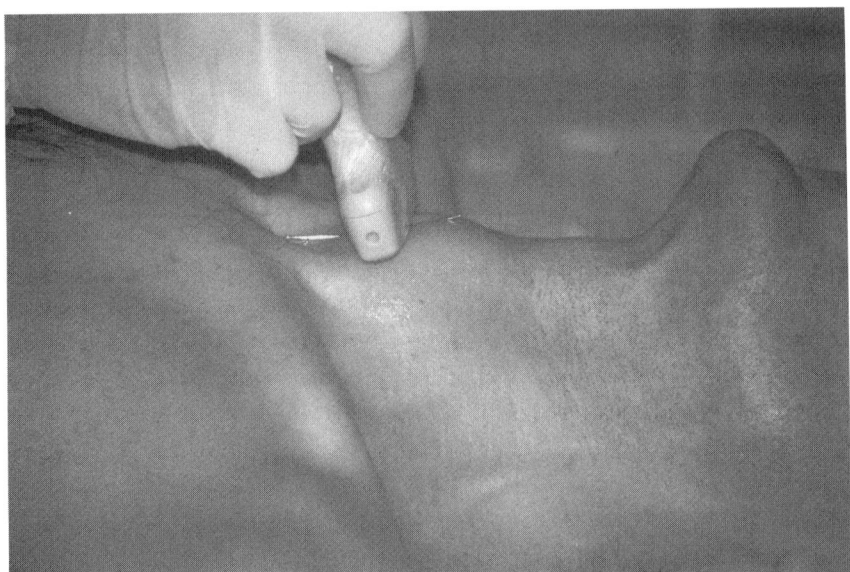

Figure 11. 3: PEI treatment of a large (40 ml) cystic lesion in a 38-year-old man. B: US identification of the center of the target lesion and determination of the point of insertion of the needle by a steel bar placed at right angle to the probe.

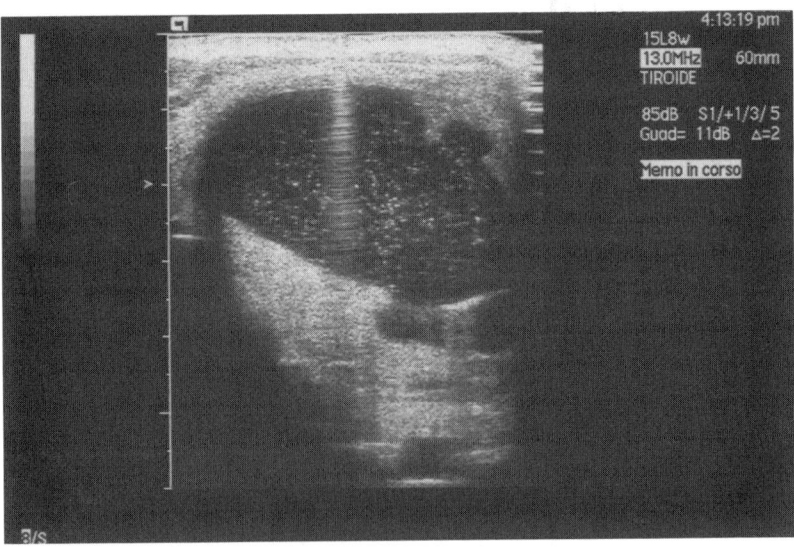

Figure 11. 3: PEI treatment of a large (40 ml) cystic lesion in a 38-year-old man. C: US image showing the acoustic shadowing projected within the cystic nodule by the bar placed on the skin.

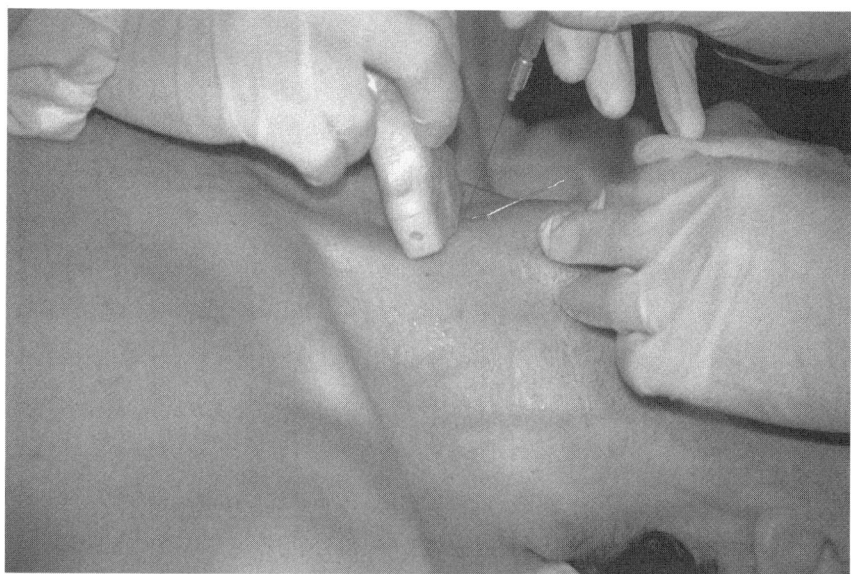

Figure 11. 4: Percutaneous drainage of the pseudocyst. A: Insertion of the needle at the right angle formed by the transversely placed US-probe and the perpendicularly placed steel bar. The needle enters the neck almost vertically.

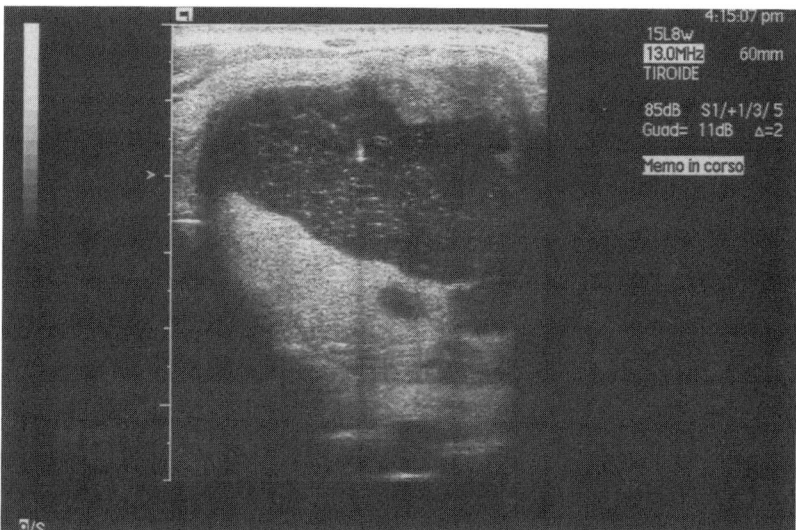

Figure 11. 4: Percutaneous drainage of the pseudocyst. B: US imaging of the needle tip (clearly observable as a hyperechoic spot within the fluid anechoic area) in the center of the cystic lesion.

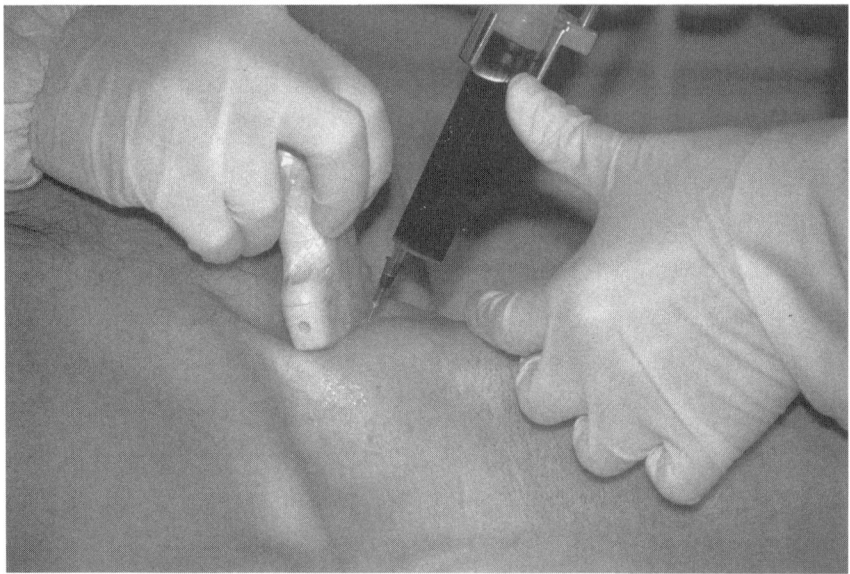

Figure 11. 4: Percutaneous drainage of the pseudocyst. C: Slow drainage of 35 ml of reddish-brown fluid from the pseudocystic thyroid lesion.

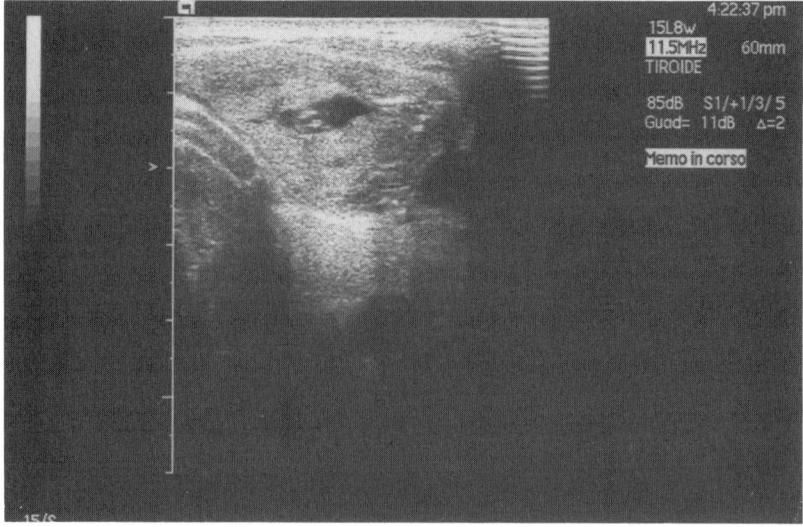

Figure 11. 5. Percutaneous sclerosis of the cavity of the pseudocystic lesion. A: A small amount of fluid is left inside the almost collapsed pseudocyst. The needle tip is kept in the center of the fluid collection

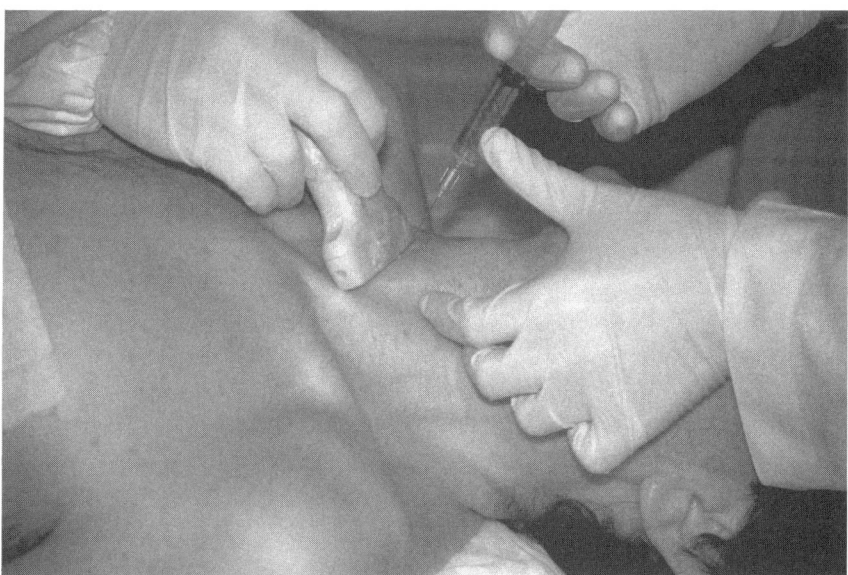

Figure 11. 5. Percutaneous sclerosis of the cavity of the pseudocystic lesion B: After the almost complete fluid drainage a syringe containing ethanol is substituted for the aspirating syringe without removing the needle.

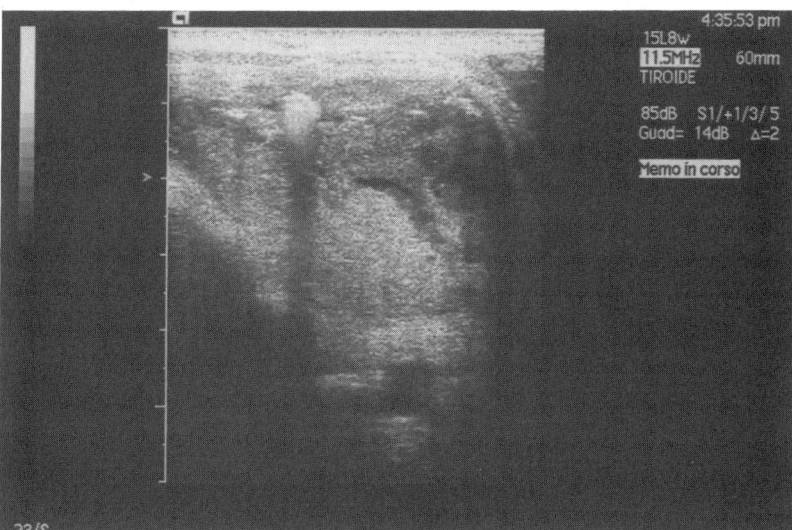

Figure 11. 5. Percutaneous sclerosis of the cavity of the pseudocystic lesion C: Ethanol injection is visualized as an inhomogeneous hyperechoic zone within the almost collapsed but rapidly refilling fluid cavity.

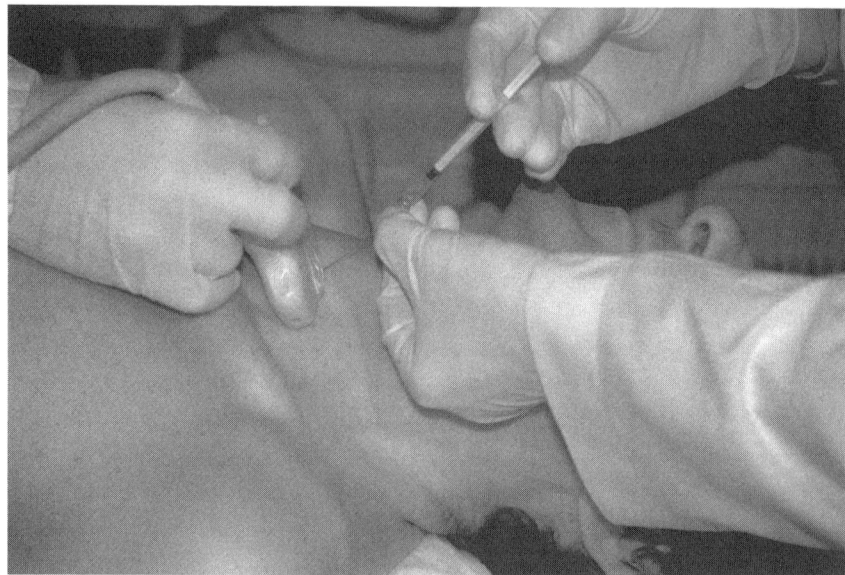

Figure 11. 6. End of PEI treatment. A: Slow injection of 1 ml of Xylocaine (which has replaced the ethanol syringe) during needle extraction.

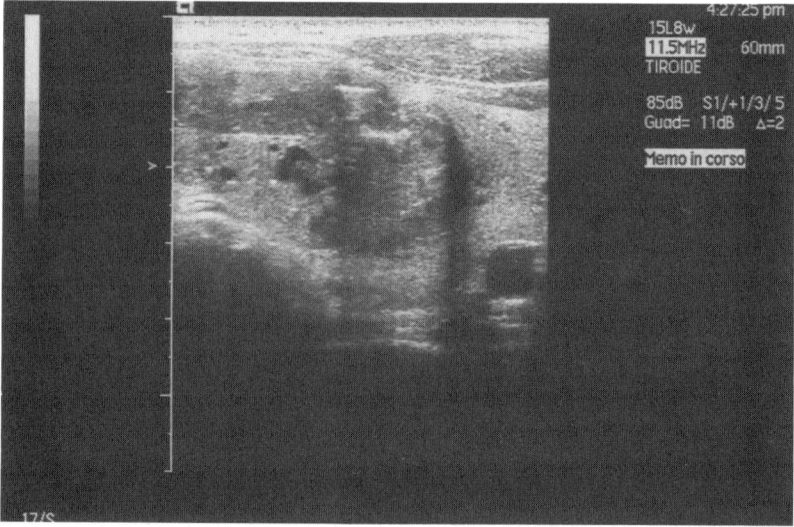

Figure 11. 6. End of PEI treatment. B: After needle withdrawal the US image shows a collapsed pseudocyst filled with scattered linear hyperechoic images due to ethanol persistence within the lesion.

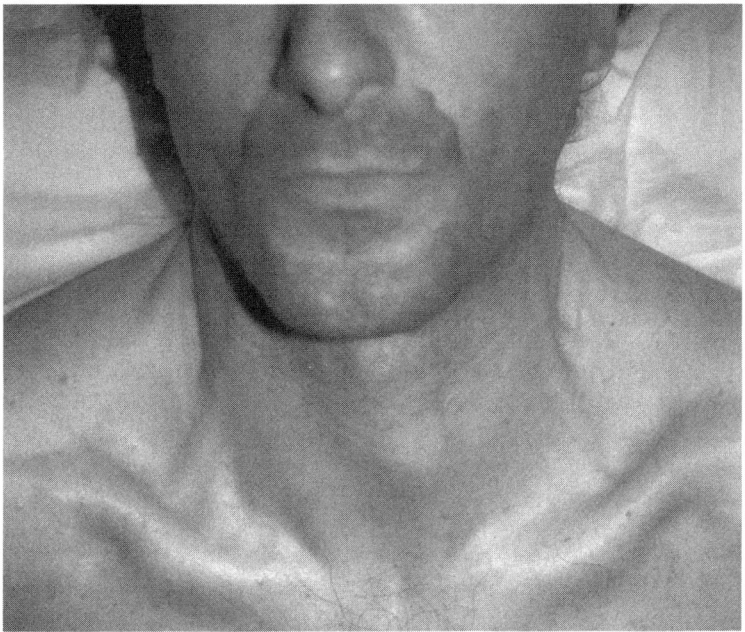

Figure 11.6. End of PEI treatment. C: A marked decrease of the cervical lump is observable at the end of treatment. The neck surface is devoid of bruising, hematoma and skin irritation.

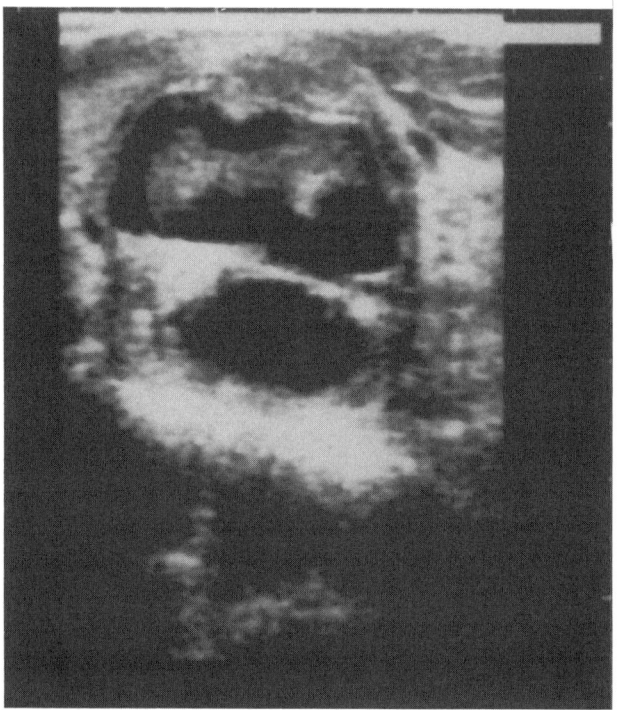

Figure 11. 7. Short-term changes after PEI. Baseline. A: Large (maximum diameter: 47 mm) multilocular pseudocyst. The lesion had recurred twice after percutaneous drainage.

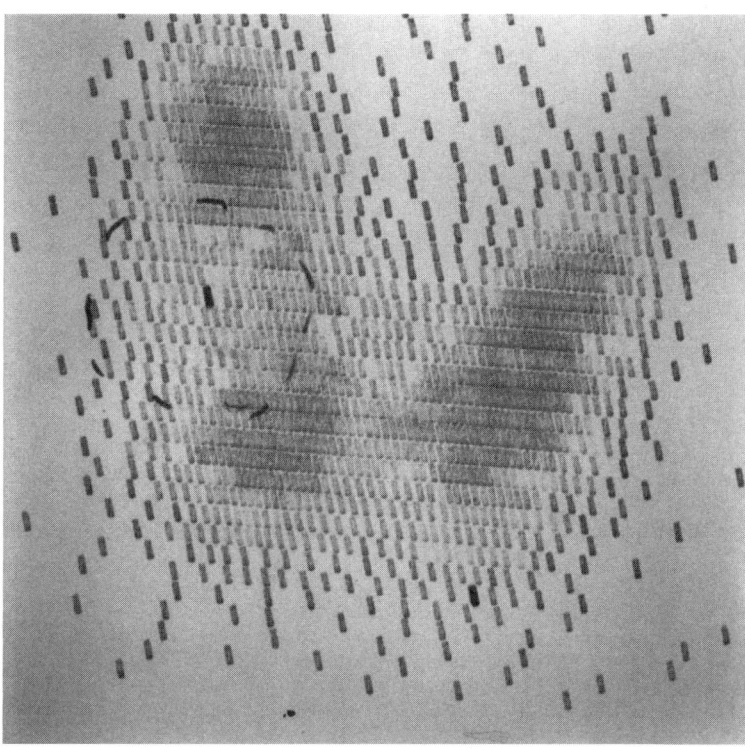

Figure 11.7 Short-term changes after PEI. Baseline. B: Thyroid scintiscan (99mTc) shows a cold area within the right lobe corresponding to the cystic lesion.

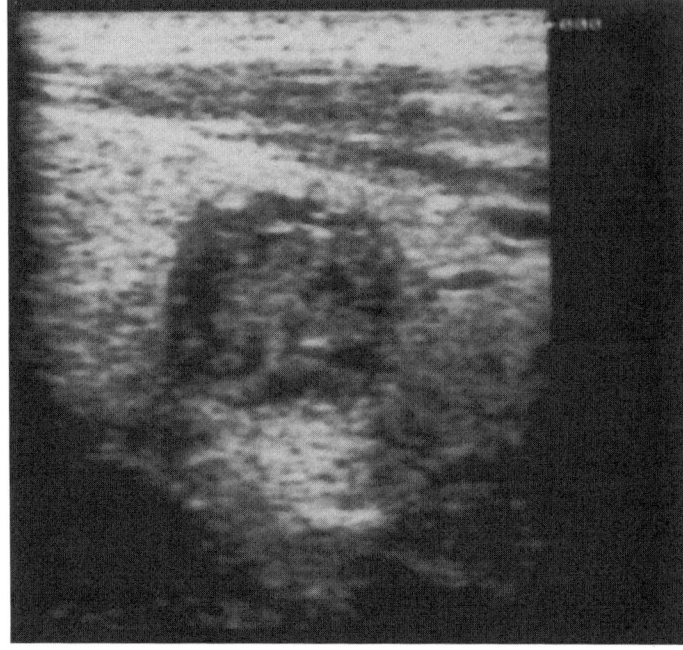

Figure 11.8 Short-term changes after PEI. After treatment. A: One month after PEI treatment (three sessions) the lesion had been transformed into a small (maximum diameter: 26 mm) mixed nodule.

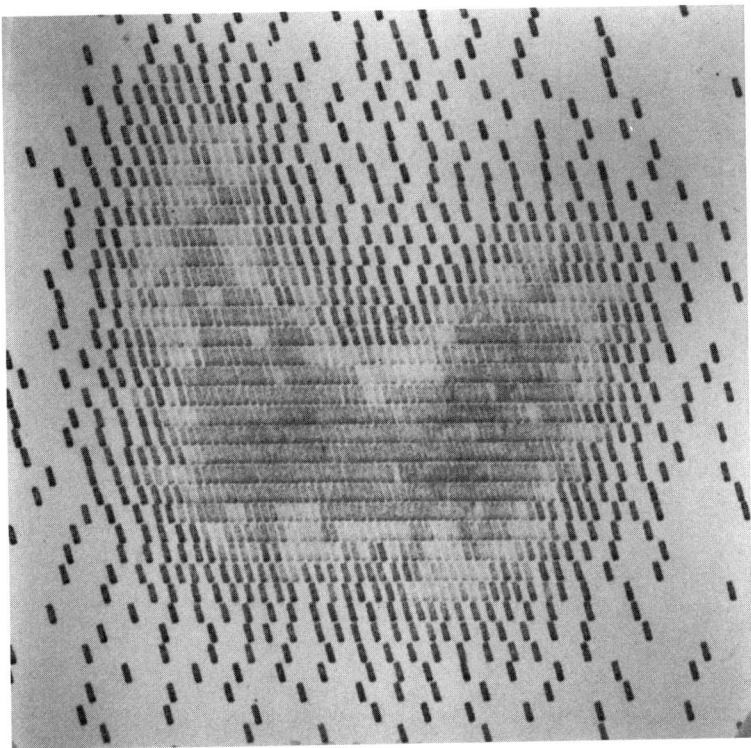

Figure 11.8 Short-term changes after PEI. After treatment. B: Disappearance of the previously observed cold area on thyroid scintiscan.

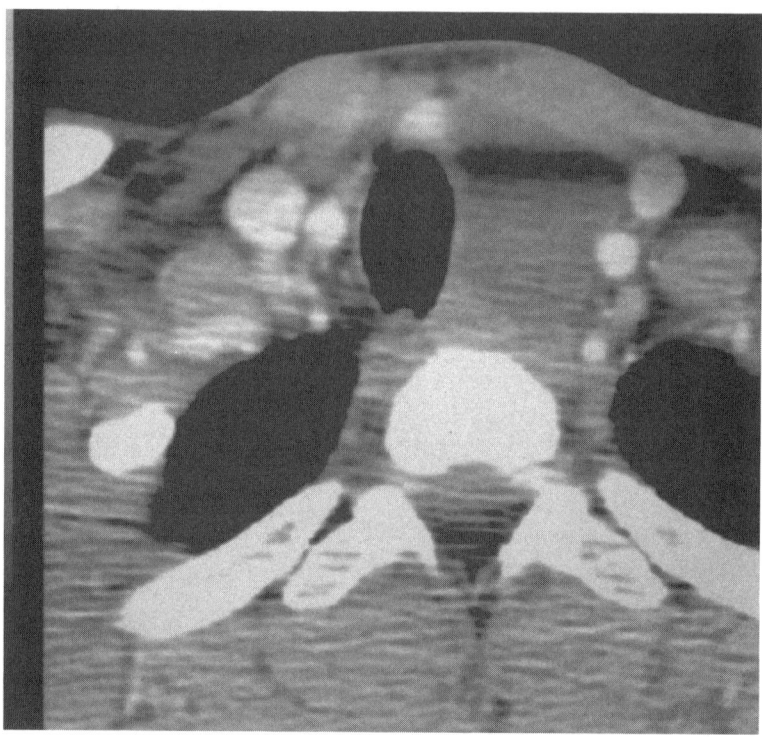

Figure 11.9 Large cervical lesion causing local compressing symptoms: baseline. A: A CT scan of the neck shows a large pseudocyst (maximum diameter: 49 mm) of the left thyroid lobe.

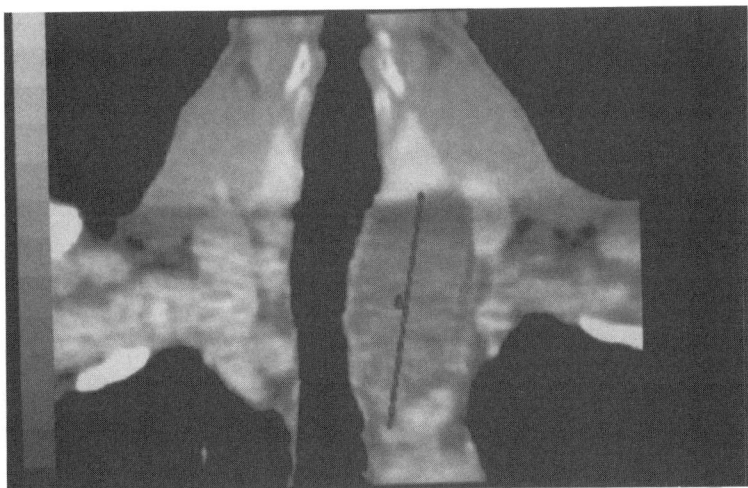

Figure 11.9 Large cervical lesion causing local compressing symptoms: baseline. B: Coronal reconstruction of the CT scan confirms the presence of dislocation and compression of the tracheal lumen.

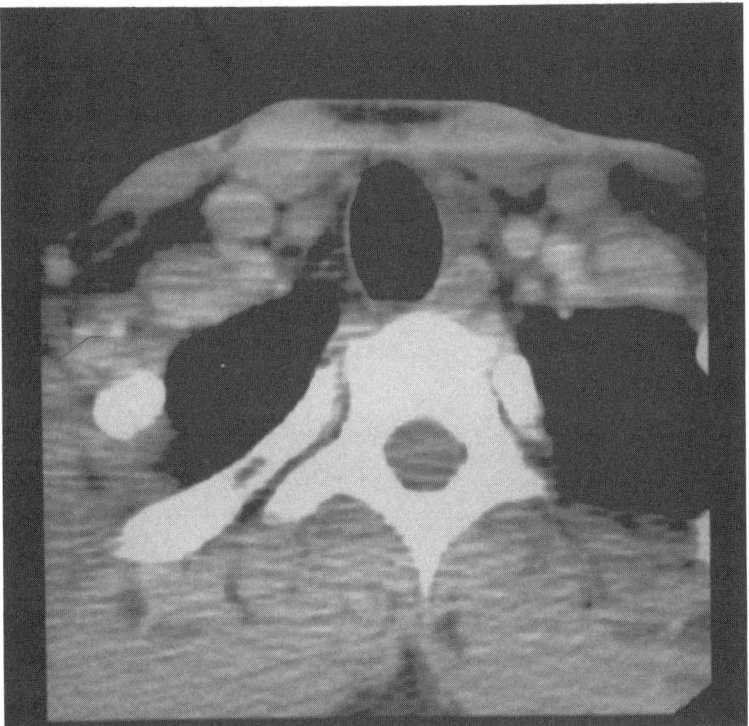

Figure 11.10 Changes after PEI. A: The CT scan performed one month after PEI treatment shows a striking reduction in nodule dimension (maximum diameter: 13 mm).

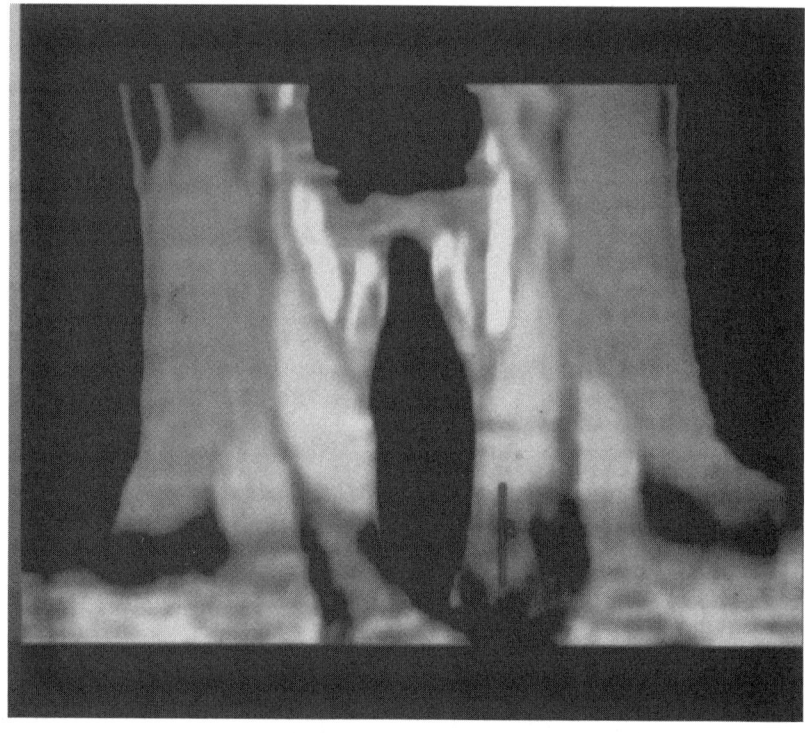

Figure 11.10. Changes after PEI. B: Coronal reconstruction of the CT scan confirms the marked improvement of the previously observed tracheal compression and dislocation.

199

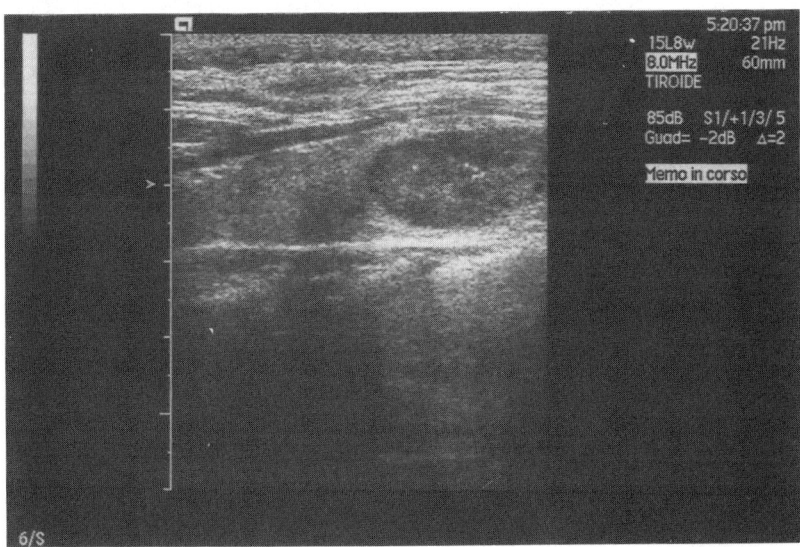

III. PEI TREATMENT OF AUTONOMOUSLY FUNCTIONING THYROID NODULES
Figure 11.11 First session of PEI treatment of an AFTN (1). A: US image of an AFTN (maximum diameter: 27 mm) of the left thyroid lobe.

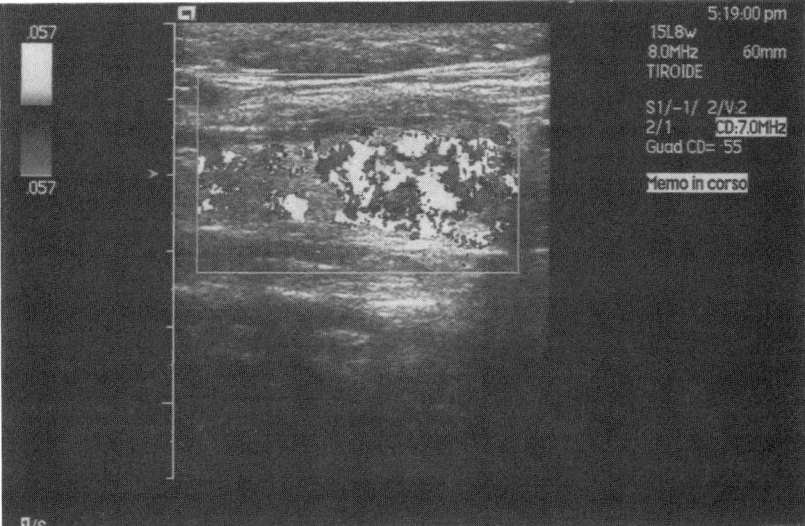

Figure 11.11 First session of PEI treatment of an AFTN (1). B: Color Doppler examination of the hyperfunctioning nodule shows several peripheral and intralesional vascular images.

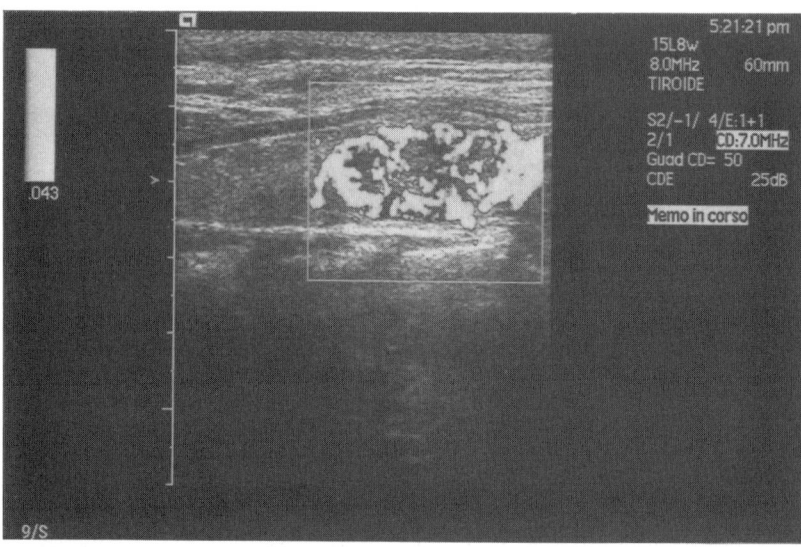

Figure 11.11 First session of PEI treatment of an AFTN (1). C: Power Doppler evaluation confirms the high degree of vascularization of the lesion.

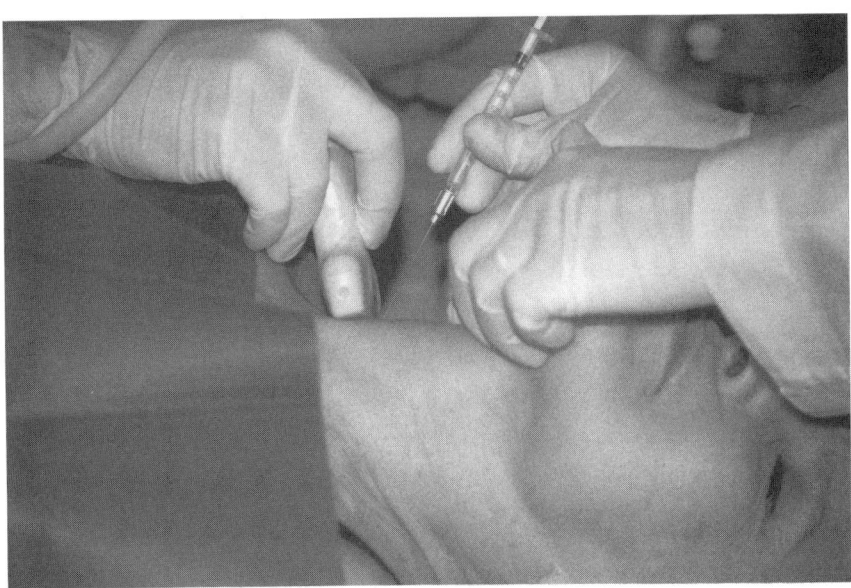
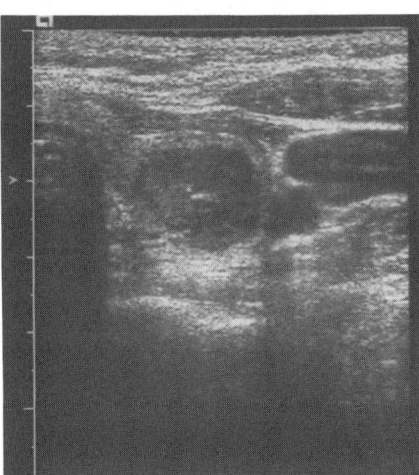
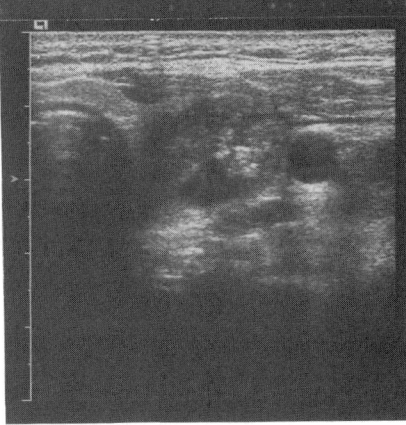

Figure 11.12 First session of PEI treatment of an AFTN (2). A: Needle insertion. Apart from fluid drainage (rarely required for AFTN), PEI treatment of the AFTN is performed as described for cystic thyroid nodules. **B**: US scan shows Xylocaine diffusion (observable as small hyperechoic spots) in the center of the lesion. **C:** US image of the ethanol bolus. Alcohol diffusion appears as an irregular, rapidly vanishing hyperechoic spot in the center of the AFTN.

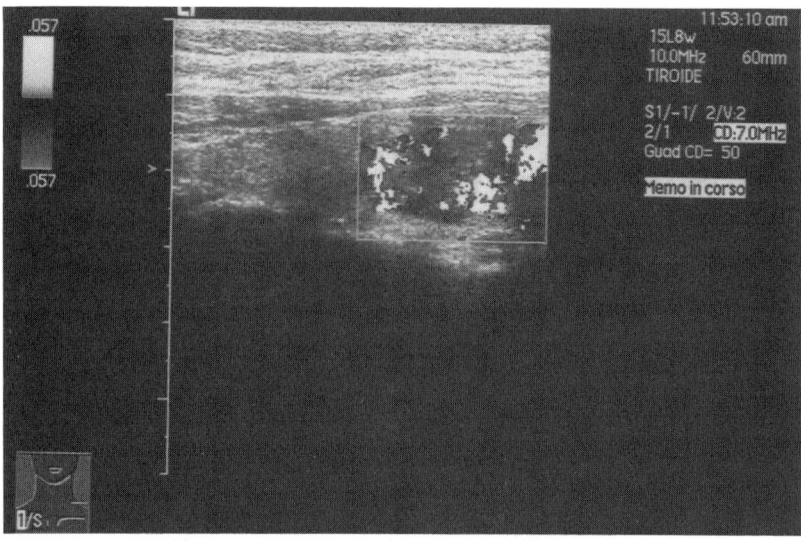

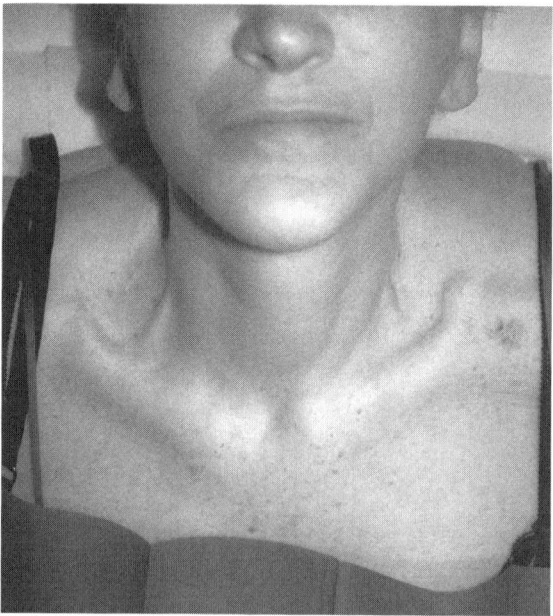

Figure 11.13 First session of PEI treatment of an AFTN (3). A: At the end of PEI session, Color Doppler examination shows a marked decrease of vascularization in the area of the AFTN perfused by ethanol. A few hyperechoic spots caused by ethanol persistence within the lesion are observable. **B:** At the end of treatment the skin surface is devoid of bruising and irritation.

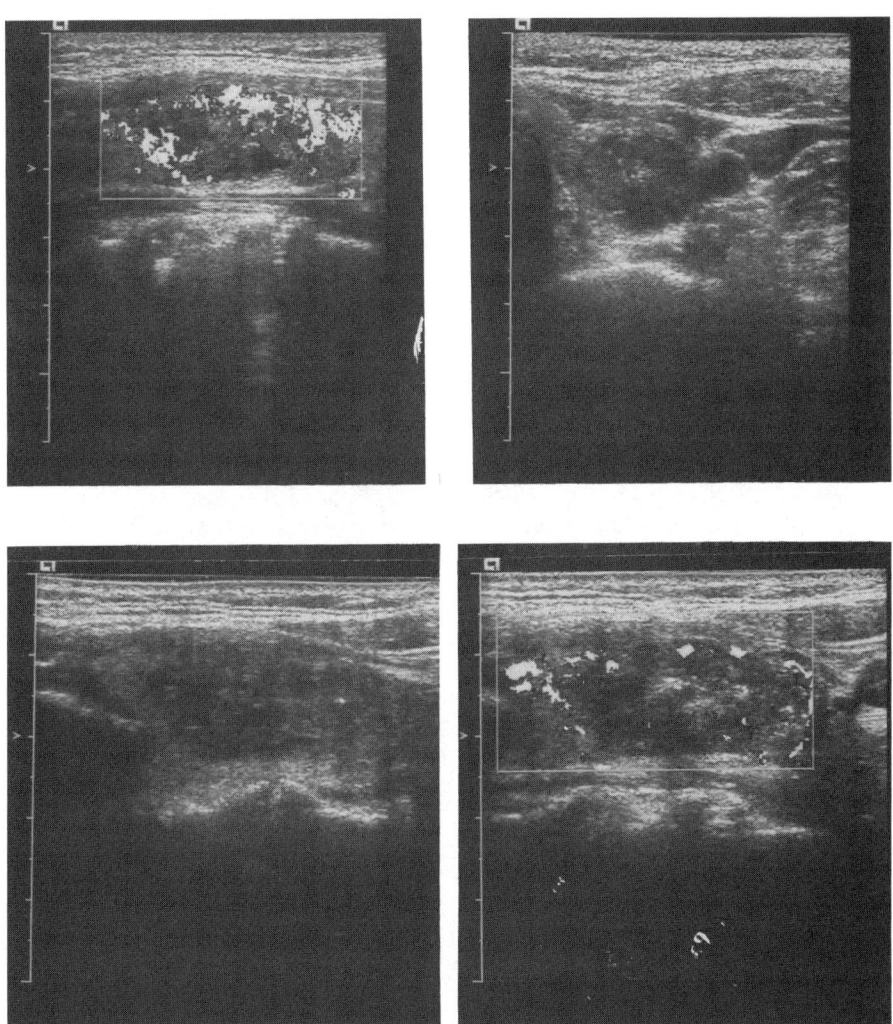

Figure 11.14 Second session of PEI treatment of an AFTN. A: Color Doppler examination (long-axis) demonstrates the persistence of vascular images in the lower pole of the lesion after the first PEI treatment. **B**: US scan (long axis) shows the tip of the needle placed precisely in the center of the still hypervascularized area. **C**: US image (short axis). Ethanol diffusion is observable within the AFTN as an irregular hyperechoic zone. **D**: At the end of second treatment Color Doppler examination shows a marked decrease of vascularization. Multiple hyperechoic spots due to ethanol diffusion are present in the lower pole of the lesion.
When, as in the case here, the needle tip is no longer clearly distinguishable it is advisable to suspend alcohol injection.

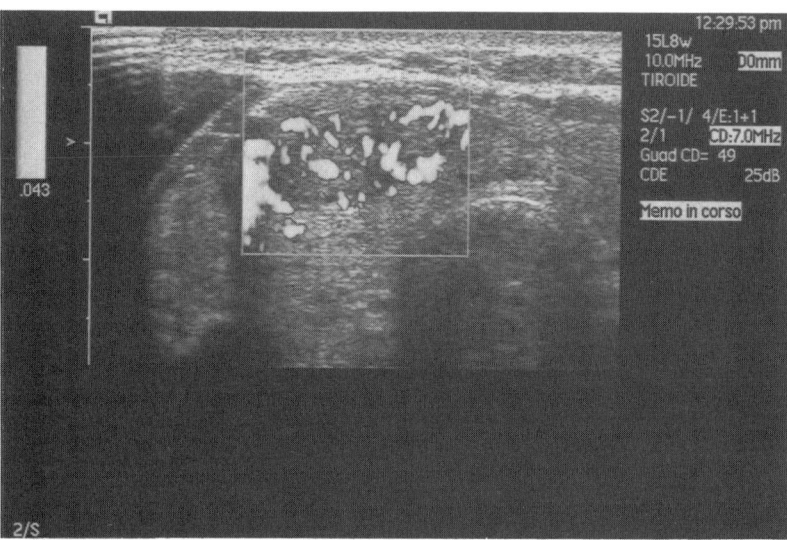

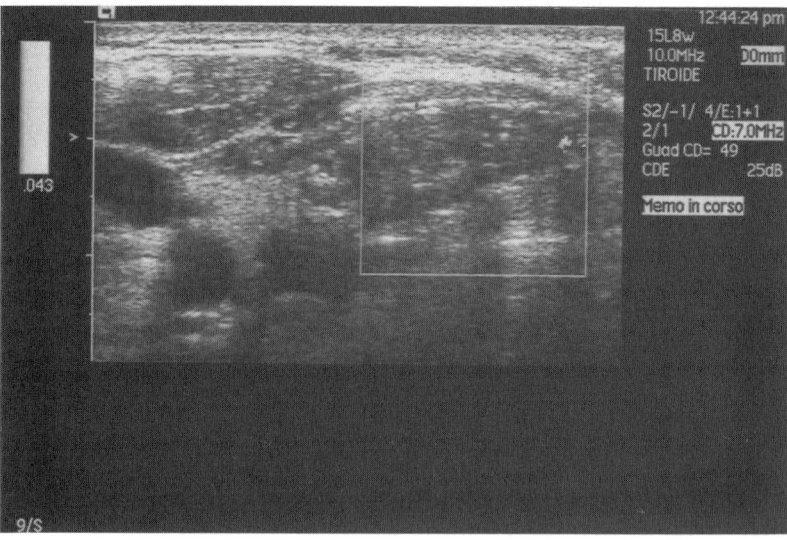

Figure 11.15 Power Doppler evaluation of an AFTN before PEI and immediately after the last session. A: Baseline US scan shows a well-defined lesion of the right thyroid lobe (maximum diameter: 29 mm) with a high degree of vascularization. **B**: After three PEI sessions (six injections of a total of 21 ml of ethanol) a complete disappearance of vascular images is observable. Several hyperechoic spots are diffused within the lesion, which shows an initial volume decrease.

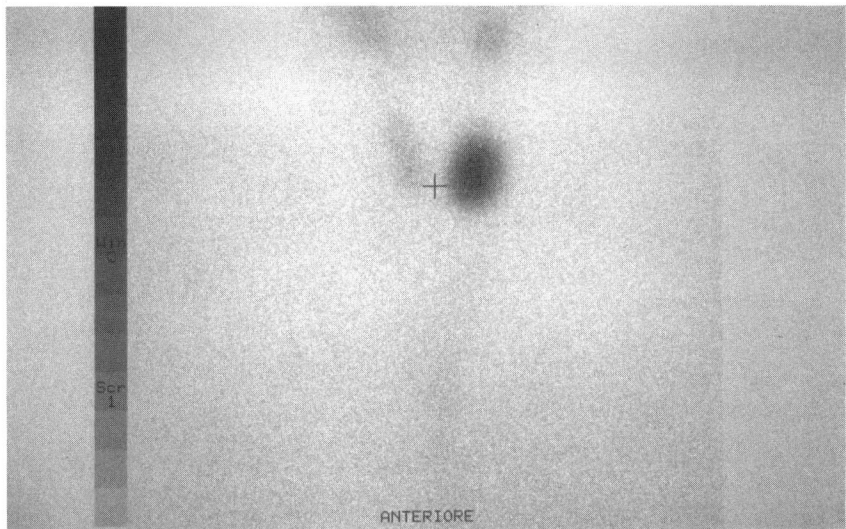

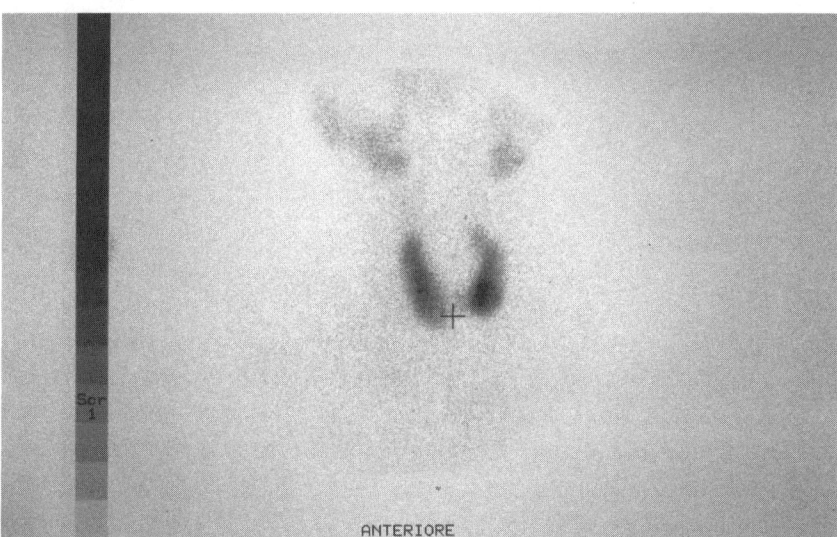

Figure 11.16 Thyroid scintiscan of an AFTN inhibiting the function of the surrounding parenchyma. A: Baseline scintiscan image of the thyroid. **B**: One month after PEI treatment a marked decrease of the hyperfunctioning area is observed. The previously suppressed lobe is now well delineated at scintiscan.

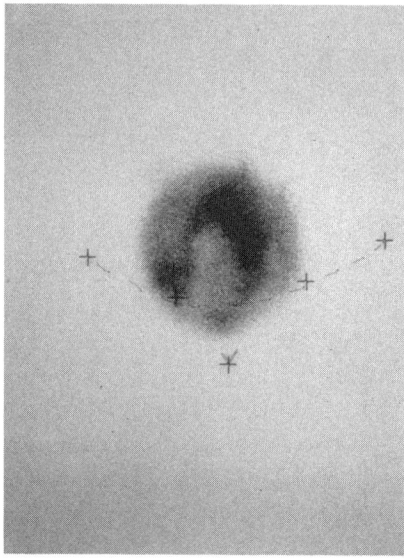

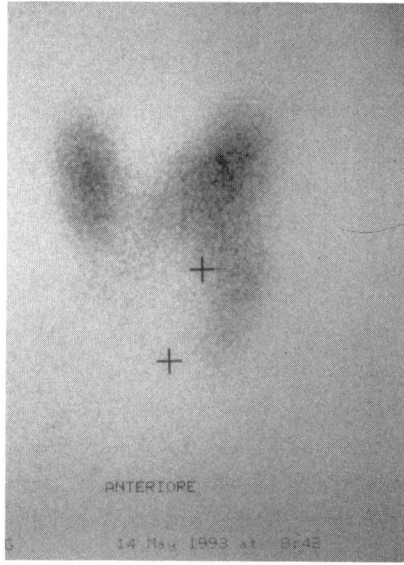

Figure 11.17 Thyroid scintiscan of a large toxic AFTN. A: A hyperfunctioning lesion of the lower pole of the left thyroid lobe completely suppresses the function of the surrounding parenchyma. **B:** Three months after PEI a complete effacement of the hyperfunctioning area is observable. The previously suppressed thyroid parenchyma is now well delineated.

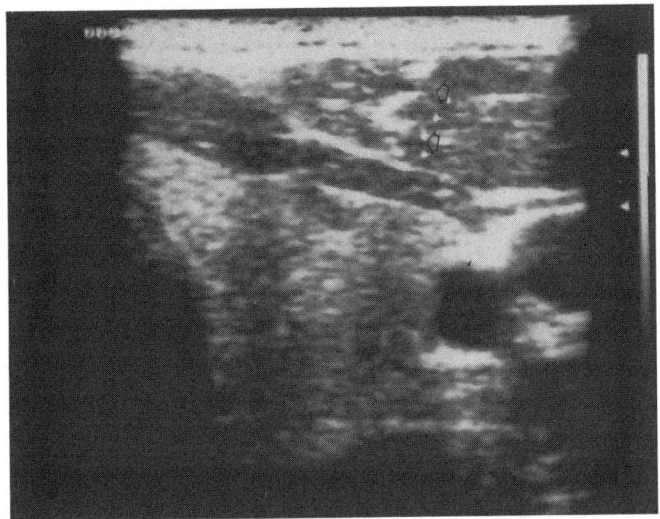

Figure 11.18 Minor complication of PEI treatment. A hematoma of the sternocleidomastoid muscle is observable as an irregular hyperechoic line (arrow). Blood extravasation along the needle track spontaneously resolved within 24 hours.

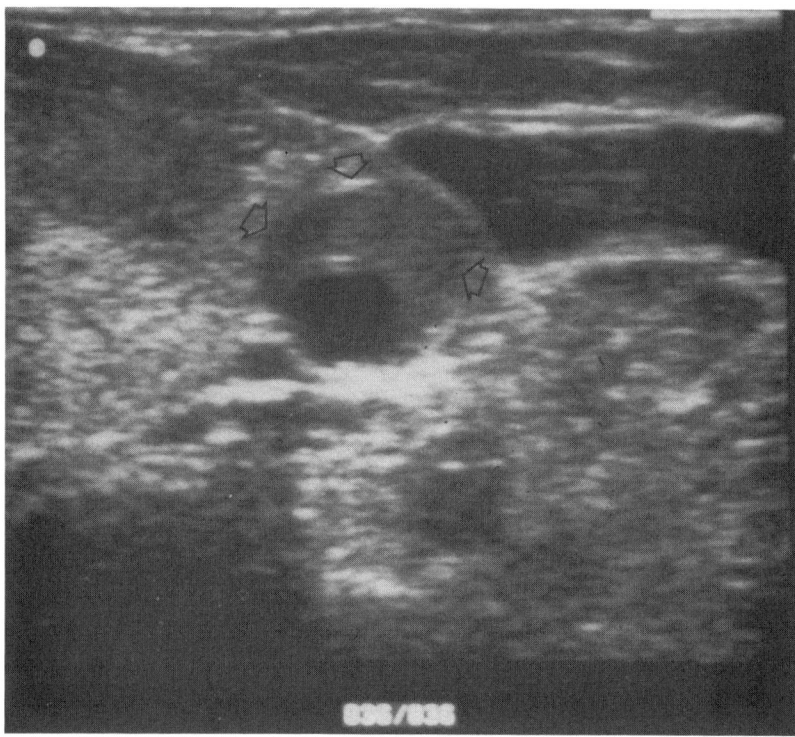

Figure 11.19 Major complication of PEI treatment. An inadvertent puncture of the carotid artery caused a blood collection dissecting the arterial wall. This serious damage of the neck vessels is not unique to PEI as it can be induced by an unskilled operator performing any procedure involving the thyroid. Hematoma was resolved spontaneously (without thrombosis of the carotid lumen) within two weeks.

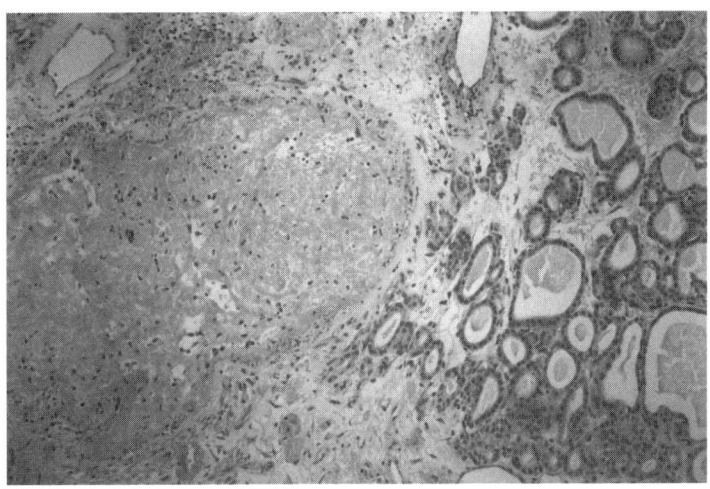

IV. MORPHOLOGICAL FEATURES RELATED TO PEI TREATMENT
Figure 11.20 Histological findings from an AFTN treated with PEI. An area of coagulative necrosis of the thyroid parenchyma induced by ethanol is observable. Ghost follicles with some spared nuclei are evident in the microscopic field.

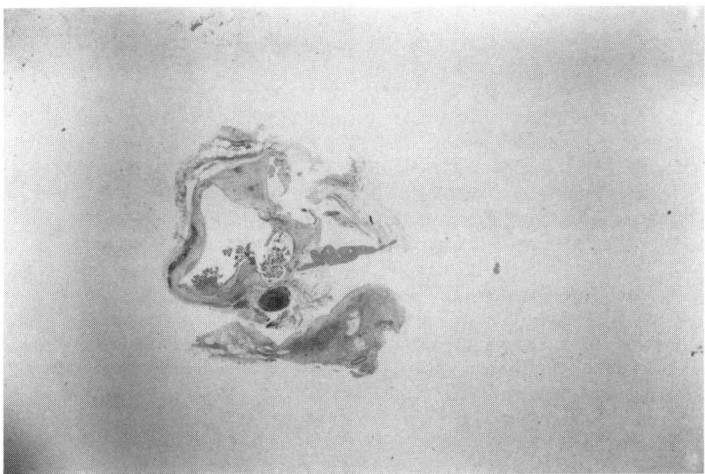

Figure 11.21 Risk of occult malignancy. The risk of overlooking a differentiated carcinoma before PEI treatment is exemplified by the present case. Small foci of papillary carcinoma are observable within the fibrous capsule of an otherwise benign cystic thyroid nodule.

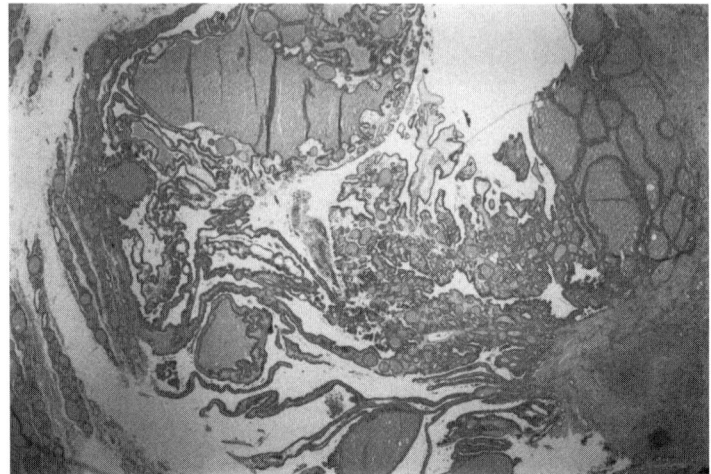

Figure 11.22 Follow-up problems after PEI. Thyroid papillary hyperplasia near a sclerotic area is observable. These changes are the most common abnormality after tissue ablation with both radioactive iodine and PEI. Papillary features may result in a microscopic picture interfering with the cytological diagnosis in FNA samples obtained after PEI treatment of benign thyroid nodules.

REFERENCES
1. Livraghi T, Festi D, Monti F, Salmi A, Vettori C. US-guided percutaneous alcohol injection of small hepatic and abdominal tumours. *Radiology* 1986; 161:309-312.
2. Karstrup S, Holm HH, Torp-Pedersen S and Hegedus L. Ultrasonically guided percutaneous inactivation of parathyroid tumors. *Br J Radiol* 1987; 60: 667 - 670.
3. Charboneau JW, Hay ID and van Heerden JA. Persistent primary hyperparathyroidism: successful ultrasound-guided percutaneous ethanol ablation of an occult adenoma. *Mayo Clin Proc* 1988; 63: 913-917.
4. Karstrup S, Transbol I, Holm HH, Glenthoj A and Hegedus L. Ultrasonically guided chemical parathyroidectomy in patients with primary hyperparathyroidism. A prospective study. *Br J Radiol* 1989; 62: 1037 - 1042.
5. Livraghi T, Paracchi A, Ferrari C, Bergonzi M, Garavaglia G, Raineri P, Vettori C. Treatment of autonomous thyroid nodules with percutaneous ethanol injection: Preliminary results. *Radiology* 1990; 175: 827 - 829.
6. Papini E, Panunzi C, Petrucci L, Picardi R, Pacella CM, Bizzarri G, Fabbrini R, Pisicchio G, Favella A, Todino V, Nardi F. Percutaneous ultrasound-guided treatment of hyperfunctioning thyroid nodules. Technique and preliminary results. *Min Endocrinol* 1991; 16: 163 -170.
7. Monzani F, Goletti O, De Negri F, Del Guerra P, Lippolis PV, Caraccio N, Chiarugi M, Federghini M, Baschieri L. Autonomous thyroid nodule and percutaneous ethanol injection therapy. *Lancet* 1991; 337: 743.
8. Paracchi A, Ferrari C, Livraghi T, Reschini E, Macchi RM, Bergonzi M, and Raineri P. Percutaneous intranodular ethanol injection: A new treatment for autonomous thyroid adenoma. *J Endocrinol Invest* 1992; 15: 353-362.
9. Goletti O, Monzani F, Caraccio N, Del Guerra P, Lippolis PV, Pucciarelli M, Seccia M, Carmassi F, Cavina E, and Baschieri L. Percutaneous ethanol injection treatment of autonomously functioning single thyroid nodules: Optimization of treatment and short term outcome. *World J Surg* 1992; 16: 784-90.

10. Monzani F, Goletti O, Caraccio N, Del Guerra P, Ferdeghini M, Pucci E, and Baschieri L. Percutaneous ethanol injection treatment of autonomous thyroid adenoma: hormonal and clinical evaluation. *Clin Endocrinol* 1992; 36: 491-497.
11. Martino E, Murtas ML, Loviselli A, Piga M, Petrini L, Miccoli P, and Pacini F (1992) Percutaneous intranodular ethanol injection for treatment of autonomously functioning thyroid nodules. *Surgery* 1992; 112: 1161-65.
12. Papini E, Panunzi C, Pacella CM, Bizzarri G, Fabbrini R, Petrucci L, Pisicchio G, and Nardi F. Percutaneous ultrasound-guided ethanol injection: a new treatment of toxic autonomously functioning thyroid nodules? *J Clin Endocrinol Metab* 1993; 76: 411-416.
13. Mazzeo S, Toni MG, De Gaudio C, caramella D, Pinto F, Lencioni R, Sanguinetti F and Bartolozzi C. Percutaneous injection of ethanol to treat autonomous thyroid nodules. *Am J Roentgenol* 1993,; 161: 871 - 876.
14. Verde G, Strada S, Delpiano S, Gallotti C, Guffanti C, Pisicchio G, Gelli D. Effectiveness of percutaneous ethanol injection in the treatment of cystic thyroid nodules. *J Endocrinol Invest* 1994; 17 (Suppl 2): 71.
15. Monzani F, Lippi F, Goletti O, Del Guerra P, Caraccio N, Lippolis PV, Baschieri L, and Pinchera A. Percutaneous aspiration and ethanol sclerotherapy for thyroid cysts. *J Clin Endocrinol Metab* 1994; 78: 800-802.
16. Verde G, Papini E, Pacella CM, Gallotti C, Del Piano S, Strada S, Fabbrini R, Bizzarri G, Rinaldi R, Panunzi C, and Gelli D. Ultrasound-guided percutaneous ethanol injection in the treatment of cystic thyroid nodules. *Clin Endocrinol* 1994; 41: 719 -24.
17. Zingrillo M, Torlontano M, Ghiggi MR, D'Aloiso L, Nirchio V, Bisceglia M and Liuzzi A. Percutaneous ethanol injection of large thyroid cystic nodules. *Thyroid* 1996; 6: 403 - 408.
18. Goletti O, Monzani F, Lenziardi M, Lippolis PV, De Negri F, Caraccio N, Cavina E and Baschieri L. Cold thyroid nodules: a new application of percutaneous ethanol injection treatment. *J Clin Ultrasound* 1994; 22: 175 - 178.
19. Bennedbaek FN & Hegedus L. Alcoholsclerotherapy for benign solitary solid cold thyroid nodules. *Lancet* 1995; 346: 1227.
20. Caraccio N, Goletti O, Lippolis PV, Casolaro A, Cavina E, Miccoli P, and Monzani F. Is percutaneous ethanol injection a useful alternative for the treatment of the cold benign thyroid nodule? Five years' experience. *Thyroid* 1997; 7: 699 - 704.
21. Bennedbaek FN, Nielsen LK, and Hegedus L. Effect of percutaneous ethanol injection therapy versus suppressive doses of L-Thyroxine on benign solitary solid cold thyroid nodules: A randomized trial. *J Clin Endocrinol Metab* 1998; 83: 830 - 835.
22. Zingrillo M, Collura D, Ghiggi MR, Nirchio V, and Trischitta V. Treatment of large cold benign thyroid nodules not eligible for surgery with percutaneous ethanol injection. *J Clin Endocrinol Metab* 1998; 83: 3905 - 3907.
23. Hegedus L, Karstrup S and Hansen JM. Ethanol injection into autonomous thyroid adenoma. *Clin Endocrinol* 1993; 38: 439 - 440.
24. Mincheva L, Simeonov S, Troev D, Mitkov M, Pavlova M, Iliev D, Botushanov N. Percutaneous ethanol sclerotherapy of autonomous thyroid nodules: preliminary results. *Folia Med (Plovdiv)*: 1997; 39: 49 - 54.
25. Zieleznik W, Sieron A, Peszel-Barlik M, Zieleznik M, Simon-Sieron M. Alcohol sclerotherapy for benign solitary thyroid nodules. *Wiad Lek* 1997; 50: 211 - 216;
26. Zbranca E, Mogos V, Vulpoi C, Bostaca T, Rusu M, Nisfoeanu G, Galesanu C, Nestor C, Natasa Macovei G. Fine needle puncture-method of treatment in nodular pathology of the thyroid. *Ann Endocrinol (Paris)* 1996; 57: 433 - 437.

27. Ozdemir H, Ilgit ET, Yucel C, Atilla S, Isik S, Cakir N. Treatment of autonomous thyroid nodules: safety and efficacy of sonographically guided percutaneous injection of ethanol. *Am J Roentgenol* 1994; 163: 929 - 932.
28. Mizurami Y, Michigishi T, Nonomura A, Yokoyama K, Noguchi M, Hashimoto T, Nakamura S and Ishizaki T. Autonomously functioning thyroid (hot) nodule of the thyroid gland. A clinical and histopathologic study of 17 cases. *Am J Clin Pathol* 1994; 101: 29 - 35.
29. Nakada K, Katoh C, Kanegae K, Tsukamoto E, Itoh K, Tamaki N. Percutaneous ethanol injection therapy for autonomously functioning thyroid nodule. *Ann Nucl Med* 1996; 10: 171 - 176.
30. Yasuda K, Ozaki O, Sugino K, Yamashita T, Toshima K, Ito K. Treatment of cystic lesions of the thyroid by ethanol instillation. *W J Surg* 1992; 16: 958 - 961.
31. Bennedbaek FN, Karstrup S and Hegedus L. Percutaneous ethanol injection therapy in the treatment of thyroid and parathyroid diseases. *Eur J Endocrinol* 1997; 136: 240 - 250.
32. Giuffrida D, Gharib H. Controversies in the management of cold, hot, and occult thyroid nodules. *Am J Med* 1995; 99: 642 - 650.
33. Pacini F, Elisei R, Di Coscio GC, Aneli S, Macchia E, Concetti R, Miccoli P, Arganini M, Pinchera A. Thyroid carcinoma in thyrotoxic patients treated by surgery. *J Endocrinol Invest* 1988; 11: 107 - 112.
34. Livraghi T, Paracchi A, Ferrari C, Reschini E, Macchi RM, Bonifacino A. Treatment of autonomous thyroid nodules with percutaneous ethanol injection: 4-year experience. *Radiology* 1994; 190: 529-533.
35. Papini E, Pacella CM, and Verde G. Percutaneous ethanol injection (PEI): what is its role in the treatment of benign thyroid nodules? *Thyroid* 1995; 5: 147 - 150.
36. Lippi F, Ferrari C, Manetti L, Rago T, Santini F, Monzani F, Bellitti P, Papini E, Busnardo B, Angelini F, Pinchera A, and the Multicenter Study Group. Treatment of solitary autonomous thyroid nodules by percutaneous ethanol injection: Results of an Italian Multicenter Study. *J Clin Endocrinol Metab* 1996; 81: 3261 - 3264.
37. Monzani F, Caraccio N, Goletti O, Lippolis PV, Casolaro A, Del Guerra P, Cavina E, Miccoli P. Five-year follow-up of percutaneous ethanol injection for the treatment of hyperfunctioning thyroid nodules: a study of 117 patients. *Clin Endocrinol (Oxf)* 1997; 46: 9 - 15.
38. Goldstein R, Hart IR. Follow-up of solitary autonomous thyroid nodules treated with 131-I. *N Engl J Med* 1983; 309: 1473 - 1476.
39. Burch HB, Shakir F, Fitzsimmons TR, Jacques DP, and Shriver CD. Diagnosis and management of the autonomously functioning thyroid nodule: The Walter Reed army medical center experience, 1975 - 1996. *Thyroid* 1998; 10: 871 - 880.
40. Wagner HE, Seiler C. Recurrent laryngeal nerve palsy after thyroid gland surgery. *Br J Surg* 1994; 81: 226 - 228.
41. Crescenzi A, Papini E, Pacella CM, Rinaldi R, Panunzi C, Petrucci L, Fabbrini R, Bizzarri GC, Anelli V, Nardi F, and Marinozzi V. Morphological changes in a hyperfunctioning thyroid adenoma after percutaneous ethanol injection: Histological, enzymatic and sub-microscopical alterations. *J Endocrinol Invest* 1996; 19: 371-376.
42. Pacella CM, Papini E, Bizzarri G, Fabbrini R, Anelli V, Rinaldi R, Valle D, Nardi F. Assessment of the effect of PEI in autonomously functioning thyroid nodules by colour-coded duplex sonography. *Eur Radiol* 1995; 5:395 - 400.
43. Miller JM, uz Zafar S, Karo JJ. The cystic thyroid nodule. *Radiology* 1974; 110: 257-261.
44. De los Santos ET, Keyhani-Rofagha S, Cunningham JL & Mazzaferri EL.

Cystic thyroid nodules. The dilemma of malignant lesions. *Arch Intern Med* 1990; 150: 1422 - 1427.

45. Papini E, Verde G, Zingrillo M, Crescenzi A, Nardi F, Guglielmi R, Rinaldi R, Petrucci L, Raponi I, Liuzzi A, Fabbrini R and Pacella CM. Percutaneous ethanol injection treatment of benign cold thyroid nodules. An effective but hazardous technique. *J Endocrinol Invest* 1997; 20 (Suppl to no. 4): 31.

46. Panunzi C, Paliotta D, Papini E, Petrucci L, Rinaldi R, Nardi F. Cutaneous seeding of follicular thyroid cancer after fine needle aspiration biopsy ? *Diagn Cytopathol* 1994; 10:156 - 58

47. Burman KD, Earll JM, Johnson MC, Wartofsky L. Clinical observations on the solitary autonomous thyroid nodule. *Arch Intern Med* 1974; 134: 915 - 919.

48. Hamburger JL. The autonomously functioning thyroid nodule: Goetsch's disease. *Endocr Revs* 1987; 8: 439 - 447.

49. Wiener JD. Plummer's disease: localized thyroid autonomy. *J Endocrinol Invest* 1987; 207 - 224.

50. Kark AE, Kissin MW, Auerbach R, Meikle M. Voice changes after thyroidectomy: role of the external laryngeal nerve. *Br Med J* 1978; 289: 1412 - 1415.

51. Jatzko GR, Lisborg PH, Muller MG, Wette VM. Recurrent nerve palsy after thyroid operations - principal nerve identification and literature review. *Surgery* 1994; 115: 139 - 144.60.

52. Holm LE, Lundell G, Israelsson A, Dahlqvist I. Incidence of hypothyroidism occurring after iodine-131 therapy for hyperthyroidism. *J Nucl Med* 1982; 23: 103 - 107.

53. O'Brien T, Gharib H, Suman VJ, Van Heerden JA. Treatment of toxic solitary thyroid nodules: surgery versus radioactive iodine. *Surgery* 1992; 112: 1166 - 1170.

54. Uzzan B, Campos J, Cucherat M, Nony P, Boissel P, and Perret GY. Effects on bone mass of long term treatment with thyroid hormones: a meta-analysis. *J Clin Endocrinol Metab* 1996; 81: 4278-4289.

55. Sawin CT, Geller, Wolf PA et al. Low serum thyrotropin concentrations as a risk factor for atrial fibrillation in older persons. *N Engl J Med* 1994; 331: 1249-1252.

56. Jensen F & Rasmussen SN. The treatment of thyroid cysts by ultrasonically guided fine needle aspiration. *Acta Chirurgica Scandinava* 1976; 142: 209 - 211.

57. Cortelazzi D, Castagnone D, Tassis B, Venegoni E, Rivolta R, ans Beck Peccoz P. Resolution of hyperthyroidism in a pregnant woman with toxic thyroid nodule by percutaneous ethanol injection. *Thyroid* 1995; 5: 473-475.

58. Studer H, Derwahl M. Mechanisms of nonneoplastic endocrine hyperplasia - a changing concept: A review focused on the thyroid gland. *Endocr Revs* 1995; 4: 411 - 426.

59. Erickson D, Gharib H, Li H, and Heerden JA. Treatment of patients with toxic multinodular goiter. *Thyroid* 1998; 8: 277 - 282.

60. Gharib H. Current evaluation of thyroid nodules. *Trends Endocrinol Metab* 1994; 5: 365 - 369.

61. Papini E, Petrucci L, Guglielmi R, Panunzi C, Rinaldi R, Bacci V, Crescenzi A, Nardi F, Fabbrini R, Pacella CM. Long-term changes in nodular goiter: A 5-year prospective randomized trial of levothyroxine suppressive therapy for benign cold thyroid nodules. *J Clin Endocrinol Metab* 1998; 83: 780-783.

62. Gharib H, Mazzaferri EL. Thyroxine suppressive therapy in patients with nodular thyroid disease. *Ann Intern Med* 1998; 128: 386 - 394.

63. Gharib H. Diagnosis of thyroid nodules by fine-needle aspiration biopsy. *Curr Opinion Endocrinol Diab* 1996; 31: 433 - 438.

12

COLOR FLOW DOPPLER SONOGRAPHY OF THE THYROID

Fausto Bogazzi, M.D.
Luigi Bartalena, M.D.
Enio Martino, M.D.
Department of Endocrinology
University of Pisa
Pisa, ITALY

INTRODUCTION

In the past, morphological evaluation of the thyroid gland relied primarily on the thyroid scan. In recent years high resolution sonography has became the first-line test in the assessment of thyroid morphology, due to its sensitivity, and easiness and because it avoids the use of radioactivity. Moreover, the ultrasonographic features of the gland may help to identify specific thyroid pathology as in the case of autoimmune thyroid disorders, characterized by diffuse hypoechogenicity (1,2).

Although scintigraphy is still considered a useful tool for thyroid functional assessment, color flow doppler sonography (CFDS) is now considered to have an important role in obtaining such functional information. CFDS is a powerful technique which combines the gray scale image of standard sonography with a color display of blood flow, and therefore allows the evaluation of thyroid vascularity, which is an indirect measure of thyroidal function (see below). Thus, conventional sonography provides information on the size and echogenic pattern of the thyroid gland, but does not unravel its functional status. Because it is easy, non-invasive and rapid, CFDS and, even, more, peak systolic velocity (PSV) (see theoretical background) can provide prompt information on thyroid status. For the interpretation of CFDS pattern and PSV values the examiner must be familiar with the basic techniques and with the pathophysiology of thyroid diseases.

THEORETICAL BACKGROUND

The doppler effect consists of a change in wavelength or frequency caused by motion; usually this is due to motion of blood flow in circulation. As pointed out in chapter 2, echoes are generated by sound-tissues interaction. Doppler-shifted echoes (i.e. the change in frequency of the returning echoes) are generated by the interaction of echoes with blood. These echoes are registered by a transducer, converted into electric impulses, analyzed by a computer-based sonography apparatus and displayed as wavelength and a color picture. The doppler shift depends on the speed of the sound, the angle between sound direction and propagation and the operating frequency. Flows toward the transducer are registered as positive waves, those away are negative. For a complete discussion on this field the reader is referred to specific textbooks (3).

We perform CFDS of the thyroid using a color doppler system with a 7.5 MHz linear transducer. The patient is first submitted to gray scale sonography; subsequently, color flow doppler information is gained. CFDS images are obtained in the transverse and longitudinal planes and color gain is adjusted to a level not associated with relevant artifacts with the probe repetition frequency at 750 Hz in the absence of filter wall. Usually the treshold for color-flow is to a level slightly above the point at which random color noise disappeared. Color flow images are depicted by red and blue spots that indicate the direction of flow toward (red) and away (blue) from the transducer. The intensity of the color is determined by the magnitude of the frequency shift. This results in a real-time, simultaneous display of the soft tissue and blood flow over the entire field of view.

For quantitative doppler evaluation, the peak systolic velocity (the doppler waveform recorded at the point with the highest frequency shift) is determined. Measurements are either performed at the level of the intrathyroid arteries or at the level of the inferior thyroid artery. Measurements at the level of the intrathyroid vessels are performed with a sampling volume of 2-3 mm. Multiple samplings are performed to account for variations, and the mean value is determined. Using these conditions, the coefficient of variation of PSV is below 10%. The angle correction is not employed due to the tortuosity of small arteries and their incomplete visualization. When the inferior thyroid artery is used (less frequently the superior thyroid artery), the sampling volume is centered in the vessel; the angle correction is parallel to the direction of flow and the angle of insonation is ≤60°. Other parameters, such as the resistive index and the blood flow, might be evaluated; they are derived from formula-based analysis of PSV and are not more useful than PSV values.

CLASSIFICATION OF COLOR DOPPLER PATTERNS

Several types of thyroid vascularity, assessed by CFDS, have been proposed (4-9). Some of these overlapp with each other, while others are restricted to the blood flow characteristics of thyroid nodules or of non-nodular thyroid tissue (Table 12.1).

Author (ref.n.)	Type	Description	Pattern
Shimamoto (6)	N	Absence of color signal	0
		Intranodular color signal of spotty or patchy appearance but lacking perinodular signals	I
		Prominent color signal at the periphery of the nodule, with or without color signals at the center	II
		Marked color flow throughout the entire nodule	III
Lagalla (7)	N-EN	Absence of color signal	I
		Perinodular color signal	II
		Perinodular and intranodular color signal	III
		Marked intraparenchimal color signal	IV
Vitti (8)	EN	Blood flow limited to the peripheral thyroid arteries or to subcapsular vessels	0
		Mildly increased color signals at the level of peripheral thyroid arteries and presence of parenchimal blood flow with patchy, uneven distribution	I
		Clearly increased color flow doppler signal with patchy distribution	II
		Markedly increased color flow doppler signals with diffuse homogeneous distribution included the "thyroid inferno"	III
Rago (9)	N	Absent color signal	I
		Perinodular color signal	II
		Marked intranodular and absent or slight perinodular blood flow	III

Table 12.1 Classification of CFDS Patterns. Type refers to thyroid nodules (N) or to non-nodular parenchyma (EN). Normal subjects have absence of color signal, rare intraparenchymal spots, or blood flow limited to the peripheral thyroid arteries.

Probably, Shimamoto's classification for thyroid nodules (6) and Vitti's classification for diffuse (non-nodular) thyroid diseases (8) are the most adequate for these two different situations. However, a detailed description of CFDS patterns and an accurate measurement of PSV values might be appropriate as well. In this chapter we will use Vitti's and Shimamoto's classification if not otherwise specified (Figure 12.1, 12.2).

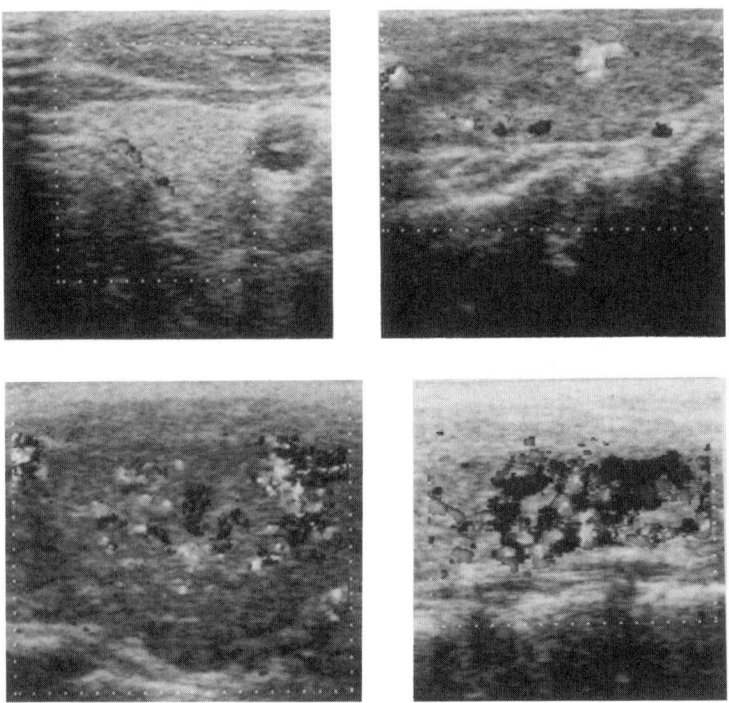

Figure 12.1 Color Flow Doppler Sonography Patterns. CFDS of diffuse (non-nodular) thyroid diseases may vary from pattern 0 (Top, Left) to pattern III (Bottom, Right).

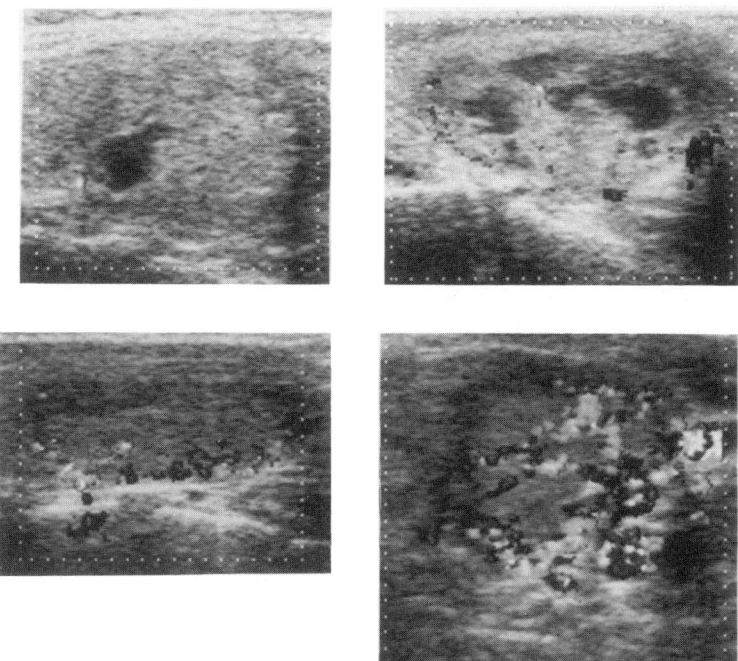

Figure 12.2 Color Flow Doppler Sonography Patterns of Thyroid Nodules. Vascularization may be minimal (Top, Left), intranodular (Top, Right), Peripheral (Bottom, Left) or peripheral and intranodular (Bottom, Right)

Normal subjects have absence of color signal, rare intraparenchymal spots, or blood flow limited to the peripheral thyroid arteries (Figure 12.3). In our Department normal PSV values are as follows: intrathyroidal arteries: 3-5 cm/s; inferior thyroid artery 15-30 cm/s.

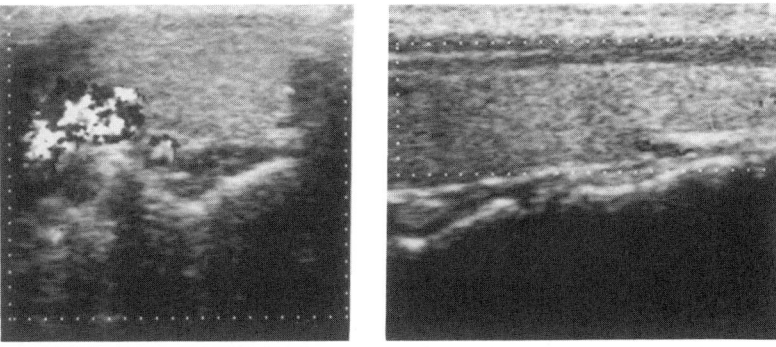

Figure 12.3 Appearance of Thyroid Vascularization in Normal Subjects as shown by CFDS.

HYPERTHYROIDISM AND THYROTOXICOSIS

Hyperthyroidism is characterized by increased serum levels of thyroid hormones (FT4 and FT3) due to thyroid hyperfunction, while in thyrotoxicosis the elevated levels are not necessarily associated with a hyperfunctioning gland. In other words, the term thyrotoxicosis refers to any increase in serum thyroid hormones, while the term hyperthyroidism is limited to the increase caused by the hyperfunction of the thyroid gland. Thyrotoxicosis, without hyperthyroidism, is most commonly due to a destructive process of the thyroid gland (subacute thyroiditis, type II amiodarone-induced thyrotoxicosis) or to the exogenous ingestion of excess thyroid hormones (thyrotoxicosis factitia, iatrogenic thyrotoxicosis) (Table 12.2).

CLASSIFICATION OF THYROTOXICOSIS
THYROTOXICOSIS ASSOCIATED WITH HYPERTHYROIDSM

Type of Thyrotoxicosis	Pathogenetic Mechanism
Graves' Disease	TSH Receptor Antibody
Toxic Multinodular Goiter	Functional Autonomy
Toxic Adenoma	Benign Tumor, TSH Receptor Mutations
TSHoma	TSH excess, Pituitary Adenoma
Trophoblastic Tumor	Chorionic Gonadotropin
Jod-Basedow	Iodine-Induced

THYROTOXICOSIS NOT ASSOCIATED WITH HYPERTHYROIDISM

Type of Thyrotoxicosis	Pathogenetic Mechanism
Subacute Thyroiditis	Release of Preformed Hormones
Painless Thyroiditis	Release of Preformed Hormones
Post-Partum Thyroiditis	Release of Preformed Hormones
Thyrotoxicosis Factitia	Excess Thyroid Hormones Ingestion
Ectopic Thyroid Tissue	Struma Ovarii, Functioning Metastatic Thyroid Cancer

Table 12.2 Classification of Causes of Thyrotoxicosis.

GRAVES' DISEASE

Graves' disease is characterized by the classical triad of goiter, hyperthyroidism and ophthalmopathy. Hyperthyroidism is due to thyroid hyperstimulation by thyrotropin receptor antibody (TRAb). Patients with Graves' hyperthyroidism usually have an enlarged thyroid gland which appears hypervascularized at CFDS. Usually, blood vascularity is markedly enhanced as well as PSV values (Figure 12.4).

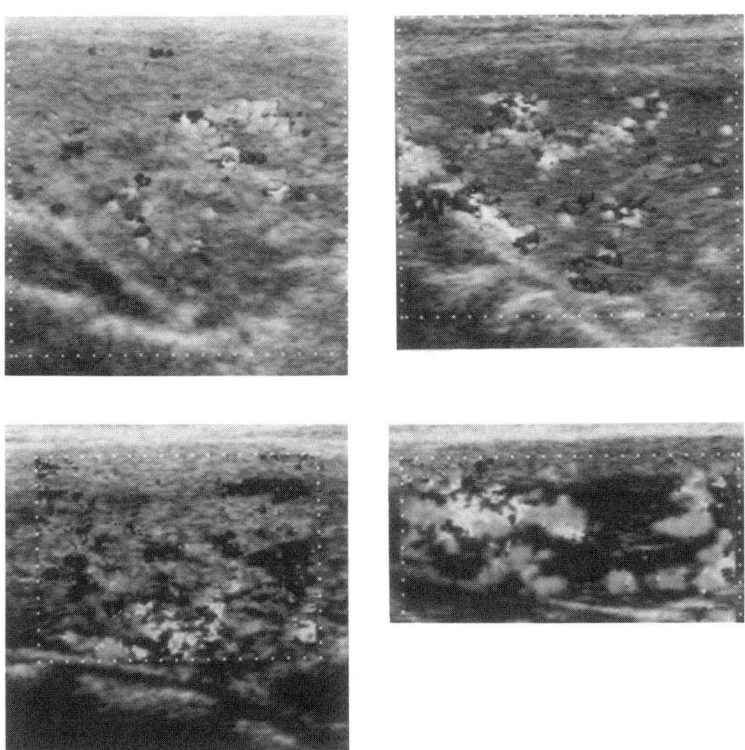

Figure 12.4 Graves' Disease. Patients with untreated Graves' hyperthyroidism have a greatly increased thyroid vascularization ranging from pattern I (Top, Left) to pattern III (Bottom).

Ralls et al. (4) used the term "thyroid inferno" to describe the extreme thyroid hypervascularization of hyperthyroid patients with Graves' disease. In several series (4, 8, 10-14) almost all untreated patients with Graves' hyperthyroidism have CFDS pattern II or III. In our own series of 49 untreated Graves' patients, 20% had CFDS pattern II and 80% pattern III (13). Castagnone et al.(10) tried to quantitate the qualitative evaluation of CFDS pattern. Intrathyroid vascularization was espressed as number of vessels per square centimeter measured on the longitudinal view using different grid scales similar to those used to count blood cells. These Authors confirmed an increased number of vessels per square centimeter in the thyroid gland of untreated patients with Graves' disease; this value significantly decreased during the remission of the disease (10). They showed that among 21 patients in remission, the 9 patients who had a relapse had a higher number of vessels per square centimeter (2.18±0.34 vs. 1.03±0.16) and higher flow on the thyroid artery (80.3±19.1 vs 10.6±2.3 ml/min) compared to the 12 patients who remained in stable remission, despite the fact that thyroid hormone levels were normal in both groups, suggesting that the CFDS pattern might help to identify patients whose hyperthyroidsm is effectively in remission (10) (Figure 12.5). Although semiquantitative, this method is less rapid and somehow cumbersome.

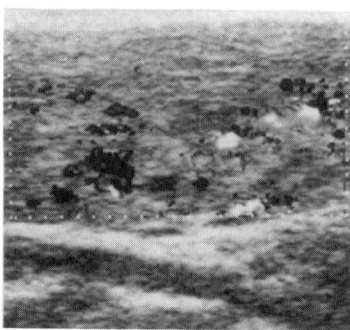 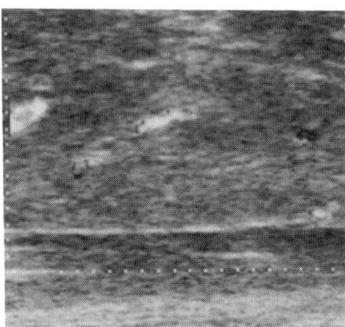

Figure 12.5 Graves' Disease. CFDS pattern of a patient with hyperthyroidism before (Left) and after methimazole treatment (Right).

Fein et al. (15) using a computer-based sonography apparatus showed that the color pixel density varies up to 50% in different sections of the same organ or tumor. Similar results were reported by Delorme et al. (16). Morosini et al. (12) correlated CFDS patterns and thyroid histology in Graves' disease. They found that patients with intraparenchymal homogeneous vascular color spots had a richly vascularized parenchyma with prevalent endothelial hyperplasia, while patients with poorly vascularized parenchymal area had fibrotic septation with prevalent vascular intimal hyperplasia. These findings suggested that changes might be due to different duration of hyperthyroidism or of thyroid stimulation by TRAb (12). It is worth noting that serum TRAb levels dropped after surgery in the latter group of patients but not in the former.

A better quantitative index is probably the peak systolic velocity (PSV) which can be easily measured at the level of the intraparenchymal vessels. Each examiner should have his/her own normal range determined in healthy subjects. In our Department normal PSV values range 3-5 cm/s, whereas Graves' patients have a mean PSV value 15 cm/s (13). PSV may also be measured at the level of the inferior thyroid artery. Also with this technique the mean PSV value is greatly increased in Graves' patients.

In conclusion, a hallmark of untreated Graves' patients detectable by CFDS is the increased number of intrathyroidal vessels independent of the technique used to show them.

TOXIC ADENOMA

This form of hyperthyroidism is generally caused by a single autonomous nodule of the thyroid. Toxic adenomas are follicular adenomas of the thyroid gland, in most cases associated with a gain of function mutation of the TSH receptor (17). This constitutive activation of the TSH receptor makes the adenoma capable of functioning without TSH stimulation. Typically, the thyroid scan shows uptake of radioiodine only by the nodule, while the extranodular tissue is suppressed and not visible.

Color flow doppler examination of patients with toxic or autonomous adenoma usually shows increased vascularity (Figure 12.6). Fobbe et al. (5) studied 25 patients, 24 of whom had a markedly increased blood flow signal, especially at the margins of the nodule; vascularity was more prominent in larger nodules than in smaller adenomas. Becker et al. (18) studied 53 patients with thyroid nodules: among the 34 patients with a nodule with internal hypervascularity at CFDS, 28 had a hot nodule at scintigraphy; among the remaining 6 with a hypervascularized nodule, 4 had cold nodules and 2 were defined as "normal". None of these "false" positive patients had thyroid cancer. In two case-reports, Barreda et al. (19) reported that a markedly increased blood flow, especially in the periphery of a nodule in the context of non-toxic goiter, suggests an autonomous nodule as confirmed by scintigraphy. Shimamoto et al. (6) reported CFDS pattern 0 in 4, pattern I in 3, pattern II in 5 and pattern III in 2 of 14 patients with follicular adenomas. However, it is not clear if all the patients of this series had autonomous nodules. Bogazzi et al. (13) described CFDS findings of 24 patients with toxic adenomas. All patients were hyperthyroid with undetectable serum TSH level and had a single hot nodule with a volume ranging 1.3 to 62.7 ml. Color flow doppler showed an increased vascularity mainly in the periphery of the adenoma: pattern I was observed in 8%, II in 70%, III in 22% (13). Mean PSV value measured at the periphery of the nodule was elevated (11 cm/s) (13). Clark et al. (20) reported that 73% of hot or warm nodules had an internal color flow; 15% showed the peripheral flow pattern and 12% had no detectable blood flow. It is worth mentioning that most, if not all, nodules were within multinodular glands.

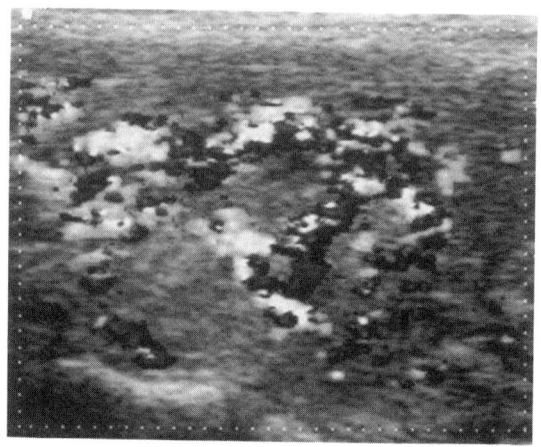
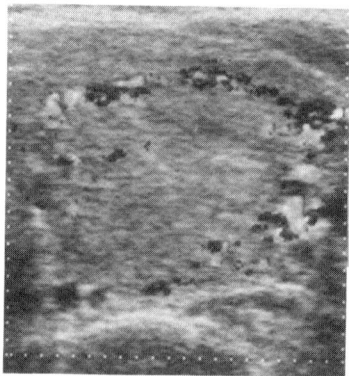
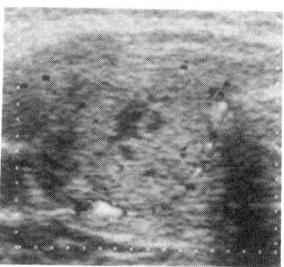

Figure 12.6 Toxic Adenoma. CFDS shows an increase of vascularity ranging from a "basket-like" appearance (Bottom) to peripheral and intranodular Blood Flow (Top).

TSH-SECRETING PITUITARY ADENOMA

Hyperthyroidism due to TSH-secreting pituitary adenoma (TSHoma) is a rare cause of hyperthyroidism. In 5 patients with TSHoma, we found increased vascularity of the thyroid gland in all cases (13) (Figure 12.7). CFDS pattern I was found in one and pattern II in four patients; PSV measured at the level of the intrathyroid vessels was elevated (mean 15 cm/s) (13). Although increased, vascularity never reached that observed in untreated Graves' patients; in particular, pattern III resembling the so-called "thyroid inferno" was not observed in patients with TSHoma. Thyroid vascularity, although diffuse, was increased particularly at the periphery of the gland (13).

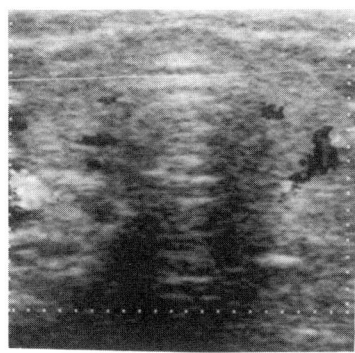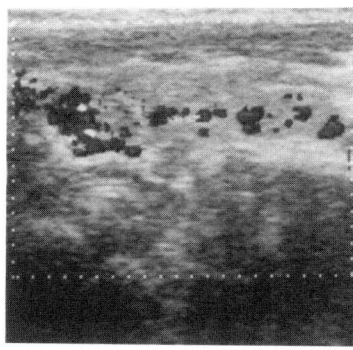

Figure 12.7 TSH-Secreting Pituitary Adenoma. Transverse (Right) and Longitudinal (Left) sections.

SUBACUTE THYROIDITIS

Subacute thyroiditis is a viral infection of the thyroid gland, characterized by gradual or sudden appearance of pain in the neck, radiated to the ear or jaw and accompanied by fever. The disease is characterized by the destruction of follicular epithelium and the leakage of preformed thyroid hormones.

In 12 patients with subacute thyroiditis during the thyrotoxic phase CFDS showed absent vascularity and normal PSV values (mean 4.2±1.1 cm/s) (13) (Figure 12.8). The results are in keeping with the concept that the increased serum thyroid hormones are not due to a hyperstimulation of the thyroid gland, but to a destructive process.

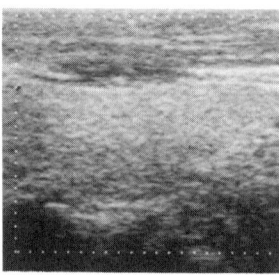
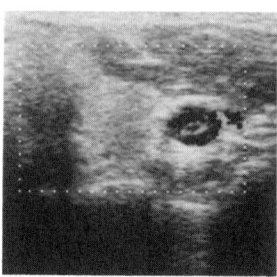
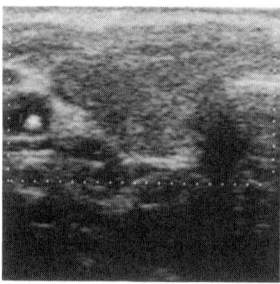
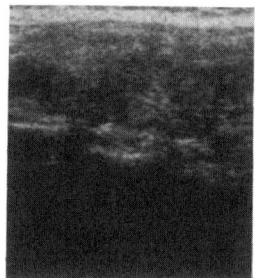
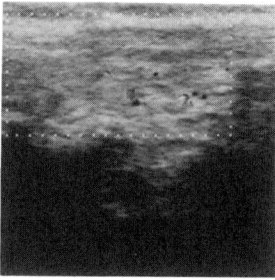

Figure 12.8 Thyrotoxicosis Factitia and Subacute Thyroiditis. Absent hypervascularization is the CFDS pattern of patients with thyrotoxicosis factitia (Top) and subacute thyroiditis (SAT) (Bottom). Note the marked heterogeneous structure of the thyroid gland of patients with SAT (particularly evident on conventional ultrasound, Bottom, Center).

At variance with our results, Clark et al. (20) reported a mild increase over backgorund flow in subacute thyroiditis, while the group of patients with various forms of "thyroiditis" studied by Fobbe et al. (5) was too small to permit an appropriate analysis. In other anecdotical reports by Anguissola et al. (21) the term "thyroiditis" was used to define either atrophic or goitrous or suppurative thyroiditis; due to the heterogeneity of these conditions, there was no typical CFDS pattern.

THYROTOXICOSIS FACTITIA

The term thyrotoxicosis factitia refers to an excess thyroid hormone condition caused by the surreptitious intake of exogenous thyroid hormone. Clinical manifestations are identical to those of spontaneous hyperthyroidism, but goiter, ophthalmopathy and thyroid autoimmune phenomena are absent. Patients deny the use of thyroid pills, and the diagnosis is often difficult. Measurement of serum thyroglobulin concentration has been shown to represent a clue in the diagnosis of thyrotoxicosis factitia since, at variance with hyperthyroidism, it is usually undetectable due to suppression of thyroid function (22). We have studied 7 patients with thyrotoxicosis factitia (14); CFDS examination showed the absence of hypervascularity or the presence of minimal intrathyroidal blood spots (pattern 0), supporting the concept of suppressed thyroid function by the exogenous thyroid hormone ingestion (Figure 12.8). PSV values measured at the level of the intraparenchymal vessels were in the normal range (mean value 4±0.8 cm/s.) (Figure 12.9).

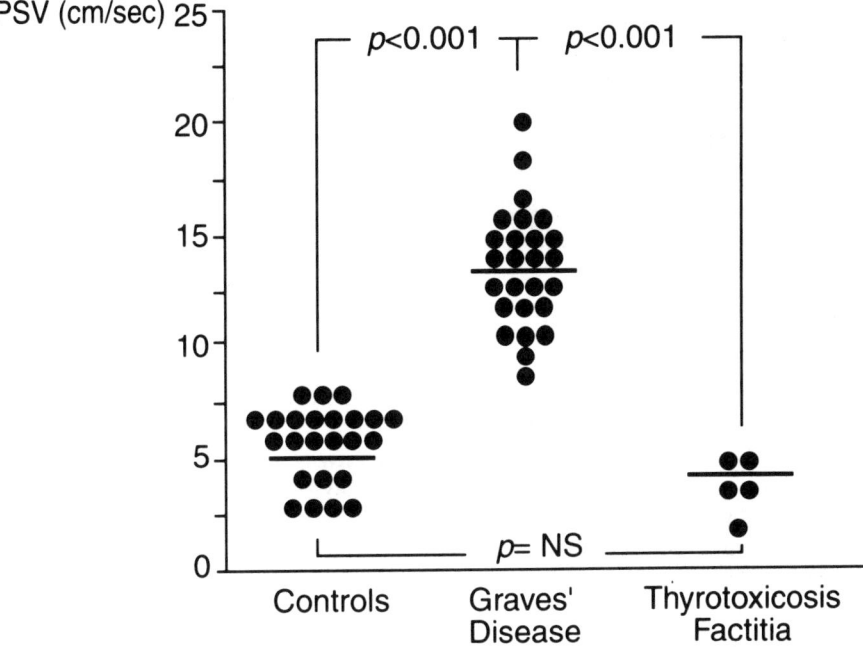

Figure 12.9 Peak Systolic Velocity (PSV) in Five Patients with Thyrotoxicosis Factitia. The horizontal line represents the mean value. From F. Bogazzi et al. (14) with permission.

AMIODARONE-INDUCED THYROTOXICOSIS

Amiodarone-induced thyrotoxicosis (AIT) occurs both in abnormal thyroid glands (nodular goiter, latent Graves' disease) (Type I AIT) or in apparently normal thyroid glands (Type II AIT). Differentiation of the two forms is crucial, because type I AIT responds well to methimazole and potassium perchlorate combined treatment, whereas type II AIT is effectively managed by glucocorticoids (23). Type I AIT is due to iodine-induced increase in thyroid hormone synthesis, whereas type II AIT is related to iodine- or amiodarone-induced damage of the gland (24). Differential diagnosis is often difficult, although RAIU is usually low-to-normal or even increased in type I, low-suppressed in type II; serum interleukin-6 levels are normal/slightly elevated in type I, markedly elevated in type II-AIT (25). All 16 patients of our series with type II AIT had a CFDS pattern 0 (i.e. absent hypervascularity) (Figure 12.10).

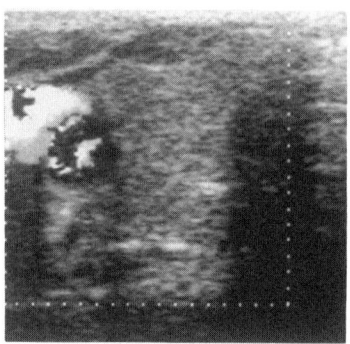 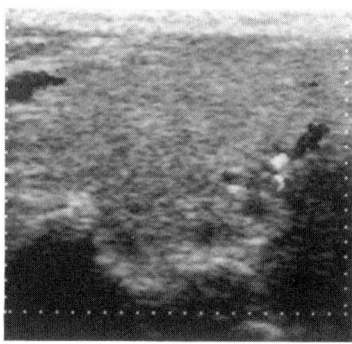

Figure 12.10 Type II Amiodarone-Induced Thyrotoxicosis. This form of thyrotoxicosis is due to a destructive process of the thyroid gland. Note the absence of hypervascularization.

Among the 11 patients with type I AIT, 64% had a CFDS pattern I, 9% a pattern II and 27% a pattern III similar to that found in patients with Graves' hyperthyroidism (26); this indicated a hyperfunctioning gland (Figures 12.11, 12.12, & 12.13). CFDS rapidly distinguishes type I and II AIT. This can avoid any delay in initiating the appropriate treatment for a rapid control of thyrotoxicosis in patients whose tachyarrhythmias or other cardiac disorders make thyroid hormone excess extremely deleterious.

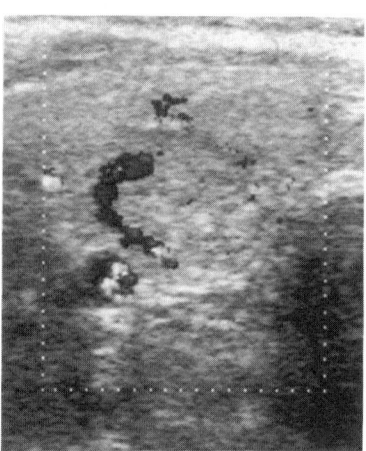 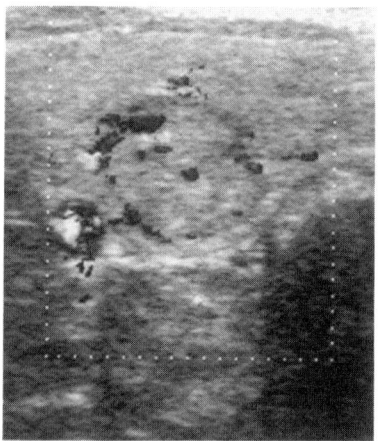

Figure 12.11 Type I Amiodarone-Induced Thyrotoxicosis. In this patient thyrotoxicosis was due to an autonomous nodule.

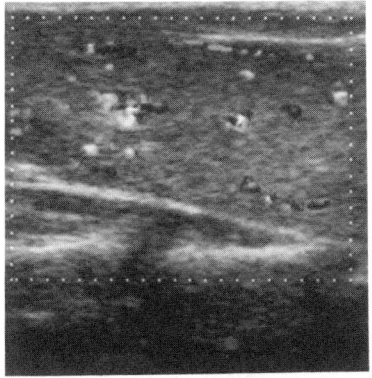
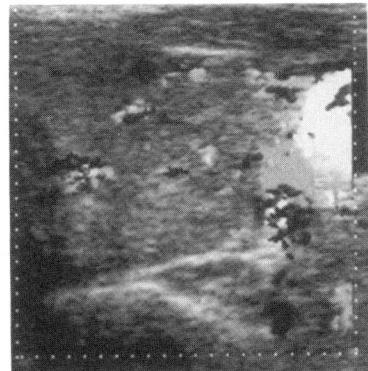
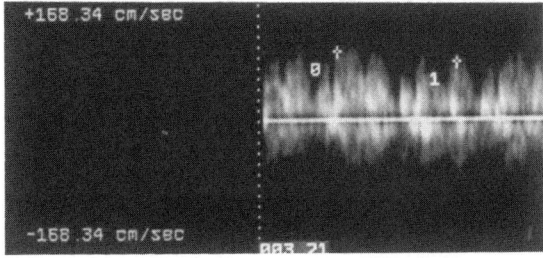

Figure 12.12 Type I Amiodarone-Induced Thyrotoxicosis. Latent Graves' Disease was the cause of hyperthyroidism in this patient under treatment with amiodarone. An increased vascularity was evident in spite of high vaules of iodine urinary excretion. High PSV values measured at the level of the inferior thyroid artery are shown at the bottom.

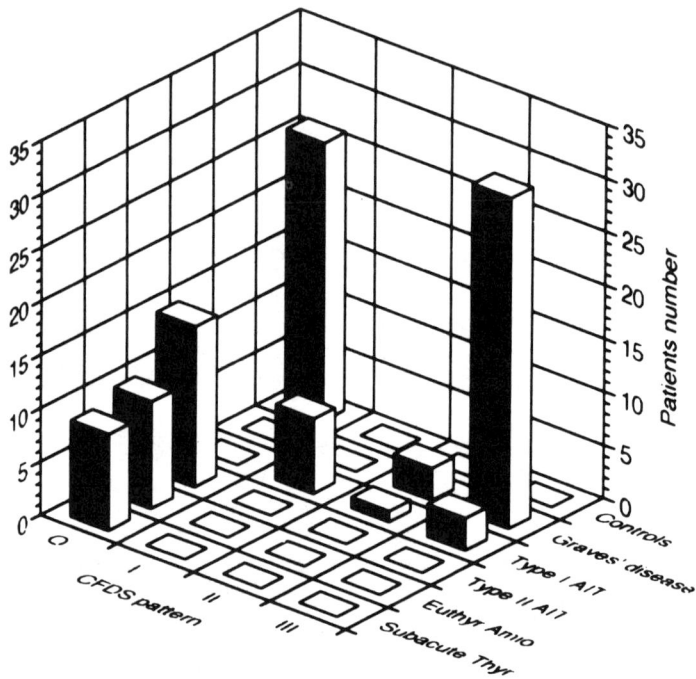

Figure 12.13 CFDS Patterns in Patients with Amiodarone-Induced Thyrotoxicosis. From F. Bogazzi et al.(26) with permission.

HYPOTHYROIDISM

Hypothyroidsm is the clinical status resulting from deficient production of thyroid hormones (Table 12.3). There is a general agreement that spontaneous goitrous hypothyroidism is characterized by increased thyroid vascularity (5, 8, 13, 27) (Figure 12.14).

Vitti et al. (8) reported that in 5 hypothyroid untreated patients the CFDS pattern was type 0 in 1, type I in 3 and type II in 1; PSV values measured at the level of the inferior thyroid artery were slightly higher than in euthyroid subjects. Lagalla et al. (27) reported the data from 20 patients with subclinical hypothyroidism of different and unknown causes: all patients had a hypervascularity of the gland with increased systolic velocity, with some degree of overlapping with untreated Graves' patients.

CLASSIFICATION OF HYPOTHYROIDISM

PRIMARY HYPOTHYROIDSM
ATROPHIC
Postablative Hypothyroidism
Primary Idiopathic Hypothyroidism (atrophic variant of Hashimoto's thyroiditis)
Sporadic Athyreotic Hypothyroidism (Agenesis or Dysplasia)
Endemic Cretinism
Unresponsiveness to TSH
GOITROUS
Hashimoto's (autoimmune) Thyroiditis
Endemic Iodine Deficiency
Iodine-Induced Hypothyroidism
Anti-Thyroid Agents
Inherited Defects of Hormones Synthesis
Riedel's Thyroiditis
Systemic disorders (Amyloidosis, Scleroderma,...)
CENTRAL HYPOTHYROIDISM
Pituitary or Hypothalamic Diseases (Secondary or Tertiary Hypothyroidism) (Sheehan's syndrome, Tumors, Infiltrative Disorders, Traumatic, Idiopathic)
Isolated TSH deficiency
TSH synthesis defect
RESISTANCE TO THYROID HORMONE ACTION (usually euthyroid)

Table 12.3 Classification of Causes of Hypothyroidism.

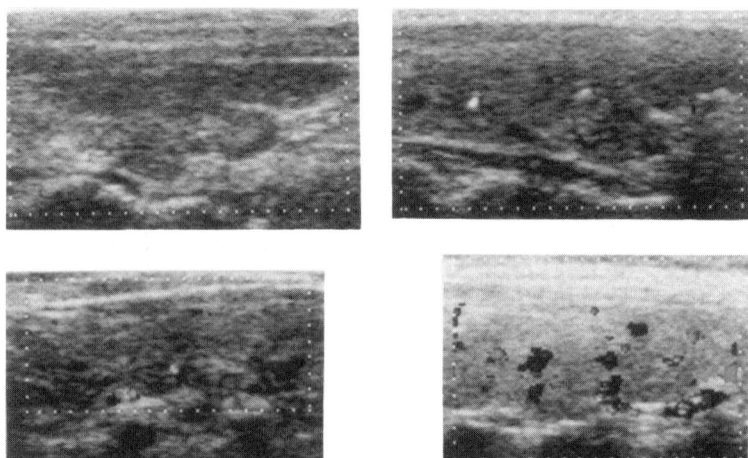

Figure 12.14 CFDS in Patients with Hashimoto's Thyroiditis. Thyroid vascularity was normal in euthyroid patients (Top, Left), and increased in untreated hypothyroid patients.

We recently reported the CFDS features of 21 untreated patients with spontaneous goitrous hypothyroidsm (13). We confirmed the increased vascularity of the thyroid gland: pattern 0 was observed in 14%, pattern I in 67% and pattern II in 19% of cases. Hypothyroid patients with goitrous Hashimoto's thyroiditis had higher PSV values than euthyroid patients with Hashimoto's thyroiditis or normal subjects suggesting a role of TSH hyperstimulation. Mean PSV value was 5.6 cm/s. The fact that the increase in PSV values was modest in hypothyroid patients, and marked in hyperthyroid patients, in spite of very high TSH values in the former group, is in keeping with the concept that a responsive (and not damaged) thyroid gland is also required to achieve a substantial increase in thyroid vascularity and blood flow. It is of interest that pattern III (the so-called "thyroid inferno") was never observed in hypothyroid patients. Our data showed that some hypothyroid patients had CFDS pattern II similar to patients with Graves' hyperthyroidsm or TSHoma (13). However, PSV values were only slightly elevated in hypothyroid patients, but greatly enhanced in hyperthyroid patients. Thus, CFDS pattern and PSV values are not always superimposable: CFDS pattern II might be found in association, for example, either with 6 cm/s PSV (hypothyroid patients with Hashimoto's thyroiditis) or with 15 cm/s PSV (Graves' hyperthyroidsm or TSHoma). For these reasons, we would like to suggest that PSV pattern represents a better index of thyroid function than CFDS pattern. High PSV values are probably indicative of hyperthyroidism, since they reflect a sustained stimulation on a thyroid gland which is capable of producing and secreting excess thyroid hormone; this does not occur in goitrous Hashimoto's hypothyroidism, in which the sustained stimulation of TSH leads only to a moderate increase in thyroid vascularity and blood velocity, due to the damage of thyroid tissue.

THYROID MALIGNANCY

The role of CFDS in predicting malignancy of thyroid nodules is still controversial, implying that the diagnostic usefulness of CFDS is presently limited (Figure 12.15). Shimamoto et al. (6) reported 13 cases of papillary carcinoma. 3 had CFDS pattern 0, 8 pattern I, 1 pattern II and 1 pattern III. In general, color signal could be depicted in 77% of papillary carcinoma and in 72% of follicular adenoma. Malignant nodules showed a greater tendency to exhibit type I flow than benign lesions. However, no specific flow pattern for malignancy could be found. Clark et al. (20) showed that the majority of "cold" nodules had a peripheral rim of color flow and no internal color flow. These authors showed that of 6 papillary carcinomas, 4 had no color flow and 2 had internal color flow. One Hürthle cell carcinoma had internal color flow. Peripheral color flow was found in 11 of 20 benign nodules, while 7 had no color and 2 had an internal color (20). They concluded that a nodule was probably benign when it had increased color flow in the context of a multinodular gland or a peripheral rim of color flow if isolated (20).

Lagalla et al. (7) reported 6 cases of thyroid carcinoma in which CFDS showed a markedly increased vascularity. However, a similar pattern was observed in 10 out of 11 cases of autonomous adenoma and in 7 cases of nodular goiter. Fobbe et al. (5) showed an increased color flow in all 6 cases of thyroid carcinoma studied; a similar pattern was described in 8 thyroid cancers by Anguissola et al. (21), by Spiezia et al. (28), and by Pacella et al. (29). Rago et al.(9) used conventional and color flow doppler sonography to differentiate benign and malignant thyroid nodules. Absent blood flow was seen in 5/30 carcinomas and 18/74 benign nodules; peripheral blood flow was evident in 5/30 cancers and 18/74 benign nodules, while intranodular blood flow was present in 20/30 cancers and 38/74 benign nodules. The Authors concluded that an internal blood flow on CFDS only slightly increased the predictivity of signs of thyroid cancer observed on conventional sonography (Table 12.4).

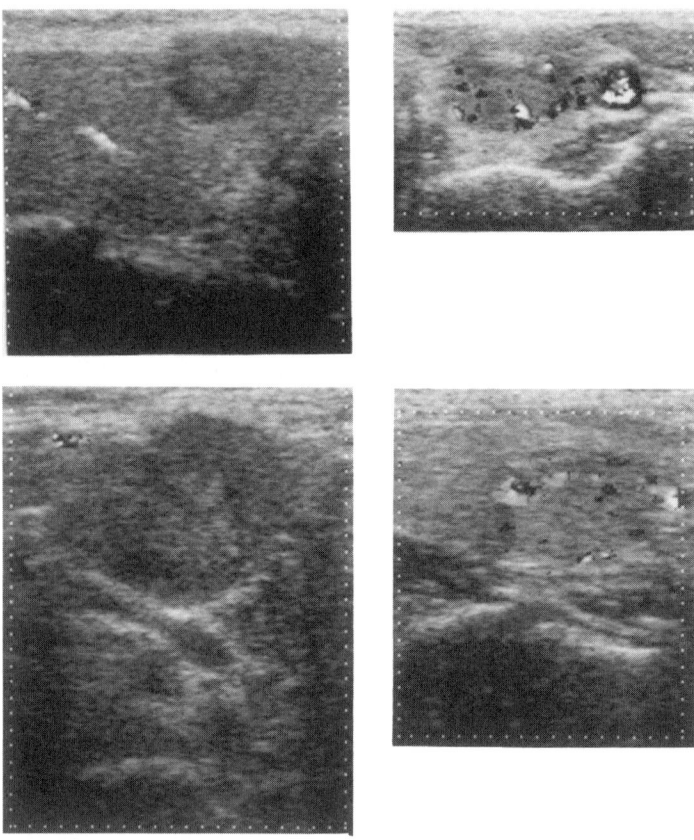

Figure 12.15 Thyroid Cancer. Papillary thyroid cancer (Top), follicular thyroid cancer (Bottom, Right), lymphonodal metastasis of papillary carcinoma (Bottom, Left). Note the variable CFDS pattern of thyroid carcinoma.

CFDS PATTERN	Carcinoma	Benign Nodules	Significance	Specificity (%)	Sensitivity (%)
Absent Blood Flow	5/30	18/74	P=0.39	75.6	16.6
Perinodular Blood Flow	5/30	18/74	P=0.39	75.6	25.0
Intranodular Blood Flow	20/30	38/74	P=0.15	48.6	34.4

Table 12.4 Color Flow Doppler Sonography and Histological Findings of Thyroid Nodules. Modified from Rago et al. (9) with permission. Statistical evaluation was performed by chi-square test.

The data available from the literature do not allow us to recommend the use of CFDS routinely as a first-line exam in the diagnosis of malignant nodules. Fine neeedle biopsy remains the best test for diagnosing thyroid malignancy.

CONCLUSIONS

Color flow doppler sonography is a rapid, informative and non-invasive technique which allows direct measurement of intrathyroidal blood flow. For the interpretation of CFDS pattern and PSV values the examiner must be familiar with basic concepts of CFDS and with the pathophysiology of thyroid disorders. The principal use of CFDS resides in its capability to discriminate between hyperthyroidism and thyrotoxicosis. In the former group of diseases, vascularity is invariably increased while in the latter vascularity is normal-to-reduced. Special forms of thyrotoxicosis, such as thyrotoxicosis factitia and type I and II AIT can be easily differentiated by CFDS. Some degree of overlap may exhists between hypothyroid patients and those who are hyperthyroid. Some hypothyroid patients have mildly increased CFDS pattern, similar to patients with Graves' hyperthyroidism or TSHoma. However, PSV values are only slightly elevated in hypothyroid patients, but greatly enhanced in hyperthyroid patients (Figure 12.16).

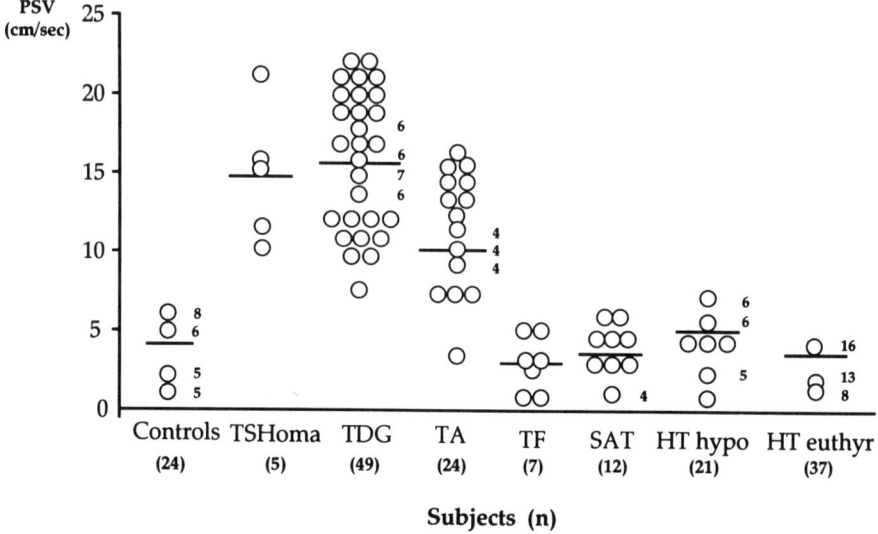

Figure 12.16 PSV Distribution in Various Thyroid Disorders. The horizontal line represents the mean value. Mean PSV in patients with elevated serum TSH or TRAb (untreated Graves' disease (TDG), TSHoma, untreated hypothyroidism due to goitrous Hashimoto's thyroiditis (HT hypo)) or with toxic adenoma (TA) was significantly higher than that found in the control group, in patients with thyrotoxicosis factitia (TF) or subacute thyroiditis (SAT) and euthyroid Hashimoto's thyroiditis (HT euthyr). Numbers refer to the number of patients having the same individual PSV value. From F. Bogazzi et al. (13) with permission.

It is likely that in the next few years we will witness a further expansion of CFDS use, which because of its rapidity might represent a first-line tool for assessment of thyroid function even at first bedside examination.

ACKNOWLEDGEMENTS

We thank Professor Aldo Pinchera and Professor Paolo Vitti for their continuous encouragement and advice. This work was partially supported by Grants from the University of Pisa (Fondi d'Ateneo) to E.M. and L.B.

REFERENCES

1. Marcocci, C., Vitti, P., Cetani, F., Catalano, F., Concetti, R., Pinchera, A. (1991) Thyroid ultrasonography helps to identify patients with diffuse lymphocytic thyroiditis who are prone to develop hypothyroidism. *J. Clin. Endocrinol. Metab.* 72: 209-213.
2. Vitti, P., Lampis, M., Piga, M., Loviselli, A., Brogioni, S., Rago, T., Pinchera, A., Martino, E. (1994) Diagnostic usefulness of thyroid ultrasonography in atrophic thyroiditis. *J. Clin. Ultrasound* 22: 375-379.
3. Kremkau, F.W. (1990) Doppler Ultrasound. Priciples and instruments. Saunders Co. Philadelphia.

4. Ralls, P.W., Mayekawa, D.S., Lee, K.P., Colletti, P.M., Radin, D.R., Boswell, W.D., Halls, J.M. (1988) Color-flow doppler sonography in Graves' disease: "thyroid inferno". Am. J. Radiol. 150: 781-784.
5. Fobbe, F., Finke, R., Reichenstein, E., Schleusener, H., Wolf, K.-J. (1989) Appearance of thyroid diseases using colour-coded duplex sonography. Europ. J. Radiol. 9:29-31.
6. Shimamoto, K., Endo, T., Ishigaki, T., Sakuma, S., Makino, N. (1993) Thyroid nodules: evaluation with color doppler ultrasonography. J. Ultrasound Med. 12:673-678.
7. Lagalla, R., Caruso, G., Romano, M., Midiri, M., Novara, V., Zappasodi, F. (1993) Eco-color-doppler nella patologia tiroidea. La Radiologia Medica 85: 109-113.
8. Vitti, P., Rago, T., Mazzeo, S., Brogioni, S., Lampis, M., De Liperi, A., Bartolozzi, C., Pinchera, A., Martino, E. (1995) Thyroid blood flow evaluation by color-flow doppler sonography distinguishes Graves' disease from Hashimoto's thyroiditis. J. Endocrinol. Invest. 18: 587-861.
9. Rago, T., Vitti, P., Chiovato, L., Mazzeo, S., De Liperi, A., Miccoli, P., Viacava, P., Bogazzi, F., Martino, E., Pinchera, A. (1998) Role of conventional ultrasonography and color flow-doppler sonography in predicting malignancy in 'cold' thyroid nodules. Eur. J. Endocrinol. 138: 41-46.
10. Castagnone, D., Rivolta, R., Rescalli, S., Baldini, M.I., Tozzi, R., Cantalamessa, L. (1996) Color doppler sonography in Graves' disease: value in assessing activity of disease and predicting outcome. Am. J. Radiol. 166: 203-207.
11. Baldini, M., Castagnone, D., Rivolta, R., Meroni, L., Pappalettera, M., Cantalamessa, L. (1997) Thyroid vascularization by color doppler ultrasonography in Graves' disease. Changes related to different phases and to the long-term outcome of the disease. Thyroid 7: 823-828.
12. Morosini, P.P., Simonella, G., Mancini, V., Argalia, G., Lucarelli, F., Montironi, R., Diamanti, L., Suraci, V. (1998) Color doppler sonography patterns related to histological findings in Graves' disease. Thyroid 8: 577-582.
13. Bogazzi, F., Bartalena, L., Brogioni, S., Burelli, L., Manetti, L., Tanda, M.L., Gasperi, M., Martino, E. (1999) Thyroid vascularity and blood flow are not dependent on serum thyroid hormone levels: studies in vivo by color flow doppler sonography. Eur. J. Endocrinol. 140: 452-456.
14. Bogazzi, F., Bartalena, L., Vitti, P., Rago, T., Brogioni, S., Martino, E. (1996) Color flow doppler sonography in thyrotoxicosis factitia. J. Endocrinol. Invest. 19: 603-606.
15. Fein, M., Delorme, S., Weisser, G., Zuna, I., van Kaick, G. (1995) Quantification of color doppler for the evaluation of tissue vascularization. Ultrasound Med. Biol. 21: 1013-1019.
16. Delorme, S., Weisser, G., Zuna, I., Fein, M., Lorenz, A., van Kaick, G. (1995) Quantitative characterization of color doppler images: reproducibility, accuracy, and limitations. J. Clin. Ultrasound 23: 537-550.
17. Tonacchera, M., Van Sande, J., Parma, J., Duprez, L., Cetani, F., Costagliola, S. (1996) TSH receptor and disease. Clin. Endocrinol. (Oxf.) 44: 621-633.
18. Becker, D., Bair, H.-J., Becker, W., Gunter, E., Lohner, W., Lerch, S., Hahn, E.G. (1997) Thyroid autonomy with color-coded image-directed doppler sonography: internal hypervascularization for the recognition of autonomous adenomas. J. Clin. Ultrasound 25: 63-69.
19. Barreda, R., Kaude, J.V., Fagien, M., Drane, W.E. (1991) Hypervascularity of nontoxic goiter as shown by color-coded doppler sonography. Am. J. Radiol. 156: 199.
20. Clark, K.J., Cronan, J.J., Scola, F.H. (1995) Color doppler sonography: anatomic and physiologic assessment of the thyroid. J. Clin. Ultrasound 23:215-233.
21. Anguissola, R., Bozzini, A., Campani, R., Bottinelli, O., Genovese, E., Guglielmoni, B., Fulle, I., Bandi, G. (1991) Ruolo della colour coded duplex sonography nello studio della patologia tiroidea. La Radiologia Medica 81:831-837.
22. Mariotti, S., Martino, E., Cupini, C., Lari, R., Giani, C., Baschieri, L., Pinchera, A. (1982) Low serum thyroglobulin as a clue to the diagnosis of thyrotoxicosis factitia. N. Engl. J. Med. 307: 410-412.

23. Bartalena, L., Brogioni, S., Grasso, L., Bogazzi, F., Burelli, A., Martino, E. (1996) Treatment of amiodarone-induced thyrotoxicosis, a difficult challenge: results of a prospective study. *J. Clin. Endocrinol. Metab.* 81: 2930-2933.
24. Brennan, M.D., Erickson, D.Z., Carney, J.A., Bahn, R.S. (1995) Non-goitrous (type I) amiodarone-associated thyrotoxicosis: evidence of follicular disruption in vitro and in vivo. *Thyroid* 5: 177-183.
25. Bartalena, L., Grasso, L., Brogioni, S., Aghini-Lombardi, F., Braverman, L.E., Martino, E. (1994) Interleukin-6 in amiodarone-induced thyrotoxicosis. *J. Clin. Endocrinol. Metab.* 78: 423-427.
26. Bogazzi, F., Bartalena, L., Brogioni, S., Mazzeo, S., Vitti, P., Burelli, A., Bartolozzi, C., Martino, E. (1997) Color flow doppler sonography rapidly differentiates type I and type II amiodarone-induced thyrotoxicosis. *Thyroid* 7: 541-545.
27. Lagalla, R., Caruso, G., Benza, I., Novara, V., Callaida, F. (1993) Eco-color-doppler nello studio dell'ipotiroidismo dell'adulto. *La Radiologia Medica* 86: 281-283.
28. Spiezia, S., Colao, A, Assanti, A.P., Cerbone, G., Picone, G.M., Merola, B. (1996) Usefulness of color echo doppler with power doppler in the diagnosis of hypoechoic thyroid nodule: work in progress. *Radiol. Med.* 921: 616-621.
29. Pacella, C.M., Guglielmi, R., Fabbrini, R., Bianchini, A., Rinaldi, R., Panunzi, C., Pacella, S., Crescenzi, A., Papini, E. (1998) Papillary carcinoma in small hypoechoic thyroid nodules: predictive value of echo color doppler evaluation. Preliminary results. *J. Exp. Clin. Cancer Res.* 17: 127-128.

INDEX

3-dimensional ultrasound, 43
Aberrant thyroid, 75
Acoustic impedance, 3,20, 33
Acoustic shadow, 170, 171
Amiodarom-induced thyrotoxicosis, 227, 228, 229
A-mode , 3, 27
Annular array, 14
Anti Tg Antibodies, 158, 166
Anticoagulants, 97, 118
Attenuation, 21
A-V malformation, 55

Beta radiation, 59
Biopsy needle guide, 128
B-mode, 3, 27
Bronchial cleft cyst, 54

Camera syringe pistol, 104
Cathode ray oscilloscope, 1
Cervical lymph nodes, 52, 91, 160
Chernobyl, 88
Colloid, 154
Complex nodule, 77
Cretinism, 157
Cystic carcinoma, 143, 145
Cystic hygroma, 54

Delphian node, 52
DeQuervan's Thyroiditis, 65; 108
Doppler shift, 214
Down Doppler, 37
Drill-spin technique, 135, 140, 141

"Eggshell" calcifications, 82
Endemic goiter, 74
Enhancement, 30, 76
Ethyl-alcohol (ethanol), 170

Focal zone, 18
Fraunhofer zone, 18
Fresnal zone, 18

Gamma radiation, 60

Halo, 81, 89
Hemiagenisis of thyroid, 74, 75
Hemotoma, 97; 205
Hilar line, 162, 165
Hockey stick sign, 75
Hürthle cell neoplasm, 108, 109
Huygen's principle, 17

Immunoperioxidose, 72, 111
"Incidentalomas", 49, 73
Indication of UG FNA, 133

Indium 111 penetrestide (octreotide), 61
intrathyroid parathyroid tumor, 91, 100, 101

Jod Basedow, 65

Lingual thyroid, 67
Lipoma, 55
Lobar mass, 73
Lymphoma, of thyroid, 149

Messenger RNA, 156
Microcalcifications, 82, 83
M-mode, 4, 27
Multinucleated giant, 108

Papanicolaou, 104
Parathyroid adenoma, 92
Parathyroid cyst , 78
Peak systolic velocity (PSV), 213
Phased array, 15
Piezoelectric, 4, 12, 34
Polyerase chain reaction (PRP), 156
Positron emission tomographs (PET), 59
Postpartum thyroiditis, 65
Psammoma bodies, 82; 110, 144
PTH, 77
Pyramidal lobe, 45, 61

Rarefaction, 10
Recombinant TSH(rhTSH), 66, 155, 156, 166
Recurrent laryngeal nerve, 89, 98, 140, 175, 176, 178
Resolution, 22
Reverberation, 32,34

Sebaceous cyst , 55
Shadowing, 30, 82
Silent thyroiditis, 41
Single photon emission tomography (SPECT), 60
Strumi cordis, 67
Strumi ovarii, 67
Superior laryngeal nerve, 89

Technetium 99^{Tm} methoxyisobutyl isonitrile (Tc^{m}IBI), 60
Technetium pertechnetate, 60
Thallium 201 (^{201}Tl), 60
Thin wall cyst, 78
Thyroglobulin, 154
Thyroglossal duct cyst, 74
Thyroglossal duct tract, 61
"thyroid inferno", 38; 173

Thyrotoxicosis factitia, 157, 220, 226, 227, 235, 236
Time-gain compensation (TGC), 26
Transducters, 4, 11, 12, 13, 14, 15, 36
TSHoma, 222

Volume, thyroid, 48

Werner suppression test, 46